Cardiology Pearls

Second Edition

BLASE A. CARABELLO, MD
Chief
Medical Service
Veterans Affairs Medical Center
Houston, Texas

PETER C. GAZES, MD
Professor of Medicine
Distinguished Clinical University Professor
 of Cardiology
Medical University of South Carolina
 (MUSC) Heart Center
Charlestown, South Carolina

Series Editors

STEVEN A. SAHN, MD
Professor of Medicine and Director
Division of Pulmonary and
 Critical Care Medicine
Medical University of South Carolina
Charleston, South Carolina

JOHN E. HEFFNER, MD
Professor and Vice Chairman
Department of Medicine
Medical University of South Carolina
Charleston, South Carolina

HANLEY & BELFUS, INC. / Philadelphia

Publisher: HANLEY & BELFUS, INC.
Medical Publishers
210 S. 13th Street
Philadelphia, PA 19107
(215) 546-7293, 800-962-1892
FAX (215) 790-9330
Website: http://www.hanleyandbelfus.com

Library of Congress Cataloging-in-Publication Data

Cardiology pearls / edited by Blase A. Carabello, Peter C. Gazes.— 2nd ed.
   p. ; cm. — (The Pearls Series®)
  Includes bibliographical references and index.
  ISBN 1-56053-403-6 (alk. paper)
   1. Cardiology—Case studies.   2. Heart—Diseases—Case studies.
 I. Carabello, Blase A. II. Gazes, Peter C., 1921– III. Title. IV. Series.
  [DNLM: 1. Cardiovascular Diseases—Case Report. 2. Cardiovascular
Diseases—Problems and Exercises. WG 18.2 C2695 2000]
RC669 .C2745 2001
616.1′209—dc21
00-023117

CARDIOLOGY PEARLS, 2nd edition   ISBN 1-56053-403-6

©2001 by Hanley & Belfus, Inc. All rights reserved. No part of this book may be reproduced, reused, republished, transmitted in any form or by any means, or stored in a database or retrieval system without written permission of the publisher.

Last digit is the print number: 9 8 7 6 5 4 3 2 1

CONTENTS

Patient   **Page**

1. A 41-year-old man with exertional chest pain 1
2. A 60-year-old woman with heaviness in both arms and weakness 4
3. A 45-year-old man with coronary artery disease and normal lipids except for low HDL 6
4. A 42-year-old man with sharp left chest pain when running 8
5. A 14-year-old girl with chest pain and rapid heart beat 10
6. A 53-year-old man with chest pain and a left bundle branch block 12
7. A 64-year-old man with congestive heart failure 14
8. A 51-year-old woman with dyspnea.. 16
9. A 63-year-old hypertensive man with a new murmur and chest pain 18
10. A 59-year-old woman with slow heart rate 20
11. A 75-year-old woman with an acute infarction and ventricular arrhythmias.................. 22
12. A 25-year-old man with dyspnea and orthostatic dizziness 24
13. A 35-year-old man an abnormal EKG... 26
14. A 46-year-old woman with abdominal pain and syncope 29
15. A 32-year-old man with recurrent syncope 31
16. A 59-year-old woman with an abnormal electrocardiogram... 33
17. A 69-year-old confused man with elevated temperature and tachycardia 35
18. A 73-year-old woman with persistent atrial fibrillation 37
19. A 56-year-old diabetic woman with an acute anterior myocardial infarction, right bundle branch block, and left anterior superior fascicular block 39
20. A 48-year-old woman with cardiomyopathy... 41
21. A 45-year-old man with no known coronary artery disease and hypercholesterolemia 43
22. A 45-year-old man with coronary artery disease and normal lipids 46
23. A 50-year-old woman with coronary artery disease and noninsulin-dependent diabetes 48
24. A 74-year-old man with an aortic valve homograft and congestive heart failure 51
25. A 45-year-old man with substernal chest pain 53
26. A 43-year-old man with end-stage renal disease on dialysis 56
27. A 50-year-old man with recurrent chest pain on exertion and at rest 58
28. A 59-year-old man with cough, dyspnea, and electrical alternans.................................. 61
29. A 64-year-old man with intermittent chest pain responsive to nitroglycerin 64
30. A 65-year-old woman with hypertension and chronic atrial fibrillation 67
31. A 22-year-old man with an abnormal electrocardiogram.. 69
32. A 55-year-old man with a complication of acute myocardial infarction........................ 72
33. An 18-year-old man with frequent premature ventricular beats 74
34. An 18-year-old man with palpitations, lightheadedness, and an abnormal electrocardiogram 76

Patient	Page
35. A 72-year-old woman on quinidine with presyncopal episodes	79
36. A 60-year-old man with an acute inferior myocardial infarction and pulmonary edema	81
37. A 60-year-old man with acute interscapular pain and a cold right hand	84
38. A 35-year-old man who received thrombolytic therapy for chest pain and ST elevation	87
39. A 26-year-old woman with headache, nausea, blurred vision, and an abnormal electrocardiogram	89
40. A 56-year-old man on digoxin with supraventricular tachycardia	91
41. A 42-year-old man with stable angina referred for a thallium stress test	93
42. A 62-year-old man with nausea and an arrhythmia	96
43. A 55-year-old woman with episodes of wide QRS tachycardia	98
44. A 60-year-old man with severe chronic obstructive lung disease and edema	100
45. A 52-year-old man with chest pain and a normal coronary arteriogram	103
46. A 63-year-old man with sudden cardiac death	106
47. A 54-year-old woman with coma and ST-segment electrocardiographic abnormalities	108
48. A 35-year-old apparently healthy man with profound T-wave abnormalities	110
49. A 34-year-old woman with a wide QRS tachycardia	112
50. A 40-year-old man with cyanosis and palpitations	115
51. A 68-year-old woman with lower-extremity weakness	118
52. A 66-year-old man with a heart rate of 38 bpm	121
53. A 40-year-old man with chronic malaise and sudden numbness in the right arm	123
54. A 52-year-old man with right bundle branch block	125
55. A 45-year-old man with hypotension following an acute inferior myocardial infarction	128
56. An 84-year-old man with chest pain and a left bundle branch block	130
57. A 36-year-old male drug abuser with chest pain	132
58. A 59-year-old man with recent onset of atrial fibrillation	134
59. A 67-year-old woman with an acute anterior myocardial infarction treated with thrombolytic therapy	137
60. A 72-year-old man with episodes of lightheadedness	140
61. A 54-year-old man with a basal systolic murmur and right bundle branch block	142
62. A 62-year-old man with syncope after voiding	145
63. A 65-year-old woman with an acute inferior infarction and premature ventricular beats	147
64. A 70-year-old woman with transient ischemic attacks and a cold right hand	149
65. A 70-year-old alcoholic man with sinus bradycardia and confusion	151
66. A 57-year-old woman with episodes of palpitations not controlled with carotid sinus message	153
67. A 60-year-old woman with sluggishness, fatigue, and chest pain	155
68. A 24-year-old man with substernal chest pain that worsened with inspiration	157
69. A 52-year-old man with early morning chest pain	159

Patient	**Page**
70. A 44-year-old man with severe chest pain and an abnormal electrocardiogram	162
71. A 32-year-old woman with episodes of rapid heart beat	164
72. A 67-year-old man with chest pain following a motor vehicle accident	166
73. A 62-year-old man with hypertension, atypical chest pain, and an abnormal electrocardiogram	168
74. A 52-year-old man with an anterior myocardial infarction managed with thrombolytic therapy	170
75. A 28-year-old man with hypotension and a continuous murmur	173
76. A 7-year-old boy with an acute myocardial infarction	175
77. A 68-year-old man with recurrent heart failure and a systolic murmur	177
78. A 45-year-old woman with exertional angina	179
79. A 30-year-old man with fever, chills, and a new heart murmur	181
80. A 45-year-old man with intractable congestive heart failure	184
81. A 23-year-old retarded woman with acute chest pain	187
82. A 25-year-old intravenous drug user with fever, chills, anorexia, and weight loss	189
83. A 51-year-old man with poorly controlled hypertension and pulmonary edema	191
84. A 56-year-old woman with palpitations and chest pain	193
85. A 54-year-old man with low voltage on electrocardiogram	196
86. A 40-year-old man with decreased exercise tolerance and a diastolic heart murmur	199
87. A 35-year-old woman with a deep venous thrombosis and a cold right arm	201
88. A 40-year-old man with dyspnea and acyanotic congenital heart disease	203
89. A 55-year-old man with an aortic valve prosthesis, fever, and first-degree atrioventricular block	205
90. A 58-year-old man with weight loss and a heart murmur	207
91. A 73-year-old man with pulmonary edema and a normal ejection fraction	209
92. A 28-year-old man with progressive fatigue, dyspnea, and cyanosis	211
93. A 24-year-old African-American woman with dyspnea on exertion and fatigue following childbirth	213
94. An 18-year-old man with dyspnea and lower-extremity cyanosis	215
95. A 71-year-old man with an acute myocardial infarction and a new heart murmur	217
96. A 46-year-old obese man with acute chest pain and dyspnea following surgery	219
97. A 52-year-old man with increasing abdominal girth and peripheral edema 10 years following a motor vehicle accident	222
98. A 72-year-old woman with hyperpyrexia on beta-blocker therapy	224
99. A 53-year-old woman with mitral stenosis and left upper- and lower-extremity weakness	226
100. A 76-year-old man with a mitral valve prosthesis and on anticoagulation who requires rectal polypectomy	228
101. A 45-year-old man with improved ventricular function after coronary bypass surgery	230

Patient	**Page**
102. A 53-year-old man with dyspnea on exertion and a heart murmur following an episode of acute chest pain	232
103. A 19-year-old woman with cyanosis and a heart murmur	234
104. A 42-year-old morbidly obese woman with dyspnea	237
105. A 44-year-old man with a heart murmur and hypertension	239
106. A 55-year-old man with an abnormal thallium scan 2 years after heart transplantation	241
107. A 30-year-old intravenous drug user with fever and acute pulmonary edema	243
108. A 62-year-old man with a systolic ejection murmur and progressive dyspnea	245
109. A 38-year-old man with a chronic murmur and rapidly progressive congestive heart failure	247
110. A 49-year-old man with congestive heart failure and weight loss	249
111. A 54-year-old man with arthralgias and dyspnea	251
112. A 49-year-old physician with congestive heart failure and acute left hemiparesis	253
113. A 28-year-old woman with chest pain and a positive stress test	256
114. A 46-year-old woman with fever and a pericardial effusion	259
115. A 65-year-old man with electrocardiographic changes following abdominal surgery	261
116. A 62-year-old man with arrhythmias, heart failure, and increasing dyspnea	263
117. A previously healthy 25-year-old man with pneumonia and shock	265
118. A 55-year-old man with a Starr-Edwards aortic valve and progressive dyspnea	268
119. A 28-year-old pregnant patient with heart failure in the second trimester	271
120. A 34-year-old man with a 10-year history of a heart murmur	274
121. A 65-year-old woman with mitral stenosis and upper right quadrant pain	277
122. A 54-year-old man in shock following a myocardial infarction	279
123. A 55-year-old renal transplant patient with hypertension, pulmonary edema, and tinnitus	281
124. A 62-year-old man with signs and symptoms of congestive heart failure and a large cardiac silhouette	283
125. A 28-year-old hunter with syncope	285
INDEX	287

FOREWORD

Present-day cardiology is replete with "high tech" diagnostic and therapeutic interventions that were only imagined a decade ago. In the face of these rapid advances in the technology of care, it is easy to forget that the roots of cardiology are in the astute use of bedside diagnostic skills. In fact, cardiology textbooks were some of the earliest purveyors of the importance of a thoughtful history and the careful gathering of diagnostic clues from the physical examination.

We are, therefore, delighted with this second edition of *Cardiology Pearls,* which presents a balanced blend of modern-day innovations and time-honored approaches to cardiac care. Presented in the format of the Pearls Series®, these case presentations challenge the reader to construct a differential diagnosis and therapeutic plan based on the patient's signs, symptoms, and basic laboratory manifestations of disease. The authors then present a comprehensive and up-to-date discussion of the underlying condition and review the patient's clinical course and outcome. The discussion is followed by Clinical Pearls, which represent the "take home" message for the busy clinician reader and student of cardiac disease. Drs. Carabello and Gazes perform their tasks eminently well in presenting challenging material in a highly readable, concise, and straightforward way.

We anticipate that *Cardiology Pearls, 2nd edition* will provide important lessons and valuable Pearls for physicians in training and experienced clinicians alike.

John E. Heffner, MD
Steven A. Sahn, MD
SERIES EDITORS

PREFACE

For many years we have lectured to medical students, nurses, housestaff, and practicing and academic physicians, with the aim of presenting in a simple and concise manner the new knowledge in cardiology. A balanced opinion is taken in all views. We strive to blend basic science with the clinical. *Cardiology Pearls, 2nd edition,* allows us to continue meeting these goals.

The large number of advances in cardiology in the past few years and the favorable response to our first edition have encouraged us to add more cases and revise the old ones for this second edition. The field of cardiac diagnosis and therapy continues to see explosive growth and change almost daily. Much of the material in this book is based on our personal experience. We have attempted to integrate new data with our experience as clinicians and academicians. The first edition's problem-oriented approach for self study and for board review is applied here, as well.

First, a brief clinical case, including physical examination and laboratory findings and often accompanied by a radiograph, EKG, echo Doppler study, catheterization data, or other pertinent illustrations, is presented. The reader is encouraged to consider the differential diagnosis and formulate a plan for diagnosis and treatment. The subsequent pages disclose the diagnosis and offer a discussion of the case, clinical pearls, and a few key references.

This book in the Pearl Series® contains 125 case presentations that provide valuable information not readily available in standard textbooks. It is aimed at primary healthcare providers in family medicine and internal medicine—including nurses, internal medicine residents, cardiac fellows, medical students, physician's assistants, cardiologists, and cardiac surgeons. It is especially useful to the cardiologist preparing for board certification. Case duplication has been eliminated, but some important facts are re-emphasized. Each case makes generous use of laboratory results and graphic illustrative material, and facilitates the reader's learning.

We have covered most of the significant cardiac problems that the physician encounters daily. The object of this book is to present actual problems encountered in daily practice in a usable format.

We would like to give special recognition to our secretary, Linda Paddock, who typed the manuscript and organized the references and art work.

Peter C. Gazes, MD
Blase A. Carabello, MD
AUTHORS

PATIENT 1

A 41-year-old man with exertional chest pain

A 41-year-old man presents with a complaint of mid-substernal tightness when he walks rapidly. The pain subsides when he slows down, and he seldom has discomfort at a slow pace. He denies pain at rest or nocturnal pain. The chest pain has not increased in frequency or duration since it started 1 year ago. He has smoked one package of cigarettes per day for 20 years and has a strong family history for coronary disease. He denies hypertension and diabetes and has never had a lipid analysis.

Physical Examination: Vital signs: pulse 70; blood pressure 110/70. Chest: lungs clear. Cardiac: normal.

Laboratory Findings: CBC: normal. Cholesterol 240 mg/dl, HDL 40 mg/dl, triglycerides 200 mg/dl, LDL 160 mg/dl. EKG: normal.

Questions: What is your diagnosis? How would you manage this patient?

Answer: Stable angina. Perform a nuclear perfusion study and then individualize management depending on the extent of disease and ischemia and the status of left ventricular function.

Discussion: Angina is considered stable when it has been present for several months without change in duration or frequency; is precipitated by a known amount of exercise and/or anxiety; and is relieved by rest and nitroglycerin. Perform coronary arteriography if a nuclear or echocardiographic stress study shows significant ischemia or left ventricular dysfunction. Over the last two decades, management of coronary artery disease has evolved significantly. The challenge today is whether **revascularization or medical therapy** should be offered to the patient with stable angina. In addition, if revascularization is to be done, should it be coronary bypass surgery (CABG), angioplasty, or placement of stents?

Optimal medical therapy includes nitroglycerin, beta-blocker or calcium blocker, aspirin, and management of risk factors such as hyperlipidemia, exercise, smoking, blood pressure, and weight loss. Many studies and meta-analyses of randomized trials show that patients with three-vessel disease, especially with a decreased ejection fraction, or left main vessel coronary artery disease, have less mortality with CABG than with medical therapy. No survival benefit has been noted in patients with one- or two-vessel disease unless two-vessel disease includes significant proximal disease of the left anterior descending artery (LAD).

Several studies compared surgery with angioplasty in patients with multivessel disease. Death or nonfatal myocardial infarctions were no different in the two groups after 5 years, but the rate of repeat revascularization was greater for the angioplasty group, and, after the first year, angina was more frequent in the angioplasty group. A subgroup with diabetes did better with CABG.

The approach to the patient with stable angina evolves around the presence of: **(1)** three-vessel disease, or two-vessel disease that includes proximal LAD disease; **(2)** significant ischemia detected by noninvasive testing; **(3)** left ventricular dysfunction. If two of these three are present, patients do better with revascularization. When only one factor is present, medical therapy is sufficient. Left main disease should be treated surgically. The use of intracoronary stents reduces the restenosis rate by one quarter to one third compared to percutaneous transluminal coronary angioplasty (PTCA), and eventually may show better results than surgery for multivessel disease. In addition, restenosis has been reduced by administration of clopidogrel (Plavix) and abciximab (Reopro) with PTCA and stents. Patients with single-vessel disease and suitable lesions should be considered for PTCA with stenting if the thallium stress test shows a large area of decreased perfusion with good redistribution or a decrease in left ventricular function either at rest or with stress.

Most of the studies comparing CABG with medical therapy, or CABG with angioplasty, or medical therapy with angioplasty, were done prior to the availability of stents and drugs such as the GP IIb/IIIa inhibitors. In addition, medical therapy has advanced especially since the introduction of the statin drugs that lower cholesterol, LDL, and triglycerides; increase HDL; and stabilize plaques. The Atorvastatin Versus Revascularization Treatment (AVERT) trial compared **atorvastatin** to angioplasty in patients with stable coronary artery disease with single- or double-vessel disease and preserved left ventricular function. Subjects who received 80 mg of atorvastatin had less angina, reduction in nonfatal myocardial infarction, and less revascularization and hospitalization. These results support an extremely aggressive approach to cholesterol lowering in patients with established coronary artery disease. The HDL Intervention Trial (HIT) of **gemfibrozil,** with a followup of 7 years, showed a significant decrease in coronary artery disease death and nonfatal infarction, compared to placebo. Aggressive medical therapy in the future may change the natural history of coronary artery disease and reduce the need for CABG and noninvasive interventions.

Some patients with persistent chronic stable angina who have failed aggressive medical therapy may not be candidates for revascularization procedures. Consider transmyocardial laser revascularization, enhanced external counter pulsation, and spinal cord stimulation in such cases. Each of these procedures offers benefits, but also limitations.

The present patient had a 95% proximal LAD lesion that showed a large area of decreased perfusion involving the lateral wall and septum. The vessel was stented with good results, and aggressive risk factor management was begun. Six months later, his thallium stress test was normal.

Clinical Pearls

1. Patients with stable angina should have a thallium-Sestimibi or echocardiographic stress test. If extensive ischemia or left ventricular dysfunction is detected, perform coronary arteriography.

2. Individualize patients with one-, two-, or three-vessel disease for medical therapy, PTCA, stents, surgery, or combinations—depending on the severity of symptoms, coronary artery pathology, extent of ischemia, and left ventricular function.

3. Perform CABG in patients with three-vessel disease and decreased left ventricular ejection fraction, or left main disease.

REFERENCES

1. Serruys PW, de Jaegere P, Kiemeneij F, et al.: A comparison of balloon-expandable-stent implantation with balloon angioplasty in patients with coronary artery disease. Benestent Study Group. N Engl J Med 1994;331;489–495.
2. Gutstein DE, Fuster V: Management of stable coronary artery disease. Am Fam Phys 1997;56:99–106.
3. ACC/AHA Guidelines for Coronary Angiography: Executive Summary and Recommendations. A report of the American College of Cardiology/American Heart Association Task Force on Practice Guidelines. Circulation 1999;99:2345–2357.
4. Whitlow PL, Dimas AP, Bashore TM, et al.: Relationship of extent of revascularization with angina at 1 year in the Bypass Angioplasty Revascularization Investigation (BARI). J Am Col Cardiol 1999;34:1744–1749.

PATIENT 2

A 60-year-old woman with heaviness in both arms and weakness

A 60-year-old woman has been experiencing heaviness in both arms and weakness for 6 months. She has been known to have hypertension for several years and currently is taking hydrochlorothiazide 25 mg daily. She denies any chest, neck, or jaw pain. The heaviness in her arms is constant and not aggravated by exercise. Her family physician referred her as possibly having coronary artery disease, because of her electrocardiogram and arm symptoms.

Physical Examination: Vital signs: pulse 60; blood pressure 150/90. Cardiac: short aortic systolic murmur, no extra sounds. Chest: lungs clear. Abdomen and extremities: normal.

Laboratory Findings: Complete blood count: normal. Chemistries: pending. EKG: see below.

Question: What is the diagnosis?

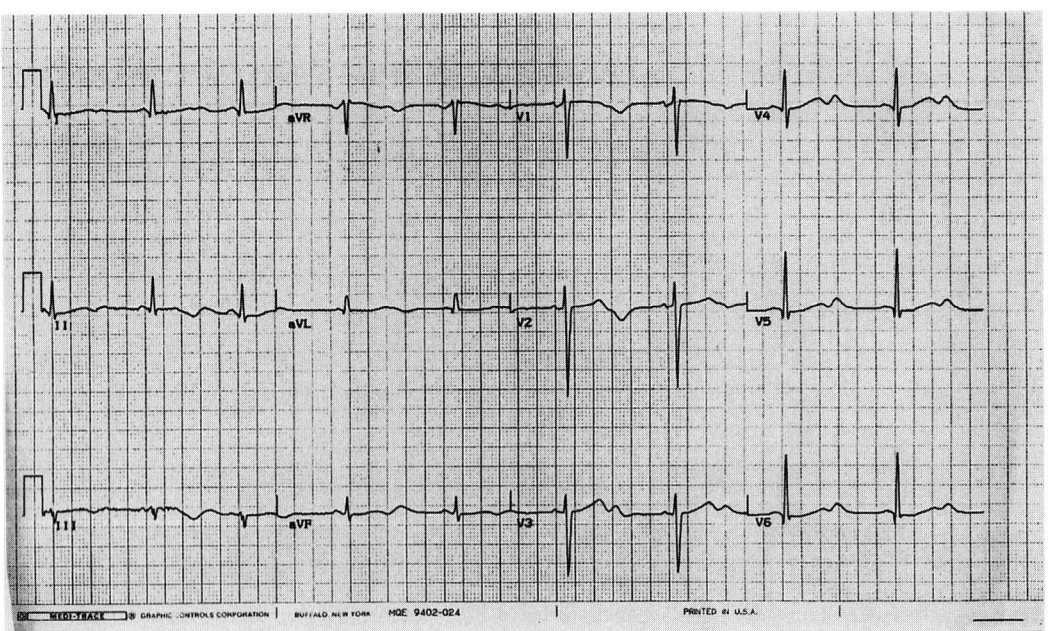

Answer: Hypokalemia with EKG changes.

Discussion: The EKG was helpful in the diagnosis of hypokalemia before the blood chemistry results were returned from the laboratory. Hypokalemia prolongs the QT interval at the expense of the T wave, which becomes low, flat or inverted, and broad. Prominent, upright "U" waves, usually taller than the T wave, often are present. Hypocalcemia prolongs the QT interval by prolonging the ST segment, and the T wave remains normal or inverted, but is not broad.

Potassium homeostasis plays an important role in the maintenance of normal cardiac function. Internal potassium homeostasis is affected by many factors, such as acid-based status, plasma insulin concentration, and plasma catecholamines. Aldosterone activity may play a minor role. Hypokalemia significantly alters the action potential curve. The resting action potential becomes more negative, phase 4 depolarization may be increased, and phases 2 and 3 of Purkinje fibers are prolonged. The delay in repolarization induced by hypokalemia **prolongs the action potential curve,** which is reflected in an increase of the QT interval and development of U waves on the surface EKG. This change can result in torsade de pointes because of early after depolarizations (during phase 3 of the action potential curve). The genesis of the U wave has not been firmly established.

Hypokalemia also has been associated with AV conduction disturbances and supraventricular arrhythmia. Hypokalemia can induce a cardiomyopathy and the risk of stroke.

There are many causes of hypokalemia, including: diuretics, alcoholism, gastrointestinal disorders with vomiting, diarrhea or gastric suction, renal tubular acidosis, primary and secondary hyperaldosteronism, antibiotics (penicillin, carbenicillin, aminoglycoside, amphotericin), magnesium depletion, trauma, drugs such as theophylline and albuterol, leukemia and bronchogenic tumors that produce adrenocorticotropic hormone, Bartter's syndrome, familial periodic paralysis, and chronic ingestion of licorice or laxatives. The glycyrrhizic acid of licorice inhibits the enzyme that catalyzes the conversion of cortisol to cortisone. The cortisol level is elevated, which results in kaliuresis and hypokalemia (licorice-induced pseudoaldosteronism). Habitual drinking of oolong tea can cause hypokalemia. It contains great quantities of caffeine, which is bound by the serum protein albumin. In patients with hypoalbuminemia, caffeine induces hypokalemia.

The present patient had a potassium level of 1.8 mEq/L. The heaviness and weakness in her arms was *not* due to myocardial ischemia, but was related to the hypokalemic myopathy. Hydrochlorothiazide, chlorthalidone, and metolazone are diuretics that typically produce hypokalemia and increase the need for potassium supplements. In addition, this patient exhibited hypomagnesemia, which also requires replacement. With potassium replacement, the present patient's EKG returned to normal, and her symptoms cleared.

Clinical Pearls

1. Thiazide diuretics frequently produce hypokalemia.
2. Prior to the return of laboratory reports, the EKG may indicate hypokalemia by demonstrating a long QT interval and prominent, upright U waves.
3. Hypokalemia can produce arrhythmias, cardiomyopathy, and skeletal myopathy.
4. Investigate unusual causes, such as large ingestion of licorice and oolong tea.

REFERENCES

1. Mandal AK: Hypokalemia and hyperkalemia. Med Clin North Am 1997;81:611–639.
2. Ascherio A, Rimm EB, Hernan MA, et al.: Intake of potassium, magnesium, calcium, and fiber and risk of stroke among U.S. men. Circulation 1998;98:1198–1204.
3. Hasagawa J, Suyama Y, Kinugawa T, et al.: Echocardiographic findings of the heart resembling dilated cardiomyopathy during hypokalemic myopathy due to licorice-induced pseudoaldosteronism. Cardiovasc Drugs Ther 1998;12:599–600.
4. Aizaki T, Osaka M, Hara H, et al.: Hypokalemia with syncope caused by habitual drinking of oolong tea. Intern Med 1999;38:252–256.

PATIENT 3

A 45-year-old man with coronary artery disease and normal lipids except for low HDL

A 45-year-old, male cigarette-smoker with known coronary artery disease has the following lipid profile:

Cholesterol = 160 mg/dl
LDL = 100 mg/dl
HDL = 30 mg/dl
Triglycerides = 150 mg/dl
VLDL = 30 mg/dl

Physical Examination: Normal.

Question: How would you manage this patient?

Answer: It is important to raise the high-density lipoprotein (HDL), even if the other fractions are normal.

Discussion: HDL is involved in a process of reverse cholesterol transport, in which it transports cholesterol to the liver from the peripheral tissues. Nascent HDL (small pre-beta) is synthesized in the liver or intestines and secreted in the blood. Its free cholesterol is esterified by lecithin-cholesterol acyl transferase, with apo A1 as a cofactor, and forms large mature particles (HDL_2). The cholesterol ester in the core of HDL_2 can be transferred by cholesterol ester transfer proteins to the triglyceride-rich lipoprotein and intermediate density lipoprotein for uptake by the low-density lipoprotein (LDL) receptors on the liver. Cholesteryl ester also can be removed from HDL by HDL receptors on the liver. As the cholesteryl ester is removed from HDL, this particle (now rich in triglycerides) is converted back to nascent HDL by the action of hepatic triglyceride lipase.

Low HDL is a predictor of increased coronary artery disease independent of all other risk factors, including hypercholesterolemia, cigarette smoking, and hypertension. Factors that caused or are correlated with low HDL levels are cigarette smoking, lack of exercise, obesity, androgenic or related steroids, beta-blockers, hypertriglyceridemia, and genetic factors. Estrogens, cessation of smoking, exercise, and low levels of red wine consumption can increase HDL. Lipid-lowering drugs also can raise HDL even if other lipid parameters are in the normal range. **Niacin** has the greatest ability to raise HDL, up to 30%. Gemfibrozil can raise it up to 12%, and statin drugs less so. For each 1 mg/dl increase in HDL, there is a 2–3% decrease in coronary artery disease.

The present patient has a normal routine lipid panel except for the low HDL. Other factors that should be considered in such instances are small LDL (type B) particles, lipoprotein (a), homocysteine, plasma fibrinogen, and C-reactive protein. In the present patient, niacin (Niaspan, a controlled-release form) and/or gemfibrozil should be considered if controlling other factors such as exercise, cessation of smoking, and weight reduction does not produce a significant increase in HDL. Niaspan also produces favorable changes in LDL, triglycerides, lipoprotein (a), and small dense particles of LDL. Adverse hepatic effects are minor, and flushing is less than that noted with other sustained-release niacin preparations.

Clinical Pearls

1. Low HDL is an important risk factor for coronary artery disease.
2. Patients can have coronary artery disease with a normal routine lipid profile except for low HDL.
3. In patients with normal traditional lipid levels except for low HDL, look to other factors such as small dense LDL (type B), lipoprotein (a), homocysteine, fibrinogen, and C-reactive protein.
4. HDL can be raised by cessation of smoking, exercise, red wine, and drugs such as niacin, gemfibrozil, and estrogens.

REFERENCES
1. Superko HR: Lipid disorders contributing to coronary heart disease: An update. Curr Probl Cardiol 1996;21:736–780.
2. Guyton JR, Goldberg AC, Kresberg RA, et al: Effectiveness of once-nightly dosing of extended-release niacin alone or in combination for hypercholesterolemia. Am J Cardiol 1998;82:737–743.
3. Genest J Jr, Marcil M, Denis M, Yu L: High-density lipoproteins in health and in disease. J Investig Med 1999;47:31–42.

PATIENT 4

A 42-year-old man with sharp left chest pain when running

A 42-year-old, long-distance runner developed left sharp chest pain while running. The pain subsided at rest and lasted only 10 minutes. He went to the emergency department.

Physical Examination: Vital signs: normal. Cardiac exam: normal. EKG: computer interpretation was anterior current of injury and left ventricular hypertrophy by voltage criteria (see below).

Question: What is the most probable diagnosis?

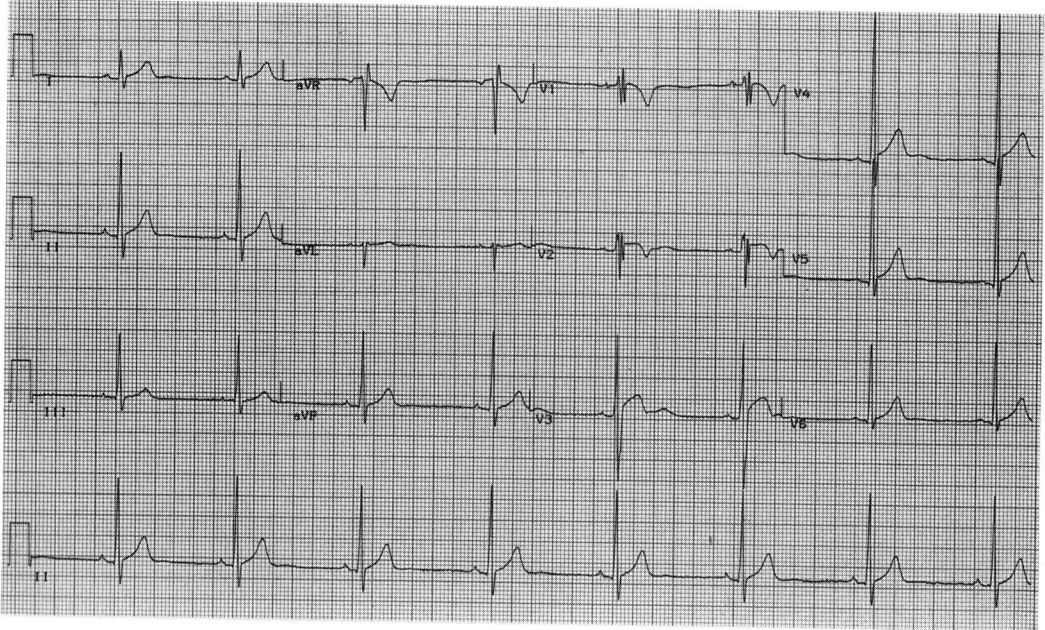

Diagnosis: Athlete's heart.

Discussion: Computer interpretations of EKGs make major errors 20% of the time and minor errors about 40% of the time. Therefore, these tracings should be overread. High levels of exercise can produce physiologic adaptations that can simulate organic heart disease. Intermittent epinephrine release with exercise can produce physiologic cardiac hypertrophy. The EKG may show high R wave voltage, and the echocardiogram can demonstrate hypertrophy. There is no evidence that this is harmful, as is the case for hypertrophy due to chronic overload conditions.

Exercise hypertrophy favors synthesis of a fast, high ATPase myosin, whereas pressure overload favors synthesis of a slow, low ATPase myosin. Relaxation is accelerated by exercise, and pressure overload slows it. In addition, chronic exercise can cause sinus bradycardia, first-degree AV block, occasional periods of Wenckebach second-degree block, junctional rhythm, accelerated idioventricular rhythm, and repolarization changes. The ST-T changes may simulate a current of injury, as noted in this patient's EKG. Most often these represent early repolarization.

It has been postulated that a strength-trained heart (weight lifting, throwing, and wrestling) and an endurance-trained heart (running) can be distinguished. The strength-trained heart develops predominantly left ventricular wall thickness with very little change in ventricular chamber size, and an endurance-trained heart develops predominantly increased left ventricular chamber size and less left ventricular wall thickness. However, this classification is not an absolute and dichotomous concept, but rather a relative concept. Overall, athlete's heart regardless of training demonstrates normal systolic and diastolic function.

Athlete's heart must be differentiated from hypertrophic cardiomyopathy. Athlete's heart does not have the usual patterns of left ventricular hypertrophy; the left atrium is not enlarged; the left ventricular cavity is normal; and with deconditioning, the hypertrophy decreases. The present patient had no evidence of cardiac disease, and he continues to run.

Clinical Pearls

1. Computer EKG interpretations always should be overread.
2. Athletes may have physiologic hypertrophy of the right and left heart chambers and many EKG changes besides hypertrophy, such as sinus bradycardia, junctional rhythm, accelerated idioventricular rhythm, first and second degree (Mobitz I) AV heart block, and repolarization changes.

REFERENCES

1. Park RC, Crawford MH: Heart of the athlete. Curr Probl Cardiol 1985;10:1–73.
2. Katz AM: Treating heart failure: Yesterday, today, and tomorrow. Adv Cardiovasc Med 1994;1:1.
3. Pluim BM, Zwinderman AH, van der Laarse A, van der Wall EE: The athlete's heart. A meta-analysis of cardiac structure and function. Circulation 2000;101:336–344.

PATIENT 5

A 14-year-old girl with chest pain and rapid heart beat

A 14-year-old girl with a subarterial ventricular septal defect and aortic leaflet prolapse with mild aortic insufficiency awoke on the morning of admission with suprasternal notch, superior mid-sternal chest pain, and a fast heart beat. The pain did not radiate, lasted up to 30 minutes, and was worse with inspiration. At times she felt warm, but her temperature was not recorded.

Physical Examination: Vital signs: temperature 100 F; respirations 20; blood pressure 130/80. Chest: clear. Cardiac: harsh systolic murmur grade IV/VI over left upper sternal border and faint diastolic murmur along lower left sternal border; regular rapid heart beat at about 250 beats per minute; no pericardial rubs.

Laboratory Findings: CBC, urinalysis, electrolytes: normal. EKGs: see below.

Question: What is your diagnosis?

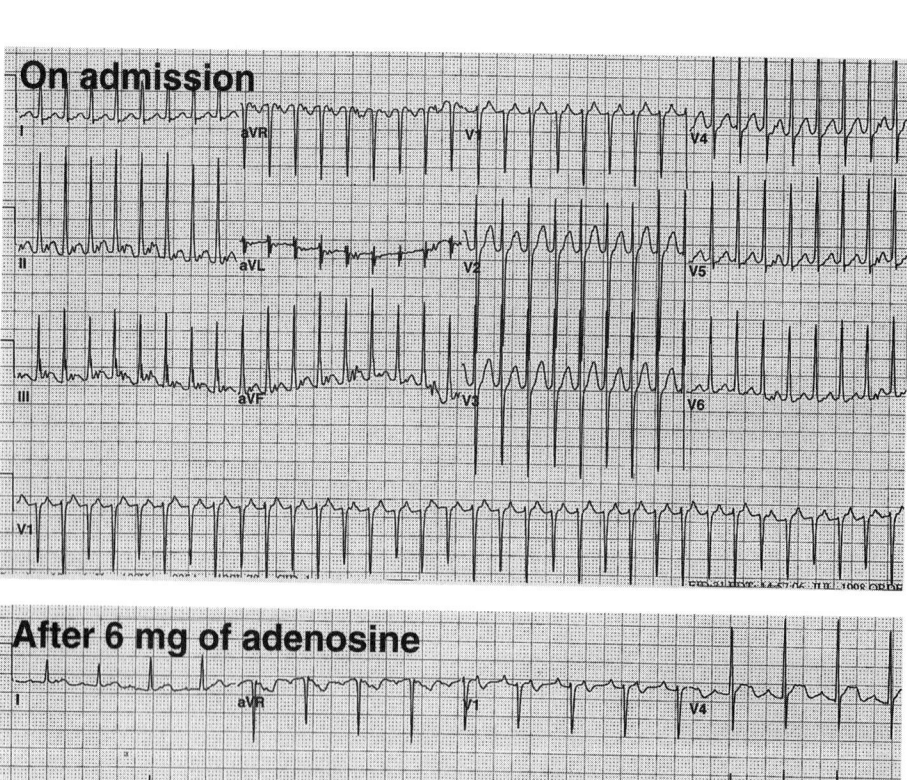

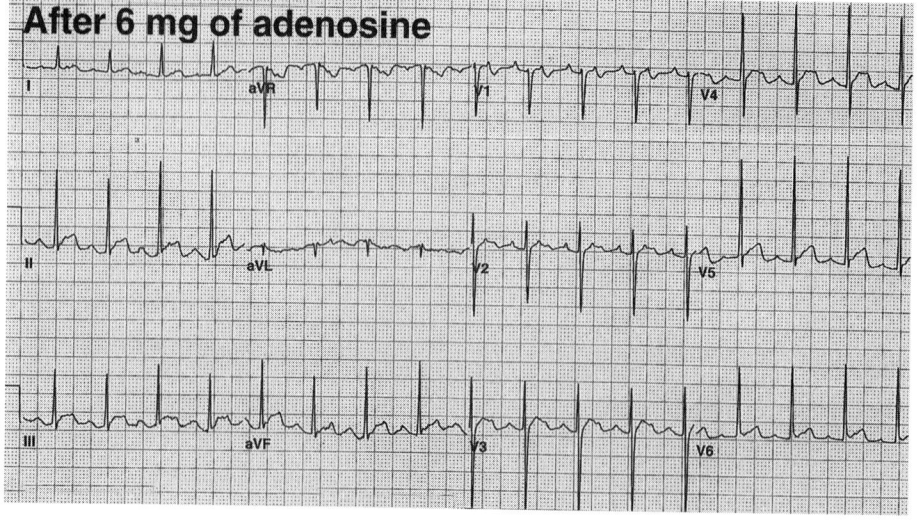

Diagnosis: Atrial flutter; ventricular septal defect with aortic leaflet prolapse and aortic insufficiency; acute pericarditis.

Discussion: Initially, the electrocardiogram in the present patient showed a rapid regular supraventricular tachycardia with a rate of 250 beats per minute (*top tracing*). A P wave with an RP interval less than 70 msec was noted after the QRS complex. This was considered to be atrioventricular nodal reentry tachycardia, and 6 mg of adenosine was given intravenously. The ventricular rate slowed, and a 2:1 atrial flutter with an atrial rate of 250 beats per minute (*lower tracing*) was clearly noted. In addition, diffuse ST elevation was present. Digoxin was given, and the patient converted to regular sinus rhythm.

Pericardial disease has been reported with atrial septal defects, but not with ventricular septal defects. The patient's symptoms were characteristic of acute pericarditis, even though no pericardial friction rub was audible. The visceral pericardial membrane has no pain fibers. Only the lower part of the parietal membrane carries pain fibers from the phrenic nerve. The afferent nerves of pain perception enter the spinal cord at the level of C3–C5 via the phrenic nerve. Involvement of the mediastinum, diaphragm, and pleura also may contribute to the pain.

One-to-one atrial flutter can occur with a rapid ventricular rate. The top tracing also shows electrical alternans that can occur with rapid heart rates. Electrical alternans is thought to be due to positional and rotational changes or aberrancy of intraventricular conduction. Often, if rapid 1:1 atrial flutter persists, congestive heart failure develops.

Adenosine was a good choice since it has a short life (1.5–10 seconds) and is specific for converting AV nodal reentry tachycardia; in the present patient, it successfully blocked the AV node. The rate of the flutter waves (*lower tracing*) is the same as the ventricular rate in the top tracing. Adenosine depresses sinoatrial activity, AV nodal conduction, atrial contractility, and ventricular automaticity. A_2 receptors present in endothelial and vascular smooth muscles mediate adenosine coronary vasodilatory effect, and A_1 receptors in cardiomyocytes mediate its negative chronotropic, dromotropic, and inotropic actions. Facial flushing, dyspnea, and chest heaviness are some side effects of adenosine. Use caution in asthmatic patients and patients taking dipyridamole (which blocks the uptake of adenosine and increases its potency). Intravenous theophylline can reverse its effect.

The present patient has atrial flutter, which could be secondary to the acute pericarditis. Arrhythmias with pericarditis usually indicate additional heart disease, but can be associated with the inflamed pericardium being contiguous to sinoatrial node or to atrial wall involvement. A pericardial friction rub was not present, but this does not exclude pericarditis. The typical history and ST elevation on the EKG confirm the diagnosis. In addition, an echocardiograph showed a small pericardial effusion. The pericarditis resolved with ibuprofen administration. Surgery for the ventricular septal defect and aortic insufficiency is planned for the future. Aortic insufficiency develops in 5–8% of patients with ventricular septal defects, because of the lack of support of the aortic root.

Clinical Pearls

1. Patients with cardiac lesions may have unrelated problems, such as acute pericarditis.
2. Atrial arrhythmias can be noted with acute pericarditis.
3. Adenosine can be used as a diagnostic tool in differentiating regular tachycardias.
4. A pericardial friction rub often is present, but its absence does not exclude acute pericarditis.

REFERENCES

1. Just H, Mattingly TW: Interatrial septal defect and pericardial disease. Coincidence or causal relationship? Am Heart J 1968;76:157–167.
2. Gazes PC: Pericarditis. Cardiovasc Dis Chest Pain 1985;1:2–8.
3. Lerman, BB, Belardinelli L: Cardiac electorophysiology of a denosine: Basic and clinical concepts. Circulation 1991;83:1499.

PATIENT 6

A 53-year-old man with chest pain and a left bundle branch block

A 53-year-old, male cigarette-smoker with hypercholesterolemia is admitted because of severe substernal chest pain radiating to his jaw and down both arms. He has been experiencing this pain for 1 hour.

Physical Examination: Vital signs: pulse 100 and regular; blood pressure 110/70. Cardiac: S_2 paradoxically split with expiration.

Laboratory Findings: Enzymes: pending. EKGs: see below.

Question: Should a thrombolytic agent be given when the first tracing is taken?

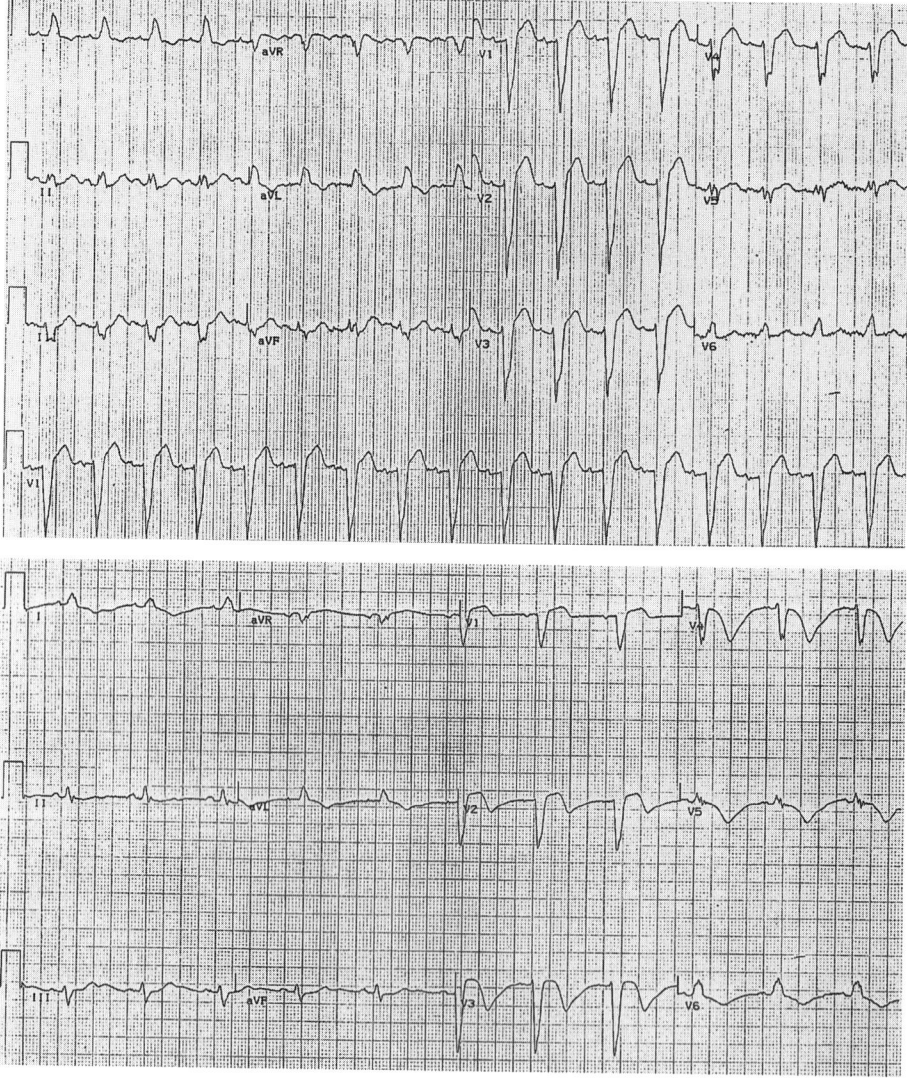

Answer: A thrombolytic agent should be given in the setting of a left bundle branch block in view of the classic history of myocardial infarction.

Discussion: It is difficult to make a diagnosis of an infarction in the presence of a left bundle branch block (LBBB), because the direction of septal activation is reversed and R waves instead of Q waves are produced in the precordial leads—especially in the presence of infarction of the free left ventricular wall. If there is ST elevation in the anterolateral chest leads or in the inferior leads concordant with the QRS complex, or 5-mm ST elevation discordant with the QRS complex, then suspect infarction. In addition, small Q waves in leads L_1, aVL, V_5, or V_6 in the setting of LBBB are suggestive. In such cases, the infarction also involves the septum.

In the present patient the diffusely inverted T waves noted in the bottom tracing were indicative of infarction, especially since the troponins and CK-MB were elevated. However, a thrombolytic agent should be given even before the second tracing or enzyme results are returned.

The top tracing shows an LBBB that could have been present previously or is new. Regardless, if LBBB is present and there is a good history for infarction, administer a thrombolytic agent. The following criteria usually are required for a patient to be eligible for thrombolytic therapy: (1) chest pain characteristic of myocardial ischemia lasting 20 minutes or longer; (2) ST elevation of 0.1 mV or more in two or more contiguous leads that persists despite sublingual nitroglycerin and with or without Q wave development; (3) characteristic chest pain with an LBBB; and (4) passage of less than 12 hours from the clinical onset of myocardial infarction.

The present patient received a thrombolytic agent and adjunctive therapy. His course was uneventful.

Clinical Pearls

1. In the setting of LBBB, myocardial infarction is suggested by ST segment of elevation of 1 mm or more concordant with the QRS complex; 5-mm ST segment elevation discordant with the QRS complex; small Q waves in L_1, aVL, V_5 or V_6; or progressive development of diffuse T wave increases.

2. In the proper history setting of significant chest pain with LBBB, do not wait for further EKG findings or enzyme results before administrating thromoblytic therapy.

REFERENCES

1. Sgarbossa EB, Pinski SL, Barbagelata A, et al: Electrocardiographic diagnosis of evolving acute myocardial infarction in the presence of left bundle-branch block. GUSTO-1 (Global Utilization of Streptokinase and Tissue Plasminogen Activator for Occluded Coronary Arteries) Investigators. N Engl J Med 1996;334:481–487.
2. Ryan TJ, Antman EM, Brooks NH, et al.: 1999 update: ACC/AHA guidelines for the management of patients with acute myocardial infarction. A report of the American College of Cardiology/American Heart Association Task Force on Practice Guidelines (Committee on Management of Acute Myocardial Infarction). J Am Coll Cardiol 1999;34(3):890–911.

PATIENT 7

A 64-year-old man with congestive heart failure

A 64-year-old man suffers a bout of acute pulmonary edema. He has dyspnea, but no chest pain. He responds to medical therapy and subsequently is seen as an outpatient. He denies having hypertension or diabetes and has no anginal symptoms. At one time he had a high alcohol intake, but he has abstained during the past 10 years.

Physical Examination: Vital signs: pulse 85; blood pressure 130/70. Cardiac: a grade II/VI murmur of aortic insufficiency is noted along the left sternal border and a high-pitched murmur of mitral insufficiency at the apex.

Laboratory Findings: EKG: left axis -30%, intraventricular conduction delay, left atrial enlargement, and nonspecific ST-T changes in the lateral leads. Echocardiogram: dilated cardiomyopathy, with an ejection fraction of 20%; left ventricular end diastolic dimension 7.20 cm, end systolic dimension 6.24 cm. Doppler study: mild mitral and aortic insufficiency. Heart catheterization: global hypokinesis with 1+ mitral insufficiency, minimal aortic insufficiency, ejection fraction 33%; first diagonal has a 30% lesion, a 40% proximal lesion in ramus, and a 30% lesion in obtuse marginal; right coronary artery normal.

Question: What is the most likely diagnosis?

Diagnosis: Alcoholic cardiomyopathy with minimal valvular and coronary artery disease.

Discussion: An examination of this patient's course is instructive. At the time of the initial event, a biopsy of the patient's right ventricle showed myofiber nuclear enlargement and angulation and cystoplasmic enlargement with nonspecific cardiomyopathy. Medications initially prescribed included captopril, lasix, and digoxin. Over 2 years, his multiple gated acquisition (MUGA) ejection fraction rose from 20% to 59%. After an additional 2 years, however, the ejection fraction dropped to 26%, and metoprolol was added. The patient began to note substernal tightness on undue exertion, which was relieved by rest. He had no further symptoms after increasing his captopril, and his ejection fraction rose to 37%. One year later, he had left arm weakness, and a duplex scan showed an 80% lesion in the right carotid artery. A carotid endarterectomy was performed. Three years passed uneventfully, but then mitral and aortic insufficiency increased, as shown by echo-Doppler studies. Heart catheterization was advised. The left main coronary artery now showed a 75% ostial lesion, confirmed by intravascular ultrasound. The proximal LAD had 50% stenosis, and the first obtuse marginal had a 90% stenosis at its takeoff. Global hypokinesis with an ejection fraction of 40% was noted, and an aortogram showed 3–4+ aortic insufficiency. The degree of mitral insufficiency could not be evaluated because of ventricular ectopy. One month later, a myocardial perfusion scan showed a dilated left ventricle, a scar in the inferior wall extending to the apex, and an ejection fraction of 18%. The patient completed 10 minutes of the Bruce protocol, with a maximum exercise heart rate of 172 and maximum blood pressure of 170/70. The EKG showed left ventricular hypertrophy with repolarization abnormality, and further ST depression occurred with stress. Upon administration of low- and high-dose dobutamine, dobutamine stress echocardiogram showed improvement in contraction of the inferolateral and posterior walls. The anteroseptal and apex areas improved only with low-dose dobutamine. The test was consistent with **hibernating myocardium.** Duplex scan showed an 80% obstruction of the left carotid artery.

After much discussion, the patient agreed to extensive surgery, including left carotid artery endarterectomy with dacron patch angioplasty, aortic valve replacement, mitral valve repair, and six-vessel coronary bypass. Since surgery, he has been asymptomatic. His ejection fraction rose from 18% to 36% in 1 year, by MUGA.

Apparently, this patient initially had *alcoholic* cardiomyopathy with minimal coronary and valvular lesions, which improved on an ACE inhibitor. At that point, the valvular disease and coronary disease were not of sufficient degree to be the primary cause of the cardiomyopathy. Subsequently, the valvular lesions worsened and the coronary disease became more severe, including an ostial left main lesion. The ejection fraction improved with surgery, indicating that hibernating myocardium was a significant factor.

Clinical Pearls

1. Cardiomyopathy can improve with medical therapy, especially with afterload reduction.
2. Patients with minimal valvular and coronary artery disease may have associated cardiomyopathy of unknown cause, yet over subsequent years the coronary disease and valvular disease may worsen.
3. Hibernating myocardium can be detected by low-dose dobutamine stress echocardiogram and can be improved with revascularization.

REFERENCES

1. Regan TJ: Alcoholic cardiomyopathy. Prog Cardiovasc Dis 1984;27:141–152.
2. Nagueh SF, Zoghbi WA: Stress echocardiography for the assessment of myocardial ischemia and viability. Curr Probl Cardiol 1996;21:445–520.

PATIENT 8

A 51-year-old woman with dyspnea

A 51-year-old woman has had progressive exertional dyspnea, sometimes occurring at rest, for many years. Tachypnea associated with hyperventilation produces lightheadedness. Frequent coughing spells productive of yellow, clear sputum occur mostly at night, and she also has a postnasal drip. Coughing produces urinary incontinence. She has frequent episodes of bronchitis and pneumonitis. Four-pillow orthopnea and peripheral edema developed over the past year. She has been known to have hypertension for many years; it recently was controlled with Lotensin. The cough was present prior to beginning Lotensin. She smoked one pack of cigarettes daily for 30 years, but stopped 2 years ago.

Physical Examination: General: short and obese. Vital signs: Pulse 82; blood pressure 160/100; temperature 98.2° F. Neck: pulsations cannot be visualized due to very short neck. Chest: normal configuration; bibasilar "velcro-type" crackles, but no wheezing. Abdomen: obese; liver not palpable. Extremities: 2+ peripheral edema just above the ankles.

Laboratory Findings: Pulmonary function studies: moderate restrictive pulmonary disease. Echocardiography: right ventricular hypertrophy and dilatation; flattening of the ventricular septum with a pressure overload of the right ventricle; moderate tricuspid insufficiency and severe pulmonary hypertension (99 mmHg); borderline left ventricular hypertrophy with ejection fraction greater than 60%. EKG: see below.

Questions: What is your diagnosis? How would you confirm it?

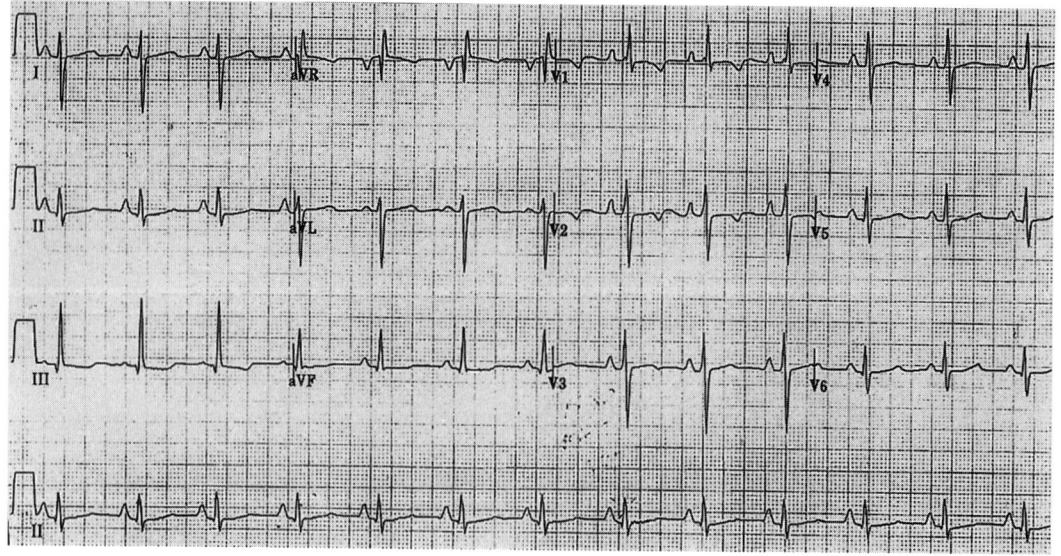

Answer: Pulmonary fibrosis with cor pulmonale. The diagnosis can be confirmed by thoracoscopic biopsy.

Discussion: Clinically, the findings of normal chest configuration and "velcro-type" bibasilar rales suggest pulmonary fibrosis rather than chronic obstructive pulmonary disease (COPD). In addition, the EKG showing right ventricular hypertrophy and right atrial enlargement favors this diagnosis. Tall R waves in the right precordial leads are unusual in COPD and are seen more often in restrictive lung diseases. Pulmonary function studies and lung biopsy confirmed the diagnosis in the present patient.

Fibrosis in such patients causes destruction of the functioning pulmonary parenchyma and reduction of the pulmonary vascular bed, with resultant pulmonary hypertension and, eventually, cor pulmonale. Patients with restrictive lung disease have a normal or low cardiac output and do not have bounding pulses as noted with COPD. At times, the high pulmonary artery pressure may produce a diastolic murmur of pulmonary valve insufficiency or a murmur of tricuspid insufficiency (both louder with inspiration). There may be a pulmonic ejection sound and a prominent venous jugular A wave. A right ventricular lift may be present over the precordium, in contrast to COPD, in which it may be felt only under the xiphoid as a downward pulsation.

With severe hypoxia, heart failure ensues; this usually is terminal and seldom reversible in patients with pulmonary fibrosis, as can be noted with COPD. Controlling the pulmonary hypertension by effective ventilation, increased oxygenation, and lowering of CO_2 reduces the load on the heart in patients with COPD, and thus can prevent or reverse heart failure. Consider unilateral or bilateral lung transplantation.

The present patient was given oxygen and adrenal corticosteroids, but he continued to worsen, and eventually expired.

Clinical Pearls

1. Consider normal chest configuration with "velcro-type" bibsaliar rales but without evidence of bronchospasm to be due to restrictive lung disease.

2. Patients with COPD do not live long enough to get severe, free-wall right ventricular hypertrophy (tall R waves in V1), as noted in patients with restrictive lung disease.

3. Restrictive lung disease can be diagnosed with pulmonary function studies and thoracoscopic biopsy.

REFERENCES

1. Padmavati S, Raizada V: Electrocardiogram in chronic cor pulmonale. Br Heart J 1972;34:658–667.
2. Vizza CD, Lynch JP, Ochoa LL, et al: Right and left ventricular dysfunction in patients with severe pulmonary disease. Chest 1998;113:576–583.

PATIENT 9

A 63-year-old hypertensive man with a new murmur and chest pain

A 63-year-old hypertensive man notes increasing dyspnea, orthopnea, paroxysmal nocturnal dyspnea, and intermittent sharp substernal chest pain 2 weeks after undergoing a laparoscopic Nissen fundoplication. The chest pain radiates to his jaw and upper back. It lasts from several seconds to 30 minutes, and it occurs both at rest and with exercise. A transthoracic echocardiogram (TTE) and Doppler study reveals concentric left ventricular hypertrophy, an ejection fraction of 50%, mild aortic insufficiency, and moderate mitral insufficiency.

Physical Examination: Vital signs: pulse 90; blood pressure 116/69; respiratory rate 21; temperature 99°F. Neck: 3 cm jugular venous distention above sternal angle of Louis at 45° position; normal carotid pulsations. Chest: clear. Cardiac: grade II/VI ejection systolic murmur in first and second intercostal space to right of sternum, with radiation to apex and into right carotid; grade II/VI high-pitched systolic murmur at apex; faint early decrescendo diastolic murmur along left sternal border at about fourth intercostal space. Extremities: pulses equal in arms and legs.

Laboratory Findings: EKG: normal sinus rhythm; left atrial enlargement; left anterior superior fascicular block, and left ventricular hypertrophy. Repeat TTE and Doppler study: ejection fraction 30%; aortic valve thickened, with normal aortic root dimensions; mild mitral and aortic regurgitation; right ventricular systolic pressure estimated at 63 mmHg.

Question: What further studies are indicated?

Answer: Transesophageal echocardiogram (TEE) to further evaluate the heart murmurs.

Discussion: TEE performed about 24 hours after admission disclosed an ascending aortic mass extending to the right coronary cusp and almost obliterating the aortic lumen. The mass had a dense, homogenous appearance consistent with a thrombus. A dissection flap was noted in the descending aorta, with spontaneous contrast in the false lumen. The patient had several episodes of substernal chest pain with ST segment depression and T wave inversion.

Prior to surgery, it was decided that the coronary arteries should be evaluated, especially in view of the low ejection fraction. **Coronary arteriography** showed minor luminal irregularities in the left anterior descending coronary artery, with ostial stenosis of the first two diagonals approaching 75%. There were minor luminal irregularities of both the circumflex and right coronary arteries. **Aortography** demonstrated a striking compression of the aorta above the aortic valve. Pressure recordings taken from the aortic root revealed ventricularization of the proximal aortic root (BP 99/32), with an intra-aortic gradient (15 mmHg) on catheter pullback across the compressed section of the ascending aorta. The ventricular cavity was not entered. A MUGA ejection fraction was 18%.

Vascular complications of aortic dissection are well recognized as stemming from the dissecting hematoma, with resultant occlusion of branch vessels or aortic rupture. Aortic lumen compression is common, but critical **supravalvular aortic lumen stenosis** is rare. Intussusception of the intimal sleeve in circumferential dissections and true lumen obliteration and expanding hematoma are the mechanisms described.

In the present patient, TEE revealed the thrombosed false lumen and intimal flap not seen on TTE. A 15-mmHg gradient across the intra-aortic stenosis was evident and, because of the aortic insufficiency, a diastolic pressure in the aorta proximal to the obstruction was approaching the left ventricular end diastolic pressure. Despite not entering the ventricular cavity, the transmyocardial perfusion pressure probably was low, resulting in the progressive drop in the ejection fraction. Before the patient could be taken to the operating room, he became bradycardic, developed electromechanical dissociation, and died. His demise suggested either global myocardial hypoxia and progressive contractile failure, or rupture of the aorta in the pericardial space and subsequent tamponade.

Clinical Pearls

1. Dissecting aneurysms can produce many complications and, rarely, supravalvular aortic lumen stenosis, as noted in this patient.
2. TEE is more sensitive and specific than TTE in the diagnosis of dissections.
3. Dissections must be recognized early, so that surgical treatment can be initiated immediately.

REFERENCES
1. Cigarroa JE, Isselbacher EM, DeSanctis RW, Eagle KA: Diagnostic imaging in the evaluation of suspected aortic dissection. Old standards and new directions. N Engl J Med 1993;328:35–43.
2. Xie SW, Picard MH, Weissman NJ: Aortic dissections masquerading as aortic valvular disease. J Clin Ultrasound 1995;23:382–387.

PATIENT 10

A 59-year-old woman with slow heart rate

A 59-year-old woman with systolic dysfunction and an ejection fraction of 30% secondary to coronary artery disease is experiencing a slow heart rate while receiving digoxin. She has chronic renal disease, with a creatinine level of 2–3 mg/dl.

Physical Examination: Vital signs: pulse 41; blood pressure 140/80. Neck: at 45° position, deep jugular pulsations rise 4 cm above sternal angle of Louis. Cardiac: cardiomegaly with diffuse PMI; slow heart rate; no murmur. Chest: bibasilar rales. Abdomen: hepatomegaly. Extremities: minimal edema.

Laboratory Findings: Creatinine 2.5 mg/dl. EKGs: see below.

Question: What type of second-degree AV block is present in the top tracing: Mobitz I or II?

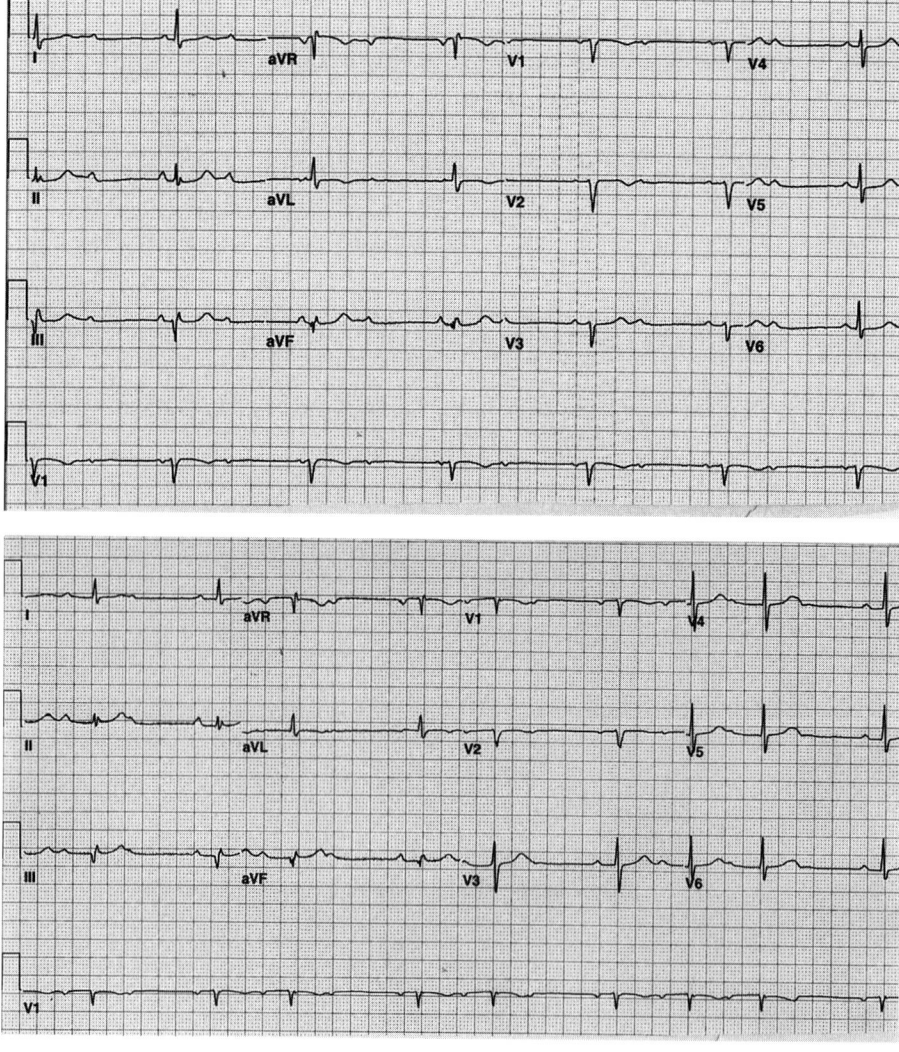

Answer: Mobitz I (Wenckebach) AV block secondary to digoxin toxicity.

Discussion: The first EKG (*top*) shows a 2:1 AV heart block, with a constant P-R interval of the conducted beat and normal width QRS complexes. It is rare to have a Mobitz II without QRS widening, since the block is infra-nodal. With a narrow QRS complex, the block usually is 2:1 AV Wenckebach (Mobitz I). Often, further monitoring shows a classic Wenckebach, as noted in the second EKG (*bottom*) taken several hours later. This tracing shows a 3:2 AV Wenckebach. Rarely, a type II AV block with a normal QRS complex can be due to intrahisian AV block. If bundle branch block is present, it could be in the AV node or the His Purkinkje system.

In the first EKG, the P-P cycles that contain a QRS complex have a shorter P-P interval than those without a QRS complex. This condition is referred to as **ventriculophasic sinus arrhythmia,** and may be due to the autonomic nervous system responding to changes in ventricular stroke volume. It also may be due to contraction of the ventricle, which in some mechanical way stimulates the sinus pacemaker to discharge slightly ahead of schedule.

The present patient's digoxin level was 2.8 ng. Renal insufficiency was a contributing factor to the elevated level and toxicity, since at least 80% of digoxin is excreted by the kidney. Such patients may have a low lean body weight and, therefore, take a lower loading dose, but *it is essential that the maintenance dose be reduced.* Follow serum levels of digoxin closely. Various degrees of AV node heart block can occur with digitalis. In most cases the block is high in the AV node, and even if third-degree AV block develops, the idiojunctional rate is adequate, and the QRS width is normal.

The present patient seldom has Adams-Stokes attacks and does not require a temporary pacemaker. Once digoxin is discontinued and fully excreted, the AV block will clear. Mobitz I (Wenckebach) is the usual type of AV block produced by digoxin, as noted in the present patient.

Clinical Pearls

1. Digitalis may produce Mobitz type I (Wenckebach) AV nodal block.
2. Mobitz I AV block can be present as a 2:1 AV block with a constant P-R interval of the conducted beat and normal width QRS complexes.
3. Further monitoring often shows a type I Mobitz 2:1 AV block going into a 3:2 typical AV Wenckebach.

REFERENCES

1. Rosenbaum M, Lepeschkin E: The effect of ventricular systole on auricular rhythm in auriculoventricular block. Circulation 1955;11:240.
2. Narula OS: Wenckebach type I and type II atrioventricular block (revisited). Cardiovasc Clin 1974;6:137–167.
3. Gonzalez MD, Scherlag BJ, Mabo P, Lazzara R: Functional dissociation of cellular activation as a mechanism of Mobitz type II atrioventricular block. Circulation 1993;87:1389–1398.

PATIENT 11

A 75-year-old woman with an acute infarction and ventricular arrhythmias

A 75-year-old woman had a lateral myocardial infarction 2 years ago. Currently, she is experiencing palpitations and weakness. Holter monitoring reveals many premature ventricular beats in a bigeminal pattern; they are multifocal and in pairs or runs of three beats. Ejection fraction by MUGA is 40%. She is given many antiarrhythmic drugs (e.g., quinidine, disopyramide, sotalol), which she cannot tolerate because of nausea.

Physical Examination: Vital signs: normal except for irregular pulse. Cardiac: premature beats, no murmurs, S_4 sound.

Laboratory Findings: EKGs (see below): first (*top*) taken before antiarrhythmic drug given; second (*bottom*) 48 hours after receiving antiarrhythmic drug.

Question: What antiarrhythmic drug was given to produce the EKG changes?

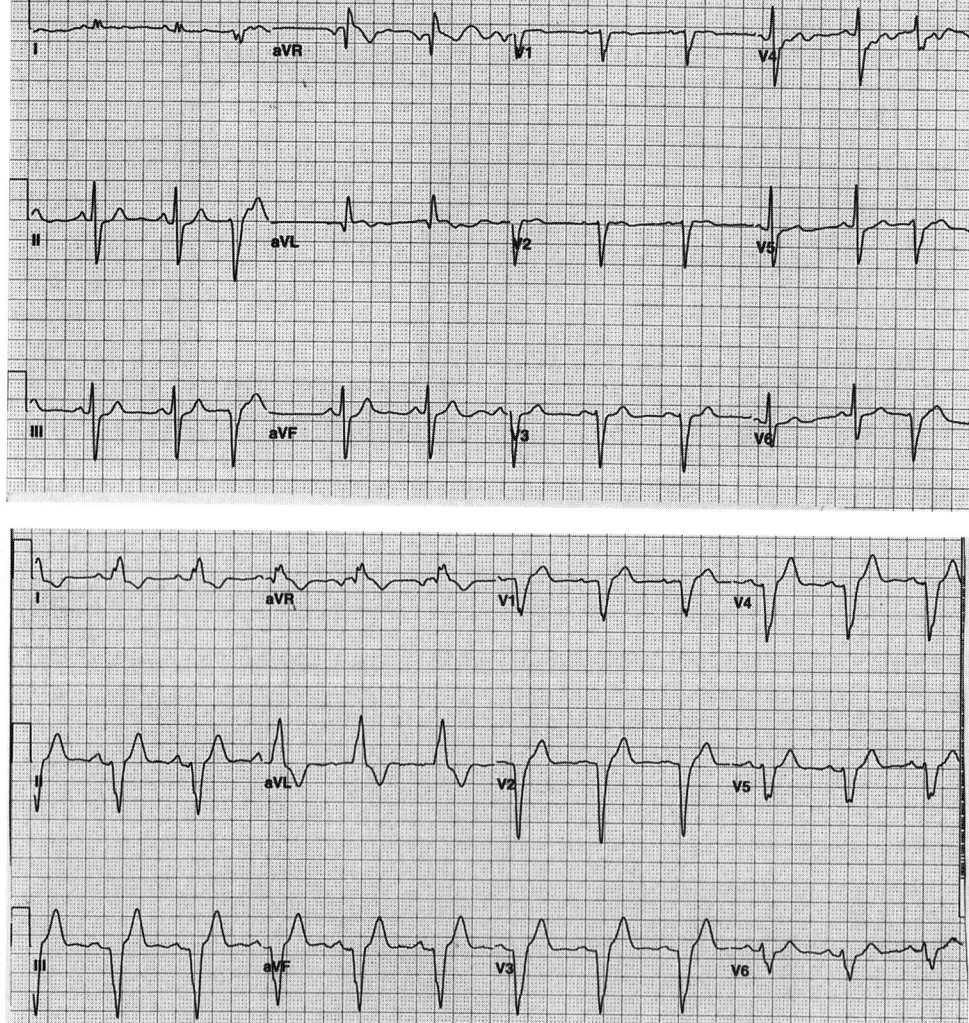

Answer: A type 1C drug, propafenone, which caused widening of the QRS complex.

Discussion: This patient was very symptomatic because of the ventricular arrhythmias. In view of this and the low ejection fraction, she was given antiarrhythmic drugs. Finally, she tolerated propafenone and the arrhythmia cleared, but after 48 hours the QRS complexes were considerably wider.

The classification of antiarrhythmic drugs is still controversial, but for clinical purposes the Vaughn Williams system is useful. Many of the newer antiarrhythmic drugs have antiarrhythmic effects that straddle the four major categories. The "Sicilian Gambit" is more complex, categorizing drugs individually based on their effect on channels, receptors, and transmembrane pumps.

The dominant action of each class of drug according to the Vaughn Williams classification is as follows: **Class 1** drugs depress the fast inward sodium current; **Class 2** drugs reduce sympathetic excitation; **Class 3** drugs prolong the action potential duration by blocking potassium channels; and **Class 4** drugs block the slow calcium channel response. Class 1A drugs (quinidine, procainamide, and disopyramide) moderately depress phase 0 (slow conduction velocity) and lengthen the action potential duration, which prolongs repolarization and increases refractoriness. These actions can prolong the QRS and QT intervals. Class 1B drugs (lidocaine and mexiletine) mildly depress phase 0 and shorten the action potential duration and repolarization. They cause no QRS or QT interval changes. Class 1C drugs (flecainide, encainide, and propafenone) markedly depress phase 0 and minimally affect the action potential duration and repolarization. They prolong the PR and QRS intervals.

Class 2 drugs are β-adrenergic receptor blockers that slow conduction and refractoriness in the AV node and prolong the PR interval. They do not change the QT interval. Class 3 drugs (amiodarone, sotalol) are potassium channel blockers that prolong the action potential duration and increase refractoriness; thus, they prolong the QT interval. Class 4 drugs (verapamil and diltiazem) are calcium channel blockers that prolong AV conduction and refractoriness, and so prolong the PR interval.

The Cardiac Arrhythmia Suppression Trial (CAST) showed that ventricular ectopy could be suppressed with flecainide, encainide, or moricizine, but these drugs increased mortality (sudden death and cardiovascular mortality) and prolonged the QRS duration—even at therapeutic levels. Propafenone also prolongs the QRS. It is not clear what degree of QRS widening warrants discontinuing therapy. However, most agree that if the **QRS widens by more than 30%,** the dose should be reduced or the drug stopped because **proarrhythmias can occur.** In the present patient, the QRS widened by 50% (*bottom tracing*), and the drug dosage was reduced.

It appears that drugs that affect conduction velocity of the action potential curve, such as types 1A and 1C, may produce proarrhythmias. The Beta-Blocker Heart Attack Trial (BHAT) showed on serial Holter recordings that β-blockers had no suppressant effect on PVBs, but reduced the occurrences of ventricular fibrillation. From these studies and those with amiodarone, it appears that antifibrillatory drugs (namely, β-blockers and amiodarone) are best post infarction, and that the antiectopic drugs (types 1A and 1C) that suppress the ventricular arrhythmias may be proarrhythmic because of effects on conduction velocity.

Clinical Pearls

1. Type 1C drugs such as propafenone prolong QRS complex duration and may be proarrhythmic.
2. β-blockers may not suppress ventricular ectopy, but can prevent ventricular fibrillation.
3. Patients who have ventricular arrhythmias post infarct should be given antifibrillatory drugs such as β-blockers and amiodarone, rather than antiectopic drugs.

REFERENCES

1. Vaughn Williams EM: A classification of antiarrhythmic actions reassessed after a decade of new drugs. J Clin Pharmacol 1984;24:129–147.
2. Morganroth J, Lichstein E, Byington R: Beta-blocker Heart Attack Trial: impact of propranolol therapy on ventricular arrhythmias. Prev Med 1985;14:346–357.
3. Antman EM, Friedman PL: Propafenone hydrochloride: a unique new antiarrhythmic. Primary Cardiology 1988;14(3):24.
4. Preliminary report: effect of encainide and flecainide on mortality in a randomized trial of arrhythmia suppression after myocardial infarction. The Cardiac Arrhythmia Suppression Trial (CAST) Investigators. N Engl J Med 1989;321:406–412.
5. Zehender M, Hohnloser S, Geibel A, et al: Short-term and long-term treatment with propafenone: Determinants of arrhythmia suppression, persistence of efficacy, arrhythmogenesis, and side effects in patients with symptoms. Br Heart J 1992;67:491–497.

PATIENT 12

A 25-year-old man with dyspnea and orthostatic dizziness

A 25-year-old man was referred because of dyspnea and orthostatic dizziness. He was told he had an abnormal EKG. He denies any chest pain or syncope. Dyspnea occurs with moderate exertion.

Physical Examination: Vital signs: pulse 70; blood pressure 120/76. HEENT and neck: negative. Cardiac: harsh ejection grade III/VI intensity systolic murmur, heard best along left sternal border at third and fourth intercostal spaces; murmur decreases in intensity on squatting, increases on standing.

Laboratory Findings: CBC, urinalysis: normal. EKG: see below.

Question: What is your diagnosis?

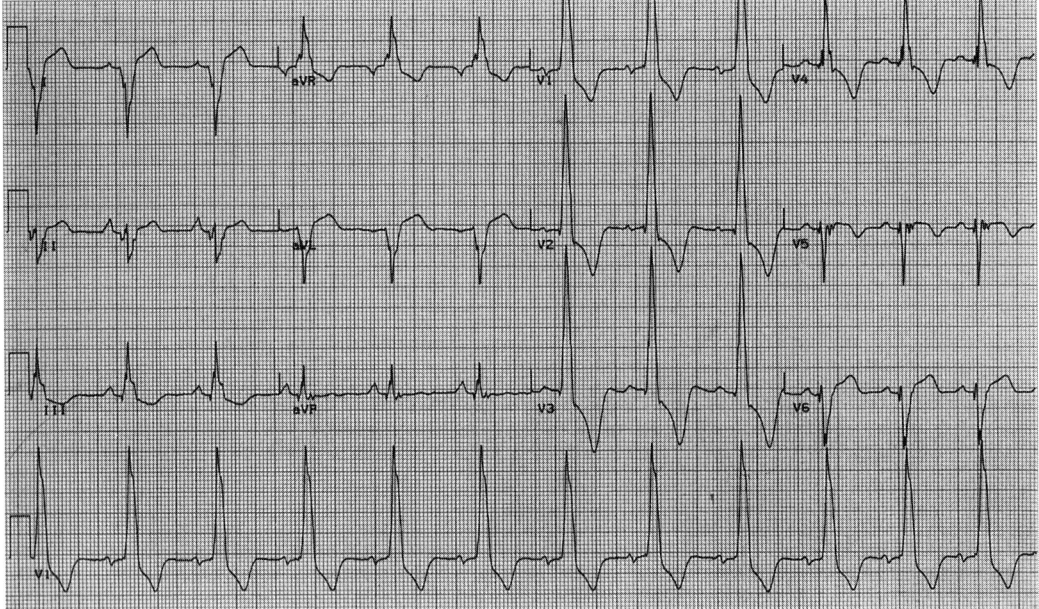

Diagnosis: Idiopathic hypertrophic subaortic stenosis (IHSS) with unusual EKG findings.

Discussion: When IHSS is present, the EKG usually reveals left ventricular hypertrophy and may simulate an infarction pattern with deep Q waves in the inferior and left precordial leads. The Q waves can be due to spetal hypertrophy and fibrosis. However, Cosio found that myopathic septal muscle has electrophysiologic properties that are different from those of the remainder of the myocardium, and this difference may account for the Q waves. The apex forms of hypertrophic cardiomyopathy (Japanese type) can have giant T wave inversion in the mid precordial leads.

The present patient's EKG is most unusual. It has features of right bundle branch block, left posterior inferior fascicular block, right atrial enlargement, right ventricular hypertrophy, and an anterolateral infarction of undetermined age. An echocardiogram confirmed the diagnosis.

There is asymmetric septal hypertrophy, with the interventricular septum measuring 2.7 cm at end diastole and the left ventricular posterior wall measuring 1.75 cm at end diastole. The left ventricular performance is normal, with an estimated ejection fraction greater than 60%. The left atrium is enlarged, measuring 5.3 cm. The cardiac valves are structurally normal. The anterior leaflet of the mitral valve during systole is displaced toward the septum (systolic anterior motion; SAM), and mid systolic closure of the aortic valve is noted since there is a gradient. The maximum velocity across the left ventricular outflow tract (LVOT) is 4.2 m/s, corresponding to a peak LVOT gradient of 71 mmHg. SAM can be found in the other conditions of left ventricular hypertrophy; in disorders featuring increased contractility; and in transposition of the great arteries.

The present patient was given a beta blocker, and he became asymptomatic.

Clinical Pearls

1. The EKG associated with hypertrophic cardiomyopathy can take several forms: narrow Q waves, left ventricular hypertrophy, bundle branch block, deeply inverted T waves, and left atrial enlargement.
2. A murmur that intensifies on standing and decreases on squatting frequently is a clue to IHSS.
3. The diagnosis of IHSS often can be made at the bedside by detecting bifid carotid pulses and heart murmur changes with maneuvers that increase or decrease ventricular volume.

REFERENCES
1. Yamaguchi H, Ishimura T, Nishiyama S, et al.: Hypertrophic nonobstructive cardiomyopathy with giant negative T waves (apical hypertrophy): Ventriculographic and echocardiographic features in 30 patients. Am J Cardiol 1979;44:401–412.
2. Cosio FG, Moro C, Alonso M, et al: The Q waves of hypertropic cardiomyopathy: An electrophysiologic study. N Engl J Med 1980;302:96–99.

PATIENT 13

A 35-year-old man with an abnormal EKG

A 35-year-old man has an abnormal EKG prior to having an open kidney biopsy. He has had no cardiovascular complaints. A diagnosis of Henoch-Schönlein purpura (HSP) was made previously by skin biopsy. In addition to prednisone, he was treated with dapsone 200 mg daily to prevent further flare-up of skin manifestations. Renal involvement is being considered because he has hematuria and proteinuria. Two percutaneous biopsies of the kidney were unsuccessful. Therefore, he is scheduled for open renal biopsy.

Physical Examination: Vital signs: normal. Cardiac: normal. Skin: no fresh petechial lesions on legs, but some modeled areas where HSP was documented by biopsies.

Laboratory Findings: CBC, electrolytes: normal. Platelets: 135,000/μl. Creatinine 1.1 mg/dl. Proteinuria. EKG and vectocardiogram: see below and next page.

Question: What do the EKG and vectorcardiogram show?

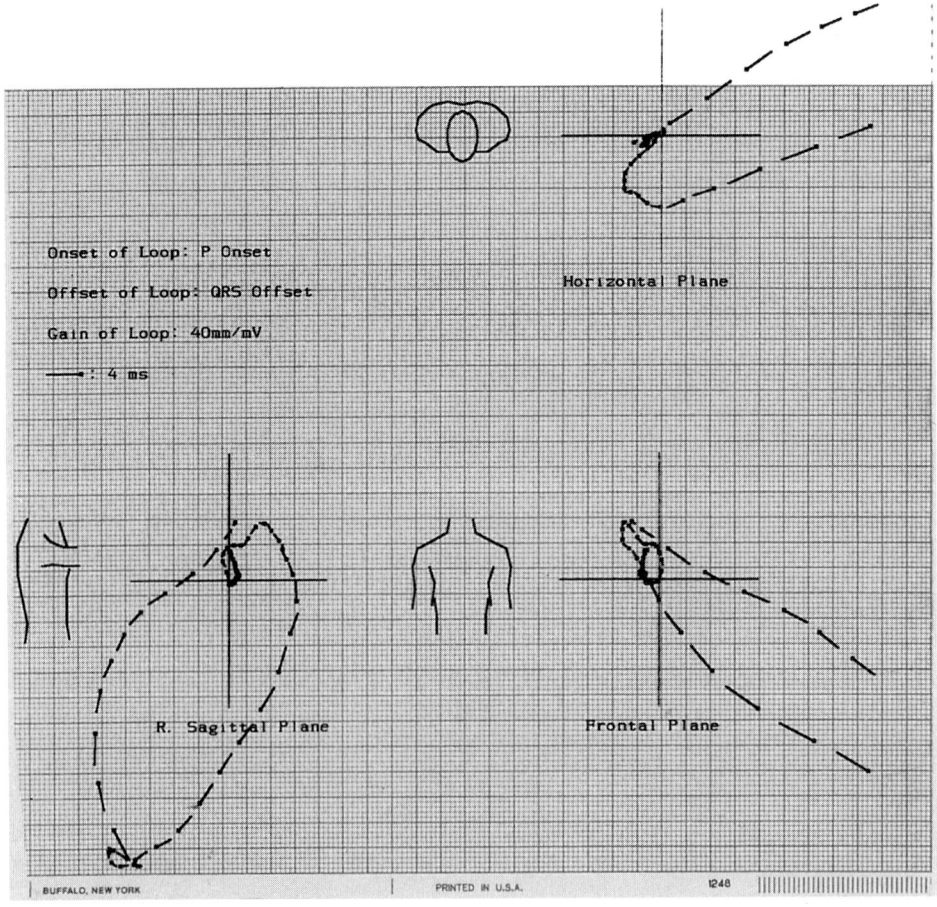

Diagnosis: Wolff-Parkinson-White syndrome (Type A)

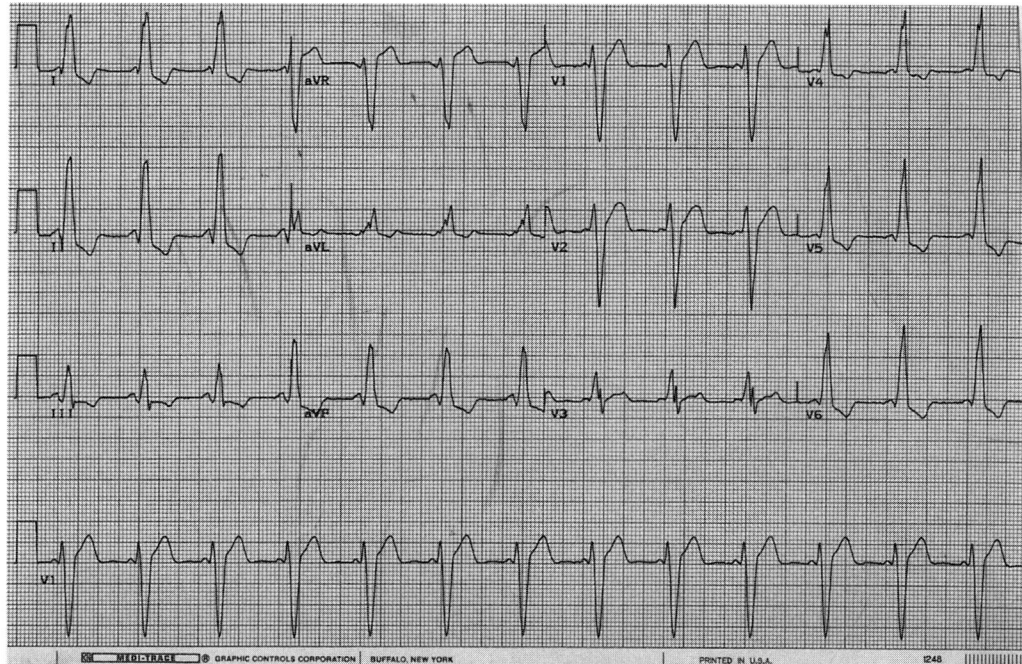

Discussion: Prior to open renal biopsy, the above EKG was taken and initially read by the computer as a short PR interval with left bundle branch block. However, a Delta wave also is present. Wolff-Parkinson-White syndrome (WPW) was confirmed in the present patient by the vectorcardiogram. The closely spaced time markings (indicative of conduction delay) in the initial and early portions of the QRS vector loops are pathognomonic of ventricular pre-excitation. In left bundle branch block, there is conduction delay in the mid portion and terminal portion of the QRS loop; in right bundle branch block, the delay is only in the terminal portion of the QRS loop. The horizontal plane vector loop in the present patient is written almost entirely anteriorly, as noted in the type A pattern of pre-excitation, and is responsible for the upright QRS deflection in all of the precordial leads of the EKG.

Activation of the ventricle over the normal AV node pathway *and* the accessory pathway produces a fusion complex whose configuration depends on the contribution of each of the two activation paths. Therefore, the classic QRS complex resembling the Eiffel Tower may not always be present. The QRS morphology can vary and may be mistaken for right bundle branch block, true posterior infarction, inferior infarction, anteroseptal infarction, left or right ventricular hypertrophy, or, as above, left bundle branch block.

ST-T changes at rest or produced by exercise often give a false positive stress EKG. Milstein et al. developed an EKG algorithm for localizing accessory pathways. A combination of this system and WPW types A and B could be as follows: **Type A (left ventricular pathways)** has positive delta and QRS complexes in V_1 for lateral and posteroseptal pathways, and the lateral pathway also has isoelectric or negative delta waves in leads I, aVL, V_5, and V_6. The posteroseptal pathway also has negative delta and QRS complexes in leads II, III, and aVF. **Type B (right ventricular pathways)** has negative delta and QRS complexes in V_1, and if located posteroseptal, there also are negative delta and QRS complexes in leads II, III, and aVF. If located anteroseptal, there is an axis of +30° or more; if located in the right ventricle free wall, there is left axis.

In the present patient, open renal biopsy of the right kidney revealed immunoglobulin A nephropathy (renal Henoch-Schönlein purpura) with minimal renal damage. The patient tolerated the renal biopsy well and was continued on prednisone and dapsone. He has never had a tachycardia.

Clinical Pearls

1. The EKG of WPW can be misinterpreted as infarction, right or left ventricular hypertrophy, or bundle branch block.
2. The WPW complex is a fusion beat produced by conduction down the normal pathway fusing with conduction down the accessory pathway.
3. Vectorcardiography can confirm the diagnosis.

REFERENCES

1. Tranchesi J, Guimarca AC, Teixeira V: Vectorial interpretation of ventricular complex in Wolff-Parkinson-White syndrome. Am J Cardiol 1959;4:334.
2. Milstein S, Sharma AD, Guiraudon GM, Klein GJ: An algorithm for the electrocardiographic localization of accessory pathways in the Wolff-Parkinson-White syndrome. Pacing Clin Electrophysiol 1987;10:555–563.
3. Yee R, Klein GJ, Guiraudon GM: The Wolff-Parkinson-White syndrome. In Zipes DP, Jalife J (eds): Cardiac Electrophysiology: From Cell to Bedside, 2nd ed. Philadelphia, WB Saunders Company, 1994, p 1199.

PATIENT 14

A 46-year-old woman with abdominal pain and syncope

A 46-year-old nurse had a number of episodes of dizziness and syncope associated with abdominal pain due to an irritable bowel. Numerous studies including electrocardiogram, echocardiogram, tilt table test, and signal-averaged EKG were normal. She wore an event recorder for 4 months and had no spells. She was seen by a psychiatrist and Zoloft and Tegretol were recommended. These did not prevent her attacks. A neurologist could not find an abnormality. Electrophysiologic studies were normal. Finally, another event recorder produced the rhythm strip below (*see figure*) during an attack of abdominal pain and syncope (*asterisk marks when recorder was activated*).

Physical Examination: Vital signs: pulse 70; blood pressure 110/60. Neck: no jugular venous distention. Chest: clear. Cardiac: normal. Abdomen: soft, no masses, slight generalized tenderness.

Laboratory Findings: CBC, SMA-7; normal. EKG: normal.

Question: What is the most likely diagnosis?

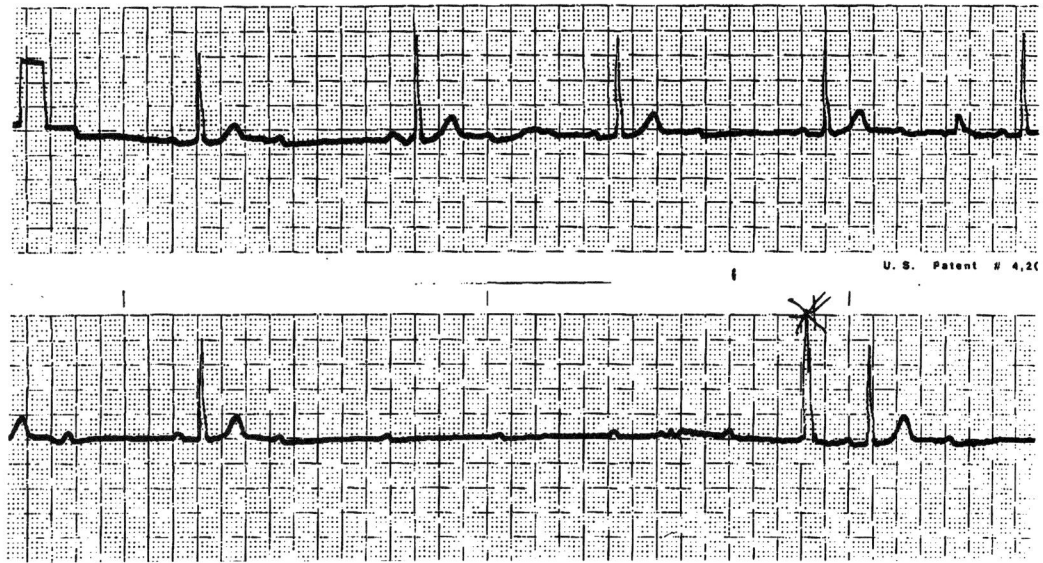

Diagnosis: Syncope with AV heart block secondary to abdominal pain and vasovagal reaction.

Discussion: Dizziness is a common complaint and is described as a weakness, vertigo, lightheadedness, and even syncope. Vertigo often is benign and positional, as noted in the elderly. Central vertigo disorder is associated with many cerebrovascular disorders. Syncope is a sudden, transient loss of consciousness that may be due to cardiovascular or noncardiovascular causes.

The **noncardiovascular classification** includes metabolic (e.g., hyperventilation, hypoglycemia, hypoxia), neurologic (e.g., cerebrovascular lesions, seizures, migraine, subclavian steal), and psychiatric (e.g., depression, hysteria) disorders. The **cardiovascular classification** is divided into disorders featuring a structurally normal heart (most reflex causes) and those of cardiac origin. When the heart is structurally normal, the differential diagnosis includes orthostatic hypotension, situational causes (coughing, micturition, sneezing, deglutition, defecation), carotid sinus syncope, vasovagal causes, drug induction, trigeminal neuralgia, glossopharyngeal neuralgia, and neurocardiogenic syncope. Cardiac causes are numerous, such as arrhythmias, cardiac tamponade, aortic stenosis, aortic dissection, hypertrophic cardiomyopathy, pulmonary stenosis, pulmonary embolism, tetralogy of Fallot, mitral stenosis, and myxoma.

The present patient had syncope due to abdominal pain and vasovagal reaction with AV heart block, determined by event recorder. Since her episode of pain could not always be controlled, a permanent DDDR pacemaker was implanted, and she has had no further syncopal episodes. However, this is not the result in all cases, since vasodepressor reactions can still occur although the pacemaker has relieved the symptoms produced by the bradyarrhythmias.

Clinical Pearls

1. There are many causes of syncope. In 50% of cases, the history and physical examination establishes the cause.

2. Numerous studies may be required to detect the cause of syncope. Monitoring with patient-activated cardiac memory loop EKG recorders may be required for long periods of time. There also are recording devices that can be implanted subcutaneously for long-term monitoring.

3. Afferent stimuli may originate from the gastrointestinal tract mechanoreceptors. The efferent pathway originates in the central nervous system medullary centers and results in hypotension and bradycardia because of parasympathetic activation.

REFERENCES
1. Isenhower WD Jr, Carter RM, Weber PC: The evaluation and diagnosis of the dizzy patient. J S C Med Assoc 1994;90:517–522.
2. Henderson MC, Prabhu SD: Syncope: Current diagnosis and treatment. Curr Probl Cardiol 1997;22:242–296.

PATIENT 15

A 32-year-old man with recurrent syncope

A 32-year-old man has had syncopal episodes since childhood. He senses the syncopal episodes coming on because he feels lightheaded, and then syncope occurs before he can take preventive action. He usually is unconscious for 4–5 minutes, and at times the episodes are associated with urinary and fecal incontinence. Neurological examinations have been normal. He is physically active, including playing basketball. Virtually all of his episodes have occurred while seated, at rest.

Physical Examination: Vital signs: normal. Neck: no bruit. Cardiac: normal. Neurologic examination: normal.

Laboratory Findings: EKG, echo Doppler, and Holter monitoring for 48 hours: normal.

Question: What test would you recommend?

Answer: Tilt table testing for the diagnosis of neurally mediated syncope, such as neurocardiogenic syncope.

Discussion: Tilt table testing often is done before electrophysiologic studies in the evaluation of syncope of undetermined origin. The procedure entails passive upright tilt from 60° to 80° for a period of 20–60 minutes, and at times is combined with isoproterenol to increase ventricular contraction. Neurally mediated syncope, also referred to as neurocardiogenic, autonomic dysfunction, vasovagal, vasodepressor, and situational, accounts for 58% of the causes of syncope. In the positive tilt test, the blood pressure drops below 80 mmHg, and the heart rate is less than 80 beats per minute. A malignant form gives asystole for 10–40 seconds.

The pathophysiology of neurocardiogenic syncope is complex. Normally, when one assumes an upright posture, approximately 500–700 ml of intravascular volume pools in the lower extremities; ventricular preload is reduced; and mechanoreceptors (C fibers in atria, ventricles, and pulmonary artery) decrease their afferent neural output to the brain. Reflex sympathetic stimulation increases the heart rate and peripheral vasoconstriction to maintain systemic arterial pressure. In neurocardiogenic syncope, the normal response is affected so that mechanoreceptors (myocardial C fibers) in the left ventricle are stimulated. This stimulation causes increased neural traffic output across afferent C fibers to the central nervous system vasomotor center, which results in increased vagal tone with resultant bradycardia, vasodilation, and syncope.

The present patient experienced asystole for 8 seconds and no blood pressure on the tilt table. Therapeutic options include: beta-adrenergic receptor blockade, volume expansion, anticholinergic agent, methylxanthines, disopyramide, amitriptyline, serotonin reuptake inhibitors, and cardiac pacing. He was begun on Lopressor 25 mg b.i.d. Two weeks later, a repeat tilt table test was positive, with asystole for 72 seconds and no blood pressure. Other measures—such as volume expansion by increasing salt intake and giving hydrofluorocortisone, and administering disopyramide—also failed to prevent his attacks; therefore, a pacemaker was inserted. Pacing can prevent the bradycardia component of hypotension, but peripheral vasodilation may still occur. Patients require pharmacologic therapy in addition to cardiac pacing to prevent the peripheral vasodilation component.

Clinical Pearls

1. Neuocardiogenic syncope is most commonly noted in young adults.
2. The diagnosis of neurocardiogenic syncope is made by a positive tilt table test.
3. There are many therapeutic recommendations, but cardiac pacing may be required for malignant asystole types.

REFERENCES
1. Kenny RA, Ingram A, Bayliss J, Suttone R: Head-up tilt: A useful test for investigating unexplained syncope. Lancet 1986;I:1352–1355.
2. Henderson MC, Prabhu SD: Syncope: Current diagnosis and treatment. Curr Probl Cardiol 1997;22:237–296.

PATIENT 16

A 59-year-old woman with an abnormal electrocardiogram

A 59-year-old woman was stung by a yellow jacket about 1 year ago. She was told she had an abnormal electrocardiogram. About 5 years ago she was told she had a slow heart rate. At times she notices that her heart beats forcefully and may skip. She has had no other cardiac symptoms.

Physical Examination: Vital signs: normal. Cardiac: no extra sounds or murmurs. Chest: lungs clear.

Laboratory Findings: Routine chemistries: normal. Electrolytes: normal. CBC: normal. Thyroid studies: normal. Echo-Doppler study: normal with normal ejection fraction; one examiner thought the mitral valve leaflets might be redundant. Thallium stress test: normal left ventricular perfusion. 24-hour Holter monitoring: PVCs, PACs at times paired. EKG: see below.

Question: What is the cause of these EKG changes?

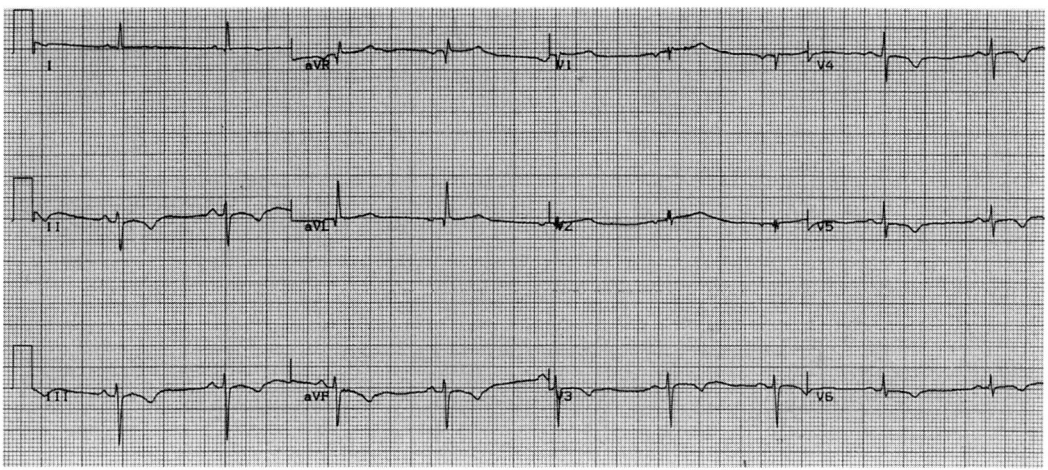

Diagnosis: Mitral valve prolapse with nonspecific EKG changes.

Discussion: According to Levine, there are 67 causes of T wave changes. T wave changes can be due to primary or secondary cardiac disease; physiologic stimuli (e.g., anxiety, hyperventilation, posture, cold, exercise, eating); pharmacologic agents (e.g., type IA antiarrhythmic drugs, digitalis, diuretics, tranquilizers, antidepressants); and reversible noncardiac disease (e.g., electrolyte disturbance, uremia, anemia, abnormalities of the thyroid, cerebrovascular lesions, acute abdominal lesions, shock). Many of these causes were excluded in the present patient.

Initially, because of the sinus bradycardia, inverted T waves, and low voltage in chest leads, myxedema was considered even though she had no clinical features. However, thyroid studies were normal. At this point, the yellow jacket sting 1 year ago was considered as the most likely cause of these persistent changes. Myocardial biopsy was entertained, but deferred for awhile, since she had no cardiac symptoms or other abnormal cardiac findings.

The patient returned 3 years later. She still had no cardiac symptoms, but now **multiple mid-systolic clicks,** which did not change on standing or squatting, were audible on auscultation. No murmur of mitral regurgitation was produced. The EKG was similar to the tracing taken 3 years ago (on the previous page), showing inferior and anterolateral T wave inversion and left anterior superior fascicular block. Echo-Doppler now showed mitral leaflets redundant with prolapse of posterior leaflet and trivial mitral insufficiency.

The clicks and murmurs in mitral valve prolapse can be variable because they depend on several hemodynamic factors, namely, left ventricular volume, contractility, and systemic blood pressure. Altering these factors can change the auscultatory findings. In approximately one-third of patients with mitral valve prolapse, the EKG shows inferior and anterolateal T wave inversion. False-positive EKG stress tests frequently occur in such patients. The QT interval may be prolonged. Most patients have some arrhythmias. There are no known causes of the EKG changes and arrhythmias. Mechanical factors such as abnormal tension on the papillary muscles and stretching of the mitral leaflets are thought to be factors in the production of these EKG changes.

Clinical Pearls

1. There are 67 causes of T wave changes.
2. Inferior and anterolateral T wave changes can occur with mitral valve prolapse.
3. The auscultatory findings can vary and at times be absent, because they depend on several hemodynamic factors, namely, left ventricular volume, contractility, and systemic blood pressure.

REFERENCES
1. Levine HD: nonspecificity of the electrocardiogram associated with coronary artery disease. Am J Med 1953;15:344.
2. Gazes PC: False-positive exercise test in the presence of the Wolff-Parkinson-White syndrome. Am Heart J 1969;78:13–15.
3. Devereux RB: Recent developments in the diagnosis and management of mitral valve prolapse. Curr Opin Cardiol 1995;10:107–116.

PATIENT 17

A 69-year-old confused man with elevated temperature and tachycardia

A 69-year-old man is brought in by his sister, who says that his behavior has been uncharacteristic. Additionally, he has had difficulty ambulating because of weakness and incoordination, and his speech has been slurred. These symptoms have progressed over several weeks, and nausea and vomiting occurred about 3 days prior to admission.

Physical Examination: Vital signs: pulse 106; blood pressure 147/60; respirations 18; temperature 100.8°. General: agitated; cannot respond well to questions. Skin: warm and dry. Cardiac: hyperdynamic precordium; grade II/VI systolic ejection murmur. Neurologic: no deficit noted.

Hospital Course: Mental state continued to decline during the next 2 days. Head CT: normal. EEG: nonspecific diffuse slowing. Cardiac enzymes: normal. Even on broad-spectrum antibiotics, his temperature spiked daily up to 101°F. Dyspnea and rapid, irregular rhythm developed. EKG: atrial fibrillation, with a rapid ventricular response up to 250 beats per minute; nonspecific ST depression.

Question: What is the most likely diagnosis?

Diagnosis: Thyrotoxic crisis (thyroid storm) and atrial fibrillation with a rapid ventricular response.

Discussion: Sudden, severe hyperthyroidism may occur as a feature of the basic disease and/or because of infection, surgery, or trauma. Such patients experience fever, mental disorientation, vomiting, and disproportionate tachycardia. Shock may occur, and the patient may drift into a coma. Mortality is very high.

Initially, the ventricular rate of the present patient was so rapid that it was unclear whether it was atrial fibrillation. He was given 6 mg of adenosine on two occasions, which slowed the ventricular rate, and it was then obvious that atrial fibrillation was present. Diltiazem and digoxin further slowed the ventricular response to 180 beats per minute. Intravenous esmolol quickly controlled the ventricular rate to between 80–100 beats per minutes. Four hours later, he spontaneously converted to regular sinus rhythm. EKG showed regular sinus rhythm with a rate of 100 and nonspecific anterolateral T wave inversion. Cardial features of hyperthyroidism such as proptosis were not present. Thyroid studies showed 6 ng/dl free T4 and 0.08 mU/mol TSH.

When atrial fibrillation occurs with a very rapid ventricular rate, consider the presence of an accessory pathway, or hyperthyroidism. In a patient with an accessory pathway and atrial fibrillation, conduction usually is antegrade by way of this pathway and retrograde to the atria by way of the AV node (antidromic). Thus, the ventricular complexes have a delta wave and the Eiffel Tower appearance. The clinical picture of confusion, agitation, fever, rapid atrial fibrillation, and positive thyroid laboratory data confirms the diagnosis of thyroid storm.

Treatment should be initiated early—even when the diagnosis is based on clinical suspicion. Besides addressing dehydration, give glucosteroids, propylthiouracil, and iodides. Beta-blockade is very effective, but may be contraindicated or should be used cautiously if cardiac failure is the dominant component of the crisis.

The present patient responded to hydration, glucosteroids, propylthiouracil, iodides, and beta-blockade.

Clinical Pearls

1. Patients with atrial fibrillation and a rapid ventricular response have either an accessory pathway or hyperthryoidism.
2. Fever, agitation, confusion, and rapid atrial fibrillation suggest thyroid storm.
3. If there is clinical suspicion, initiate therapy early—even before confirmatory laboratory studies return.
4. Beta-blockers are very effective in a thyroid crisis, but may be contraindicated or should be administered cautiously if cardiac failure is the dominant component of the crisis.

REFERENCES
1. Skelton CL: The heart and hyperthyroidism. N Engl J Med 1982;307:1206–1208.
2. Woeber KA: Thyrotoxicosis and the heart. N Engl J Med 1992;327:94.

PATIENT 18

A 73-year-old woman with persistent atrial fibrillation

A 73-year-old woman has had known hypertension and frequent episodes of palpitations with weakness and dyspnea for approximately 10 years. She has had frequent cardioversions with DC shock and with various antiarrhythmic drugs. During the past year, her attacks were more frequent and persistent, in spite of quinidine, procainamide, disopyramide, beta-blockers, sotalol, propafenone, diltiazem, verapamil, and flecainide administered on different occasions. She refused to take amiodarone. She has been on warfarin for the past 2 years. During the attacks, her ventricular rate cannot be slowed below 110–120 beats per minute—even with high doses of beta-blockers and combinations with diltiazem, verapamil, and digoxin.

Physical Examination: Vital signs: pulse irregular (110–120 bpm); blood pressure 150/90; no jugular venous distention. Chest: scattered bibasilar rales. Cardiac: no murmurs or extra sounds; irregular rhythm. Abdomen: no hepatomegaly. Extremities: no peripheral edema.

Laboratory Findings: CBC, urinalysis, and thyroid profile: normal. EKG: atrial fibrillation with ventricular response of 120 beats per minute. Echocardiogram: all chambers of normal size; valves normal; ejection fraction greater than 50%.

Question: What would you recommend now?

Answer: Pacemaker implant and atrioventricular junction ablation.

Discussion: Atrial fibrillation can be divided into three groups: **paroxysmal**—episodes are self-terminating and usually last less than 48 hours; **persistent**—episodes continue indefinitely, but can be converted to sinus rhythm; and **permanent**—conversion to sinus rhythm either is impossible or rapidly reversed. The present patient has the persistent type. Many antiarrhythmic drugs have been used to prevent atrial fibrillation after cardioversion. Generally, the drug is tailored to the patient's problem. If there is no structural heart disease, propafenone and flecainide are the usual choices. Beta-blockers, sotalol, and amiodarone are preferred for those with structural heart disease. If coronary artery disease is present, then sotalol is the main choice. Amiodarone is given if congestive heart failure is present. Type 1A drugs such as quinidine can be used if there is no cause for a long QT interval.

All of these drugs were tried in this patient, except amiodarone, which she refused. In addition, verapamil was combined with the antiarrhythmic drugs to prevent **atrial remodeling.** Pretreatment with verapamil has been shown to prevent remodeling, which seems to be due to intracellular calcium overload. The effect of calcium overloading is shortening of the atrial refractory period. This remodeling may account for high rates of recurrences of atrial fibrillation during the first week after cardioversion. Thyrotoxicosis was ruled out, and the present patient had no evidence for an accessory pathway (Wolff-Parkinson-White syndrome). These two conditions often are associated with rapid ventricular rates.

A DDDR pacemaker was implanted, and then atrioventricular junction ablation was performed. About half of patients with a history of drug-refractory atrial fibrillation do not develop permanent atrial fibrillation after atrioventricular junction ablation and dual-chamber pacemaker implantation, even in the absence of antiarrhythmic drug therapy. The present patient has remained in sinus rhythm for 1 year since the ablation and is asymptomatic.

Atrial pacing and implantable atrial defibrillators have been effective in some cases. Radiofrequency ablation has been successful for many supraventricular arrhythmias, but is still under investigation for atrial fibrillation. A few studies show that there may be focal sources (i.e., in the right atrium, near the ostium of the coronary sinus, in the left atrium at the ostia of the pulmonary veins), and these have been successfully ablated. Clinically, such patients may be selected when they have episodes of monomorphic atrial tachycardia or monomorphic premature atrial beats similar to the P waves during tachycardia. The electrophysiologic characteristics of pulmonary vein premature atrial beats are different from those in the atria. Ectopic beats from pulmonary veins can initiate atrial fibrillation, and their elimination by ablation can cure atrial fibrillation. Note that extensive linear ablation of atrial tissue and at the ostia of the pulmonary veins entails risk of pulmonary vein stenosis, cardiac tamponade, cerebral emboli, or death.

Clinical Pearls

1. Persistent atrial fibrillation in spite of antiarrhythmic agents may require pacemaker implantation and atrioventricular junction ablation.

2. Focal sources of atrial fibrillation may be abolished by the use of endocardial radiofrequency catheter ablation. Future studies may expand the use to other types of atrial fibrillation, especially with the advent of radio frequency application, by creation via sophisticated mapping systems of long, continuous linear lesions needed to compartmentalize the atria.

REFERENCES

1. Shih-Huang L, Chen S-A, Tai C-T, et al: Comparison of quality of life and cardiac performance after complete atrioventricular junction ablation and atrioventricular junction modification in patients with medically refractory atrial fibrillation. J Am Coll Cardiol 1998;31:673–644.
2. Chen S-A, Hsieh M-H, Tai C-T, et al.: Initiation of atrial fibrillation by ectopic beats originating from the pulmonary veins. Electrophysiological characteristics, pharmacological responses, and effects of radiofrequency ablation. Circulation 1999;100:1879–1886.
3. DeSimone A, Stabile G, Franco Vitale D, et al: Pretreatment with verapamil in patients with persistent or chronic atrial fibrillation who underwent electrical cardioversion. J Am Coll Cardiol 1999;34:810–814.
4. Pappone C, Oreto G, Lamberti F, et al: Catheter ablation of paroxysmal atrial fibrillation using a 3D mapping system. Circulation 1999;100:1203–1208.

PATIENT 19

A 56-year-old diabetic woman with an acute anterior myocardial infarction, right bundle branch block, and left anterior superior fascicular block

A 56-year-old diabetic woman is admitted to the hospital because of severe, crushing substernal chest pain. The pain is not radiating. Thrombolytic therapy is administered in the emergency department, and she is admitted to the critical care unit.

Physical Examination: Vital signs: pulse 105; blood pressure 100/70. Cardiac: no murmurs or extra sounds.

Laboratory Findings: CBC and urinalysis: normal. Enzymes: total CK and MB fractions and troponins elevated. EKGs: see below.

Question: How would you manage this patient?

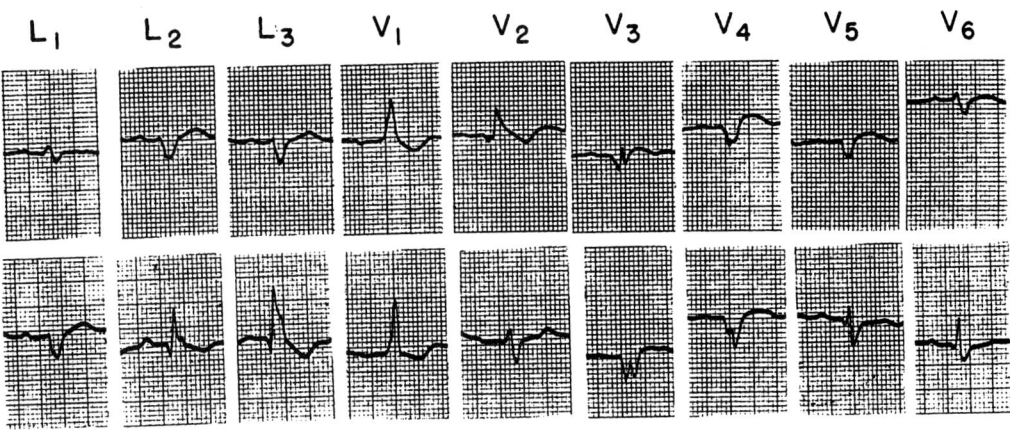

Answer: A pacemaker should be placed to manage this anterior myocardial infarction with bifascicular block.

Discussion: An anterior infarction can involve the septum and produce heart block (infranodal block). Third-degree block often is preceded by conduction impairments in various combinations involving the right bundle (RBBB) and two fascicles of the left bundle. Trifascicular block is impending if RBBB with left axis (about $-60°$ or more to the left) or right axis (about $+120°$ or more to the right) occurs in the patient with an anterior infarction. The left axis indicates block of the left anterior superior fascicle of the left bundle (LAFB), and the right axis indicates block of the left posterior inferior fascicle of the left bundle (LPFB). Insert a pacemaker when anterior infarction with any of these left fascicular blocks plus an RBBB is present, even if sinus rhythm is present. Trifascicular block can occur suddenly in such patients, and they may have a very slow idioventricular rate and suffer Adam-Stokes attacks, making it difficult to insert a pacing catheter. At times, an external Zoll transcutaneous-type pacer can be used until the transvenous type is inserted.

Other indicators for pacing in anterior infarction are as follows: new or indeterminate age bifascicular block (RBBB with LAFB or LPFB, or LBBB) with first-degree AV block; bilateral BBB (alternating RBBB and LBBB, or RBBB with alternating LAFB/LPFB; any age); Mobitz II second-degree AV block. New or age-indeterminate RBBB with first-degree AV block can be observed, and if instability occurs, a pacemaker may be inserted. Patients that have an anterior infarction and develop Mobitz II or third-degree AV block—even if these blocks are transient—should be considered for a permanent pacemaker, since sudden late deaths are common in such patients.

Consider an electrophysiology study to access the site and extent of heart block in uncertain cases. Since the advent of thrombolytic therapy or primary angioplasty with or without a stent for myocardial infarction, the incidence of AV heart block has declined.

Patients with inferior infarction and second- or third-degree AV node block due to edema of the AV node seldom require temporary pacing, because QRS complexes are narrow, the idiojunctional rhythm is adequate, and the AV block usually is transient. A temporary pacing catheter is inserted in such patients only if the ventricular rate is below 45, or if hypotension, heart failure, ischemia, ventricular arrhythmias, dizziness or syncope, or complete heart block exists with a wide QRS complex. The catheter is especially indicated if the patient does not respond to atropine. Lidocaine can cause aystole by depression of conduction in ischemia or partly depolarized myocardium, and thus block the impluse from the escape focus. Therefore, if complex ventricular ectopy is present with third-degree AV block, insert a temporary pacing catheter *before* giving lidocaine. A pacing catheter usually is removed after several days, when sinus rhythm occurs. Such patients with an inferior infarction and AV node block seldom require permanent pacing.

The first tracing (*top*) from the present patient, taken on admission, shows RBBB with LAFB and an anterior infarction. A temporary transvenous pacing catheter was inserted. Several hours later RBBB was still present, but new LPFB (*bottom tracing*) was noted. She did not develop Mobitz II or third-degree AV block, and the catheter was removed. She subsequently did well.

Clinical Pearls

1. Anterior infarction can involve the septum and bundle branches.
2. Insert a pacing catheter if an anterior infarction is associated with second- (Mobitz II) or third-degree AV block; RBBB and left anterior or left posterior fascicular block; any type of bundle branch block with first-degree AV block; or alternating right and left bundle branch blocks.
3. Inferior infarctions have edema of the AV node or His bundle and seldom require pacing unless unstable.

REFERENCES

1. Kuo C-S, Reddy CP: Effect of lidocaine on escape rate in patients with complete atrioventricular block. B. Proximal His bundle block. Am J Cardiol 1981;47:1315–1320.
2. Harpaz D, Behar S, Gottlieb S, et al: Complete atrioventricular block complicating acute myocardial infarction in the thrombolytic era. J Am Coll Cardiol 1999;34:1721–1728.
3. Ryan TJ, Antman EM, Brooks NH, et al: 1999 update: ACC/AHA Guidelines for the Management of Patients with Acute Myocardial Infarction: Executive Summary and Recommendations. A Report of the American College of Cardiology/American Heart Association Task Force on Practice Guidelines (Committee on Management of Acute Myocardial Infarction). Circulation 1999;100:1016–1030.

PATIENT 20

A 48-year-old woman with cardiomyopathy

A 48-year-old woman is admitted with a persistent cough, paroxysmal nocturnal dyspnea, orthopnea, right lower lobe infiltrate, and bilateral pleural effusions, and is treated with antibiotics. During the hospitalization, ventricular fibrillation develops, and she is resuscitated. Echocardiogram reveals four-chamber dilatation and severe global hypokinesis. She is treated aggressively for congestive heart failure, and her symptoms improve. Subsequent cardiac catheterization reveals normal coronary arteries, 3+ mitral insufficiency, and an ejection fraction of 14%. She is transferred for urgent transplant evaluation. Full evaluation shows no contraindications to transplant. MUGA ejection fraction is 9%.

Physical Examination: Vital signs: pulse 120; respirations 26; blood pressure 110/70. Neck: deep jugular vein pulsation 6 cm above angle of Louis at 45°. Cardiac: apical high-pitched murmur of II/VI intensity and S_3 gallop. Lungs: bibasilar rales. Extremities: 2+ peripheral edema. Abdomen: hepatomegaly. EKG: see below.

Question: What is the cause of the cardiomyopathy?

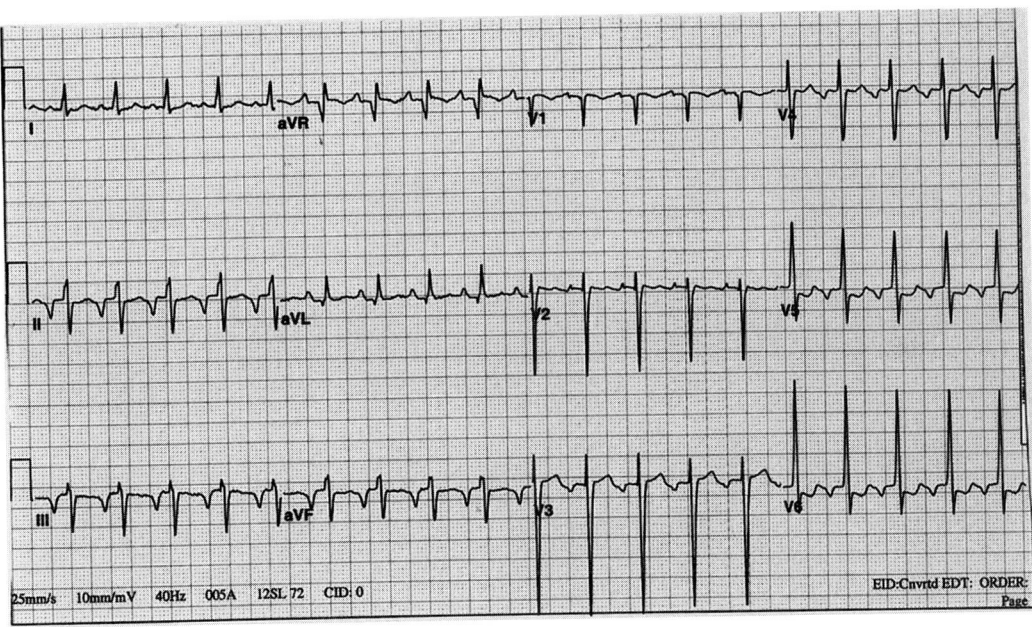

Diagnosis: Cardiomyopathy secondary to supraventricular tachycardia.

Discussion: The EKG in the present patient showed a long RP type of supraventricular tachycardia. This incessant tachycardia had been present for a long time: EKGs dating back at least 15 years showed this arrhythmia. The diagnosis of ectopic atrial tachycardia, intra-atrial reentry, or atypical AV nodal reentry tachycardia was entertained. Electrophysiologic studies revealed that this was an atypical AV-nodal reentry tachycardia.

The AV node in patients with AV nodal reentry tachycardias manifests **two pathways** on electrophysiologic studies. The alpha pathway conducts slowly and has a short refractory period, and the beta pathway conducts fast and has a long refractory period. The most common type of AV nodal reentry tachycardia conducts down to the alpha pathway and goes retrograde up the beta pathway, producing a short RP type. Rarely, the tachycardia can conduct down the beta pathway and then retrograde up the alpha pathway, producing a long RP type or atypical type, as noted in the present patient.

Radiofrequency catheter ablation was performed on this patient with great success. Heart failure cleared, and the ejection fraction by MUGA rose to 58%.

Clinical Pearls

1. Incessant supraventricular tachycardia can produce a cardiomyopathy.
2. Some long RP types of supraventricular tachycardia can be clarified only by electrophysiologic studies.
3. Radiofrequency ablation of a supraventricular tachycardia can cause reversal of a tachycardia cardiomyopathy.

REFERENCES

1. Chen SA, Chiang CE, Yang CJ, et al.: Sustained atrial tachycardia in adult patients. Electrophysiological characteristics, pharmacological response, possible mechanisms, and effects of radiofrequency ablation. Circulation 1994;90:1262–1278.
2. Pieper SJ, Stanton MS: Narrow QRS complex tachycardia. Mayo Clin Proc 1995;70:371–375.

PATIENT 21

A 45-year-old man with no known coronary artery disease and hypercholesterolemia

A 45-year-old man with no known coronary artery disease and no other risk factors has the following lipid values:

$$\text{Cholesterol} = 340 \text{ mg/dl}$$
$$\text{LDL} = 277 \text{ mg/dl}$$
$$\text{VLDL} = 30 \text{ mg/dl}$$
$$\text{HDL} = 35 \text{ mg/dl}$$
$$\text{Triglycerides} = 140 \text{ mg/dl}$$

Maximum dietary therapy does not reduce his LDL below 190 mg. He takes vitamin E and folate, and drinks red wine.

Physical Examination: Normal.

Question: How would you manage this patient?

Answer: A patient with no coronary artery disease, less than two risk factors, and abnormal lipids who is not responding to diet should receive a statin drug.

Discussion: If parents have high cholesterol or primary relatives (parents, grandparents, or siblings) have premature coronary artery disease, their children and young adults between the ages of 2 and 19 should be screened for abnormal lipids. Otherwise, screening should begin for those 20 years or older. The National Cholesterol Education Program (NCEP) guidelines recommend that dietary therapy be started in individuals with an LDL >160 mg/dl, no coronary artery disease, and fewer than two risk factors. If, in spite of dietary therapy, the LDL remains >190 mg/dl, then drug treatment should be started. If the patient has no coronary artery disease but has two or more risk factors, dietary therapy is recommended if the LDL is >130 mg/dl, with drug treatment added if it remains >160 mg/dl. Those *with* coronary artery disease should be started on dietary therapy if the LDL is >100 mg/dl, and started on drug therapy if it remains >130 mg/dl.

Recently, the American Heart Association set a new goal, aiming for about 30% of the calories to be from fat and placing more emphasis on the type of fat rather than the overall fat intake. Very-low-fat and high-carbohydrate diets can reduce HDL and raise fasting levels of triglycerides. There is a suggestion that excessive intake of polyunsaturated fats (omega-6) may decrease HDL and increase LDL oxidation and platelet aggregation, both of which contribute to coronary obstruction. Most of the fat intake should be from **monounsaturated fats** (canola and olive oil), less from **omega-6 polyunsaturated fats** (corn and soybean oil), and the least from **saturated and transfats.** Most of the oil in fish (omega-3 fatty acids) is unsaturated fat that may lower LDL cholesterol and raise HDL. The most notorious source of transfats is margarine. Partially hydrogenated vegetable oil is on the labels of items that contain transfats. There is some evidence that sito-stanol-ester margarine (Benecol) may reduce cholesterol when used as part of a low-fat, low-cholesterol diet. Caloric intake is also important and should be individualized depending on the patient's weight. Recently, obesity has been listed as one of the important risk factors along with smoking, lack of exercise, and poor lipid and hypertension control.

Since the present patient could not reduce his LDL below 190 mg/dl by diet, a statin drug was recommended. In men and women with minimal carotid atherosclerosis who are free of symptomatic cardiovascular disease, but have elevated LDL cholesterol, lovastatin reversed progression of carotid artery disease, major coronary events, and mortality in the Asymptomatic Carotid Artery Progression Study. The West of Scotland Coronary Prevention Study was a 5-year study of 6595 subjects thought to be clinically free of coronary heart disease. Treatment with pravastatin reduced LDL by 26% and definite coronary events by 30%.

Many statin drugs are available—namely, lovastatin, simvastatin, atorvastatin, pravastatin, fluvastatin, and cerivastatin. They appear to be similar, but dose-response relationships may vary. Atorvastatin is the most potent; fluvastatin is the least potent. Lovastatin and simvastatin are more lipid soluble—the significance of this is not clear. The statin drugs may stabilize a plaque and have antiatherothrombotic properties besides their effects on lipids.

The Cambridge Heart Attack and Antioxidant Study showed a significant reduction in nonfatal myocardial infarctions in the **vitamin E** group compared to placebo in patients with coronary disease. **Red wine and grape juice** have platelet-inhibitory properties and antioxidant effects. Red wine is more effective because it is more easily and rapidly absorbed by the intestine than grape juice. Long-term consumption of red wine inhibits neointimal hyperplasia in cholesterol-fed rabbits more so than white wine. This response may be due to red wine's higher antioxidant capacity. It would be interesting to see if it might alter the restenosis rate after angioplasty.

The present patient was treated with a statin drug, and all levels normalized. Followup of CK and liver function studies showed no abnormalities.

Clinical Pearls

1. Perform cholesterol screening in persons 2–19 years of age with a family history of premature coronary artery disease, or with parents who have a high cholesterol level. Otherwise, start screening at 20 years of age.

2. Even individuals with less than two risk factors and an LDL over 190 mg should receive a statin drug, if dietary therapy alone is insufficient.

3. Thirty percent of dietary calories should come from fat, with monounsaturates making up most of the percentage, less from polyunsaturates, and the least from transfats and saturated fats. *Types of fat* are more effective in preventing coronary heart disease than reducing overall fat intake.

REFERENCES

1. Ascherio A, Hennekens CH, Buring JE, et al: Trans-fatty acids intake and risk of myocardial infarction. Circulation 1994;89:94–101.
2. Furberg CD, Adams HP Jr, Applegate WB, et al: Effect of lovastatin on early carotid atherosclerosis and cardiovascular events. Asymptomatic Carotid Artery Progression Study (ACAPS) Research Group. Circulation 1994;90:1679–1687.
3. Shepherd J, Cobbe SM, Ford I, et al: Prevention of coronary heart disease with pravastatin in men with hypercholesterolemia. West of Scotland Coronary Prevention Study Group. N Engl J Med 1995;333:1301–1307.
4. Hu FB, Stampfer MJ, Manson JE, et al: Dietary fat intake and the risk of coronary heart disease in women. N Engl J Med 1997;337:1491–1499.
5. Feng A-N, Chen Y-L, Chen Y-T, et al: Red wine inhibits monocyte chemotactic protein-1 expression and modestly reduces neointimal hyperplasia after balloon injury in cholesterol-fed rabbits. Circulation 1999;100:2254–2259.

PATIENT 22

A 45-year-old man with coronary artery disease and normal lipids

A 45-year-old man with known coronary artery disease has mild hypertension. For many years, he smoked a package of cigarettes daily. He has the following lipid profile:

>Cholesterol = 170 mg/dl
>LDL = 95 mg/dl
>HDL = 45 mg/dl
>Triglycerides = 150 mg/dl
>VLDL = 30 mg/dl

Physical Examination: Blood pressure 150/90. Cardiac: normal.

Question: How would you manage this patient?

Answer: Look beyond cholesterol and total LDL for other disorders such as elevated Lp(a), homocysteine, LDL subclass pattern B, apo E polymorphism, apo B, and fibrinogen. Control hypertension and eliminate the smoking habit.

Discussion: About 30% of patients with coronary artery disease have normal lipid patterns on routine studies, such as those noted on the previous page. According to the Framingham Study, 80% of patients with coronary artery disease have the same blood cholesterol values as those who do not have coronary artery disease. Laboratory tests more sophisticated than the common lipid profile are now available.

LDL has up to four major subclasses. Small, dense LDL particles are markers for a metabolic defect that increases coronary artery disease risk. The defect may be associated with insulin resistance, low HDL_2, and elevated triglycerides. The lipid profile of patients with a predominance of small LDL particles has been termed **LDL subclass pattern B.** These particles can be elevated, yet the total LDL can be normal. LDL subclass B can be measured by gradient gel electrophoresis, analytic ultracentrifugation, or nuclear magnetic resonance (NMR) spectroscopy.

Other disorders that can be risk factors are elevated Lp(a), homocysteine, fibrinogen, and apo E4. Apo A1 is a major apolipoprotein attached to HDL and triglyceride-rich lipoproteins. Lower levels of apo A1 have been reported in patients with cardiovascular disease. Apoprotein B is the major apoprotein associated with LDL and may increase the risk for coronary artery disease even when LDL is normal.

The present patient with normal routine lipids may have one of these disorders, which are easy to treat. LDL subclass pattern B responds to diet, exercise, niacin, and fibrates, but not to statin drugs. Lp(a) responds to niacin and estrogens. Elevated homocysteine responds to folate and B6. Hyperfibrinogenemia responds to niacin and fibrates, and apo E4 responds to a reduced-fat diet. The Familial Atherosclerosis Treatment Study (FATS) showed significant reduction in apoprotein B with niacin plus colestipol, or lovastatin plus colestipol. In addition, coronary lesions showed less progression and some regression as compared to the placebo group.

Recently, an elevated C-reactive protein has been described as a risk factor for coronary artery disease. Infectious organisms such as *Chlamydia pneumoniae* or cytomegalovirus could be the cause of the chronic inflammation detected in studies with elevated C-reactive protein and vascular risks. Antibiotic therapy has been considered as a prevention for coronary artery disease. Randomized studies are needed to test this hypothesis.

A final consideration in the present patient is to give a statin drug even though the traditional lipids are normal, since it may stabilize a plaque and has antiatherothrombotic properties. In addition, the present patient should stop smoking and control his hypertension.

Clinical Pearls

1. Patients may have coronary artery disease despite a normal traditional lipid profile.
2. Seek disorders beyond cholesterol, such as small, dense LDL (pattern B); elevated Lp(a), homocysteine, fibrinogen, and apoproteins E4 and B; and a decrease in apo A1.
3. Elevated C-reactive protein may indicate that inflammation is a factor in coronary artery disease.
4. Vitamin E (antioxidant) should be considered for patients with coronary artery disease.

REFERENCES
1. Gardner CD, Fortmann SP, Krauss RM: Association of small low-density lipoprotein particles with the incidence of coronary artery disease in men and women. JAMA 1996;276:875–881.
2. Superko HR: Did grandma give you heart disease? The new battle against coronary artery disease. Am J Cardiol 1998;82(9A):34Q-46Q.

PATIENT 23

A 50-year-old woman with coronary artery disease and noninsulin-dependent diabetes

A 50-year-old woman with known coronary artery disease and diabetes presents with hypercholesterolemia, hypertriglyceridemia, and low HDL. She is 30 pounds overweight and postmenopausal. Her lipid panel is:

$$\text{Cholesterol} = 245 \text{ mg/dl}$$
$$\text{Triglycerides} = 350 \text{ mg/dl}$$
$$\text{VLDL} = 70 \text{ mg/dl}$$
$$\text{HDL} = 25 \text{ mg/dl}$$
$$\text{LDL} = 150 \text{ mg/dl}$$

Physical Examination: General: obese. Vital signs: normal. Cardiac: normal.

Question: How would you manage this patient?

Answer: The diabetes should be controlled, and she should lose weight. Estrogen can be considered as well as a fibrate or statin drug, if necessary.

Discussion: Obesity, noninsulin-dependent diabetes, and dyslipidemia are common metabolic disorders. Insulin resistance is a major factor responsible for noninsulin-dependent diabetes. Often in such patients the triglycerides are elevated, the HDL is low, and there is a predominance of small LDL (pattern B) particles. Initially, the present patient should undertake dietary modification, weight loss, and exercise—all of which can reduce insulin resistance. Weight loss also can reduce triglycerides and elevate HDL.

Obesity is now considered by the American Heart Association as a major risk factor for coronary artery disease. Body mass index (BMI) is defined as weight in kilograms divided by height in meters squared (kg/m^2). A BMI of 25–30 is considered overweight; >30 is considered obese. Statistics in the U.S. show that 50% of Americans are overweight, and 25% are obese. Twenty percent of children are overweight. Walking at a pace of one mile in 15 minutes burns up to 300 calories during a three-mile walk. To lose one pound of body fat, 3500 calories must be expended. Therefore, one pound can be lost every 12–15 days by walking three miles per day, even without any dietary changes.

Next, the present patient should be considered for **hormonal replacement.** Many observational studies state that postmenopausal estrogen has a protective effect from coronary artery disease. Estrogen can improve endothelial dysfunction, decrease cholesterol, and increase HDL. The HERS Trial (Heart and Estrogen/Progestin Replacement Study) randomized patients to either hormonal combination or placebo. The hormonal replacement lowered the LDL and increased the HDL, yet did not prevent further myocardial infarction, coronary artery disease, or death in these postmenopausal women with coronary artery disease. However, there was a risk-reduction trend after 2 years. This study does not apply to women without heart disease, those using estrogen alone, or women using a different progestin than medroxyprogesterone, which was used in the study. In addition, patients had a mean age of 67 years at entry and were 18 years postmenopausal.

Estrogen lowers Lp(a), may increase triglycerides, and can have a direct antiatherosclerotic, anticoagulatory, and vasodilatory effect. Other randomized studies are needed. At present, we must individualize patients' needs for hormonal replacement. The present patient should be considered for hormonal therapy since it is relatively soon after menopause. Raloxifene, a selective estrogen receptor modulator, has similar effects to estrogen, but does not stimulate the endometrium. Future studies will determine its value.

After these measures, a statin drug and/or a fibrate should be considered. **Statin drugs** reduce LDL and triglycerides and raise HDL. **Fibrates** reduce triglycerides and increase HDL. **Niacin** reduces small, dense LDL particles, increases HDL, and reduces triglycerides and Lp(a). It should be used cautiously in diabetics because it may increase the mean fasting glucose level. Niaspan is an extended-release form of niacin that has less hepatic toxicity and flushing than former controlled-release forms.

Triglycerides are now considered a risk factor. HDL is involved in a process of serum cholesterol transport in which it transports cholesterol to the liver from peripheral tissues (reverse cholesterol transport). HDL can be moderately increased by smoking cessation, exercise, red wine, and statin drugs. It also can be raised with gemfibrozil. The Veterans Affairs HDL Intervention Trial showed that gemifibrozil produced no changes in LDL, a 24.5% reduction in triglycerides, a 7.5% increase in HDL, and a 22% reduction in nonfatal myocardial infarction and coronary heart disease.

The present patient lost weight and controlled her diabetes. She was started on estrogen and a statin drug. Her lipids began to normalize.

Clinical Pearls

1. Obesity, noninsulin-dependent diabetes, and dyslipidemia are common metabolic disorders.
2. Obesity and hypertriglyceridemia are now listed as definite risk factors for coronary artery disease.
3. Since the HERS Trial (the first hormonal randomized study), hormonal replacement has become controversial; its use should be individualized.
4. HDL can be increased by smoking cessation, weight loss, exercise, red wine, statin drugs, estrogens, niacin, and fibrates.

REFERENCES

1. Eckel RH, Kraus RM: American Heart Association call to action: Obesity as a major risk factor for coronary heart disease. AHA Nutrition Committee. Circulation 1998;97:2099–2100.
2. Hulley S, Grady D, Bush T, et al: Randomized trial of estrogen plus progestin in secondary prevention of coronary heart disease in postmenopausal women. Heart and Estrogen/Progestin Replacement Study (HERS) Research Group. JAMA 1998;280:605–613.
3. Papademetriou V, Narayan P, Rubins H, et al: Influence of risk factors on peripheral and cerebrovascular disease in men with coronary artery disease, low high-density lipoprotein cholesterol levels, and desirable low-density lipoprotein cholesterol levels. HIT Investigators. Department of Veterans Affairs HDL Intervention Trial. Am Heart J 1998;136:734–740.
4. Rosenson RS, Tangney CC: Antiatherothrombotic properties of statins: Implications for cardiovascular event reduction. JAMA 1998;279:1643–1650.

PATIENT 24

A 74-year-old man with an aortic valve homograft and congestive heart failure

A 74-year-old man has his calcific aortic stenotic valve replaced with a homograft. Three days after surgery, heart block occurs, and a VVI pacemaker is inserted. Over the next 3 months he has increasing exertional dyspnea, peripheral edema, and fatigability. He does not have nocturnal dyspnea or orthopnea, but is experiencing insomnia. He denies chest pain or syncope. Hypertension was noted several years ago, and an ACE-inhibitor (Zestril) was begun.

Physical Examination: Vital signs: pulse 69; respirations 20; blood pressure 160/70. General: pale appearance. Neck: at 45-degree position, deep jugular vein pulsates up to earlobe; filling of the external jugular veins; carotid pulsations bounding and collapsing. Chest: bibasilar rales. Cardiac: PMI diffuse at 5th intercostal space just left of mid clavicular line; grade II/VI systolic aortic ejection murmur, heard best in primary aortic area, radiates up both sides of neck; grade III/VI murmur of aortic insufficiency along left sternal border and down to apex; second sound very loud in pulmonic area; grade III/VI high-pitched murmur of mitral insufficiency at apex, followed by a third heart sound. Abdomen: liver 12 cm in depth. Extremities: pitting edema up to knees; pistol shot sounds heard over femoral arteries.

Laboratory Findings: RBC 3.96; hemoglobin 7.1; hematocrit 23. EKG: paced ventricular rhythm. Echocardiogram: left atrium enlarged; concentric LV hypertrophy and dilatation, with estimated ejection fraction >50%; moderate aortic and mitral insufficiency; tricuspid regurgitation with normal pulmonary pressures; calculated aortic valve 1.3 cm^2; left ventricular end-systolic dimension 4.38 cm.

Question: What is the cause of the patient's congestive heart failure?

Answer: Mild degeneration of the aortic valve homograft. Anemia is a major contributing factor.

Discussion: After admission, the patient mentioned that he lost considerable blood recently after having his upper teeth extracted. Stools were negative for occult blood, and there was no evidence of hemolysis. After receiving two units of blood, he had no further dyspnea, and his edema began clearing. Lasix was added, and the Zestril was continued. One month later, he was asymptomatic and riding his bicycle 10 miles daily. No venous distention was noted, his lungs were clear, and heart rhythm was regular. Blood pressure was 130/80. The aortic systolic and diastolic murmurs and the mitral systolic murmur decreased in intensity. Echo-Doppler showed only mild aortic and mitral insufficiency. Anemia was certainly the main factor in precipitating his congestive heart failure.

Anemia can be recognized at the bedside by comparing your palm with the patient's. If the patient's palmar lines are pale, the hemoglobin probably is 7 g or less. Pallor of the conjunctivae is not a helpful clinical finding for anemia because they may be injected and not look pale. Anemia causes an increase in cardiac output and can result in heart failure, especially if there is underlying cardiac abnormality. Systemic vascular resistance is reduced due to tissue hypoxia and reduced blood viscosity. Anemia can produce peripheral vessel findings (i.e., Corrigan's collapsing pulse, Traube's pistol shot sounds over femorals, and capillary pulsations known as Quincke's sign) similar to aortic insufficiency. In addition, it can produce or aggravate insufficiency murmurs.

Since this patient responded to transfusions, homograft deterioration was not the cause of his failure, and heart catheterization was not performed. Homografts are taken from cadavers and inserted directly in the aortic position without a stent. The hemodynamics are superior to stented porcine valves. Their thrombogenicity is low, but they structurally deteriorate as do the porcine xenografts. They usually need reoperation by 10 to 15 years.

Clinical Pearls

1. Anemia can produce increased cardiac output and precipitate heart failure—especially if there is an underlying cardiac disorder.
2. Homograft valves degenerate over 10–15 years.
3. Anemia can worsen insufficiency murmurs. In addition, anemia can produce peripheral findings as noted with aortic insufficiency, which complicate clinical differentiation of the degree of aortic insufficiency that may be due to homograft aortic valve deterioration.
4. Correction of the anemia can clarify whether the anemia or underlying cardiac problem caused the heart failure.

REFERENCES
1. Varat MA, Adolph RJ, Fowler NO: Cardiovascular effects of anemia. Am Heart J 1972;83:415–426.
2. Grunkemeier GL, Bodnar E: Comparison of structural valve failure among different "models" of homograft valves. J Heart Valve Dis 1994;3:556–560.

PATIENT 25

A 45-year-old man with substernal chest pain

A 45-year-old man arrives at the emergency department with severe substernal chest pain with left arm radiation. His only risk factor is cigarette smoking. The pain is partially relieved by sublingual nitroglycerin.

Physical Examination: Vital signs: pulse 90; blood pressure 130/80. Cardiac: regular rhythm; no murmurs or extra sounds.

Laboratory Findings: CBC: normal. Cardiac enzymes: moderately elevated CK-MB and troponins. EKG: on first day, diffuse ST depression of 2 mm; on second day—see below.

Question: How would you manage this patient?

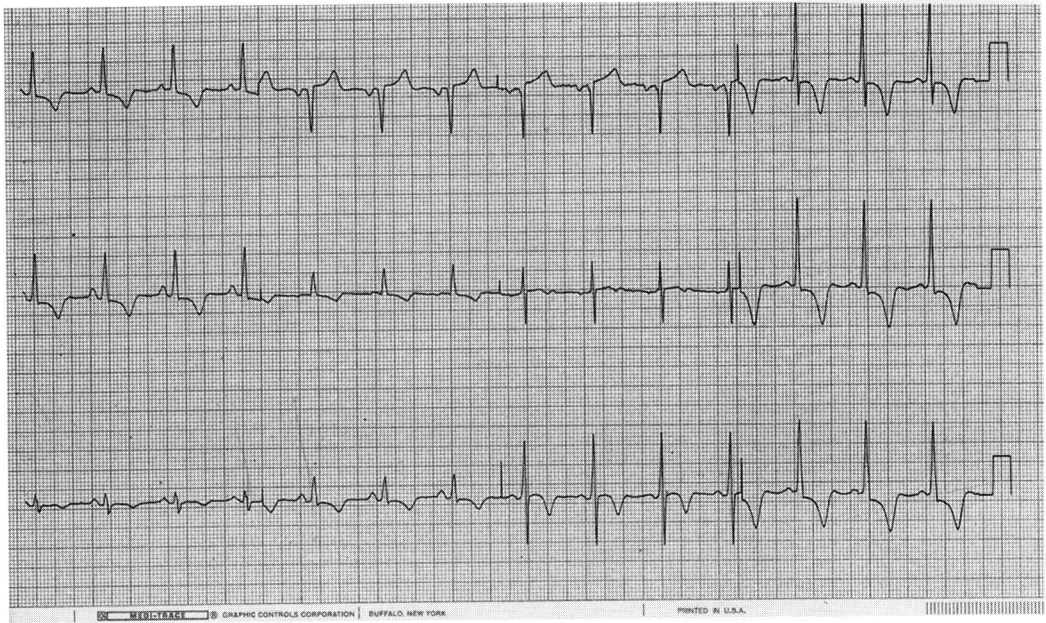

Answer: Non-Q-wave infarction requires intensive medical management, but no thrombolytic agent. Determine risk stratification to assess need for an interventional procedure.

Discussion: Unstable angina and non-Q-wave infarction are part of a spectrum, and even if we try to make a distinction between them, the major point is to distinguish the highest risk patients. The history, electrocardiographic changes, biochemical markers, and, at times, angiographic findings help, and also suggest the path of therapy to pursue. Unstable angina (UA), non-Q-wave infarction (NQMI), and Q-wave infarction (QMI) make up the entities termed the **acute coronary syndromes,** which represent different stages of plaque rupture and thrombosis. Newer diagnostic serum markers, new antiplatelet agents, electrocardiographic changes, and newer interventional devices have now changed the course of therapy.

Fuster describes UA as mild plaque rupture with labile thrombus and vasoconstriction that occludes the artery for 10 to 20 minutes. The duration of occlusion is longer in NQMI due to more plaque damage and more enzyme rise. Reperfusion occurs in NQMI to prevent QMI developing. Extensive collateral circulation often is present.

Some features of NQMI predict an adverse outcome. Post-hospital angina is noted more often in NQMI than QMI. Persistent ST depression, congestive heart failure, and life-threatening arrhythmias are predictors of increased mortality in NQMI. The troponins T and 1 are more specific markers than the CK-MB enzyme, and may indicate more complex lesions.

There has been considerable debate about whether routine coronary arteriography should be done in all patients with NQMI. The VANQWISH study randomized patients to an early invasive strategy or to an early conservative strategy with angiography only if symptom-limited stress testing was positive. Morbidity and mortality were higher in the invasive group. Early invasive management may be better for QMI with occluded vessels than NQMI with open vessels. It may be safer to perform coronary intervention after the patient with NQMI has been stabilized with medical therapy. The FRISC II study compared invasive with noninvasive treatment in unstable coronary artery disease. Half of the patients in each group were randomly assigned to long-term treatment with subcutaneous dalteparin, which is a low-molecular-weight heparin (LMWH), or placebo for 3 months. The early invasive approach resulted in less death and myocardial infarction independent of the randomized dalteparin treatment, especially in those who had signs of ischemia on electrocardiography or raised biochemical markers of myocardial damage. This study contrasts with the results of the TIMI IIIb trial and the VANQWISH trial.

The treatment for NQMI traditionally has been aspirin, intravenous heparin, and intravenous nitroglycerin. The role of beta-blockers in NQMI has been controversial. Diltiazem is effective if left heart failure is not present. LMWH and glycoprotein IIb/IIIa receptor blockers are effective, especially in medium- and high-risk groups. These agents as well as stents may become the procedures of choice.

Currently, it is suggested that these patients be risk stratified. **High-risk patients** have ST depression with prolonged pain at rest or hemodynamic instability. High-risk patients should receive IV heparin, aspirin, and early GP IIb/IIIa receptor blockers; cardiac catheterization should be performed, as well as an invasive intervention if indicated. **Medium-risk patients** have T wave inversion; their pain has subsided; and they are stable. If the troponin levels are significantly elevated, these patients should receive cardiac catheterization, as in the high-risk groups. If the troponin levels are low, then the medium-risk group should have a thallium stress test to evaluate the extent of ischemia before proceeding with angiography. **Low-risk patients** have chest pain, which may not be anginal, and normal EKGs. Such patients should be treated as outpatients with nitrates, aspirin, and diltiazem. Patients with NQMI do not benefit from thrombolytic therapy.

The present patient was considered high risk due to moderately elevated enzymes and evolving T wave changes (see EKG). Coronary arteriography and angioplasty were performed, and stents were placed in two vessels with high-grade lesions.

Even though in academic centers emphasis is placed on risk stratification, the community hospital physician generally chooses the invasive approach in all patients with NQMI. Their reasoning is that such patients may initially do well, but later have a high incidence of recurrent angina and infarction. At present, physicians in rural areas should become familiar with the use of LMWH and GP IIb/IIIa receptor inhibition. In the future, these agents may become first-line drugs, along with aspirin or clopidogrel, before patients are referred to a center for more specialized care. Aggressive management of risk factors should follow.

Clinical Pearls

1. The acute coronary syndromes are unstable angina, non-Q-wave infarction, and Q-wave infarction.
2. Patients with NQMI should be risk stratified, and invasive studies should be performed for those at acute risk.
3. The adjunctive use of LMWH and glycoprotein IIb/IIIa receptor blockers appears very promising.
4. In view of the newer changes and better invasive procedures such as stents, the future will continue to show improved outcome in such patients.

REFERENCES

1. Boden WE, O'Rourke RA, Crawford MH, et al.: Outcomes in patients with acute non-Q-wave myocardial infarction randomly assigned to an invasive as compared with a conservative management strategy. N Engl J Med 1998;338:1785–1792.
2. Gutstein De, Fuster V: Management of stable coronary artery disease. Am Fam Physician 1997;56:99–106.
3. Cannon CP: Diagnosis and management of patients with unstable angina. Curr Probl Cardiol 1999;24:681–744.
4. Invasive compared with noninvasive treatment in unstable coronary-artery disease: FRISC II prospective randomised multicentre study. Fragmin and fast revascularisation during Instability in coronary artery disease investigators. Lancet 1999;354:708–715.
5. Zaacks SM, Liebson PR, Calvin JE, et al.: Unstable angina and non-Q-wave myocardial infarction: Does the clinical diagnosis have therapeutic implications? J Am Coll Cardiol 1999;33:107–118.

PATIENT 26

A 43-year-old man with end-stage renal disease on dialysis

A 43-year-old man with end-stage renal disease who is on dialysis presents with substernal chest pain, weakness, and dyspnea. These symptoms have been intermittent for 1 week. He has a history of cocaine abuse. Prior to this admission, coronary arteriography indicated significant three-vessel disease with a normal ejection fraction. Several days before this admission, he was dialyzed.

Physical Examination: Vital signs: temperature 98.2°; pulse 82; respirations 18; blood pressure 152/93. Neck: no jugular vein distention. Lungs: clear. Cardiac: grade II/VI systolic ejection murmur along the left sternal border.

Laboratory Findings: EKG: see below.

Question: What has caused these EKG changes?

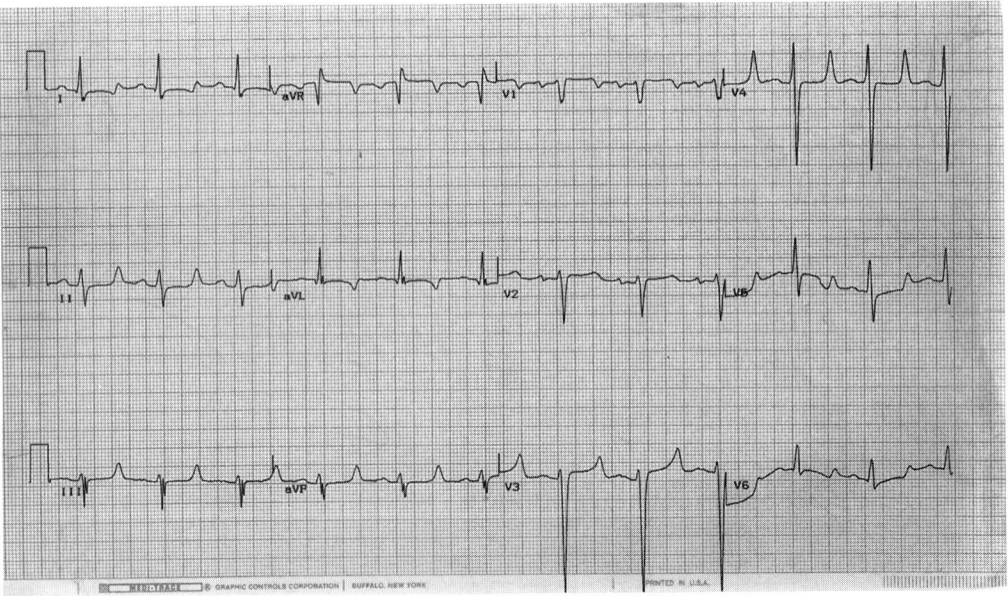

Diagnosis: Hyperkalemia and hypocalcemia.

Discussion: T wave peaking with narrow bases is an indicator of hyperkalemia. The QT interval usually is short. However, in this patient, the QT is prolonged due to the ST segment elongation that occurs with hypocalcemia. The T wave may remain normal or may become inverted when hypocalcemia is the only electrolyte abnormality. This patient with end-stage renal disease had a potassium level of 7.5 mEq/L, creatinine of 13.9 mg/dl, and calcium of 7.0 mg/dl. After dialysis, these levels improved.

The earliest sign of potassium increase is peaking of the T waves. Later, the PR interval is prolonged, and the QRS complex widens. Occasionally, there may be an acute current of injury resembling early myocardial infarction. Next, the P waves may disappear, and there is further QRS widening until ventricular fibrillation or cardiac arrest occurs.

Even though the P waves are not seen, SA node activity continues. Despite atrial paralysis, sinus impulses can proceed to the AV junction via specialized internodal conducting tracts, and then to the ventricle, without recording P waves.

The electrocardiogram often can show changes due to other electrolyte abnormalities. Hypokalemia depresses the ST segment and prolongs the QT interval, but at the expense of the T wave, which becomes broadened and often is followed by an upright "U" wave. Hypercalcemia produces a very short QT interval. The proximal limb of the T wave has an abrupt slope to its peak.

The present patient was considered for coronary bypass surgery, but he had a positive urinary screen for cocaine, and the surgeons wanted this problem addressed before surgical intervention.

Clinical Pearls

1. The electrocardiogram often shows changes diagnostic of electrolyte imbalance.

2. The early change of hyperkalemia is manifested by T wave peaking. After this, the QRS widens, and the P waves disappear—even though sinus node activity is still present. With further widening, ventricular fibrillation or cardiac arrest can occur.

3. Hypocalcemia prolongs the QT interval due to elongation of the ST segment.

4. Hypercalcemia produces a very short QT interval. Hypokalemia depresses the ST segment and prolongs the QT interval with a widened T wave, which often is followed by a tall "U" wave.

REFERENCES

1. Surawicz B: Electrolyte and the electrocardiogram. Am J Cardol 1963;12:656.
2. Sherf L, James TN: A new electrocardiographic concept: Synchronized sinoventricular conduction. Dis Chest 1969;55,127–140.
3. Huang TC, Cecchin FC, Mahoney P, et al: Corrected QT interval (QTc) prolongation and syncope associated with pseudohypoparathyroidism and hypocalcemia. J Pediatr 2000;136,404–407.

PATIENT 27

A 50-year-old man with recurrent chest pain on exertion and at rest

A 50-year-old man has had substernal heaviness on exertion as well as 20-minute episodes at rest for several days. At presentation, he has chest pain and EKG findings of 2-mm horizontal ST segment depression. Sublingual nitroglycerin relieves his chest pain; however, the attacks continue intermittently at rest until IV nitroglycerin is started. He is a cigarette smoker and has a strong family history of coronary artery disease.

Physical Examination: Vital signs: pulse 80; blood pressure 110/70. Lungs: clear. Cardiac: normal.

Laboratory Findings: CBC: normal, slight elevation of troponin 1. EKG: normal; with chest pain, ST segment depression occurred.

Question: How should this patient be managed?

Answer: Patients with unstable angina should be risk stratified and, initially, intensive medical therapy should be started. Some patients can then be selected for percutaneous interventions.

Discussion: When an atherosclerotic plaque ruptures, with subsequent intimal hemorrhage and thrombus formation, unstable angina occurs. The pathologic lesion found in the coronary arteries is commonly a platelet-rich, nonocclusive "white thrombus" overlying fissured or active plaque. In acute myocardial infarction, fibrin-rich "red thrombus" occluding the vessel completely is a more common finding.

The Agency for Health Care Policy and Research (AHCPR) has issued clinical practice guidelines for the diagnosis and treatment of unstable angina. The following are the signs and symptoms of unstable angina reported by the AHCPR: rest angina within 1 week of presentation; new-onset angina when walking less than two blocks, or with minimal activity, or at rest within 2 months of presentation; increasing angina when walking less than two blocks, or with minimal activity, or at rest; variant angina; and angina more than 24 hours after myocardial infarction. The certainty of diagnosis, hemodynamic state, and severity of symptoms determine the choice and timing of drugs for each patient.

Evaluate patients for short-term risk of death or nonfatal myocardial infarction, and divide them into the following categories: high risk, intermediate risk, and low risk. **High-risk patients** are those who have at least one of the following: prolonged pain (>20 minutes) at rest; pulmonary edema, angina with new or worsening mitral regurgitation; rest angina with ST changes greater than 1 mm; angina with S3 gallop or rales; and angina with hypotension. **Intermediate-risk patients** must have any of the following: rest angina now resolved; rest angina greater than 20 minutes, or relieved with rest or nitroglycerin; angina with T wave changes; nocturnal angina; new-onset angina when walking less than two blocks, on minimal activity, or at rest; Q waves or ST depression equal or greater than 1 mm in multiple leads; or age greater than 65 years. **Low-risk patients** have no high- or intermediate-risk features, but may have any of the following: increased angina frequency, severity, or duration; angina provoked at lower threshold; new-onset angina within 2 weeks to 2 months; or normal or unchanged EKG.

Patients with unstable angina in the low-risk category for adverse outcomes can be managed as outpatients. Give them aspirin or, if hypersensitive to aspirin, clopidogrel; sublingual nitroglycerin prn; oral beta-blocker; long-acting topical or oral nitrates; and at times a calcium blocker (diltiazem or verapamil), especially if hypertension is present. If the patient is asymptomatic in 72 hours, perform an exercise or pharmacologic stress nuclear perfusion study. If there are significant perfusion defects, refer for cardiac catheterization.

Begin intensive medical treatment in the emergency department for those in intermediate- or high-risk categories, and admit them to a hospital monitoring area. Start aspirin, intravenous nitroglycerin, β-blocker, and intravenous heparin. Add calcium channel blockers if significant hypertension is present (systolic blood pressure ≥ 150 mmHg); in patients who have refractory ischemia on a beta-blocker; and in those with variant angina.

Consider coronary arteriography for the high-risk group. Appropriate adjunctive therapy may be necessary prior to catheterization in some cases. Consider pulmonary artery pressure monitoring, inotropic therapy for shock, antiarrhythmic therapy for malignant ventricular arrhythmias, pacemaker for high-grade AV block, and, in those who remain unstable, insertion of an intra-aortic balloon pump prior to cardiac catheterization. Depending on the catheterization results, some type of revascularization procedure may be necessary.

The management of the intermediate-risk patients is the same, but less urgent. If the intermediate group has high troponin levels, perform cardiac catheterization. If the levels are low, then order a nuclear stress test once the patient is stable to evaluate the extent of ischemia prior to proceeding with angiography.

In the past few years, other important drugs such as low-molecular-weight heparin (LMWH) and GP IIb-IIIa inhibitors have become available. Extensive investigation is ongoing for direct anti-thrombins (hirudin, hirulog, and others) and LMWHs (enoxaparin, dalteparin, nadroparin, and others). Several trials have shown superior efficacy of LMWH compared to unfractionated heparin. In addition, LMWHs are easily given subcutaneously, do not need laboratory monitoring, have a more stable and reliable anticoagulant effect, produce less thrombocytopenia, do not inhibit platelet function, and have a high bioviability based on anti-factor Xa activity. LMWHs cannot be used interchangeably because of significant differences in their relative proportions of anti-factor Xa and anti-factor IIa activity.

Glycoprotein IIb/IIIa receptor blocking agents also are very promising. These block the final pathway to platelet receptors. Abciximab, epitifibatide, and tirofiban are available. Most experience has been with abciximab.

At present, it is not entirely clear when LMWHs and GP IIb/IIIa inhibitors should be used in unstable angina, and in which combinations.

The other important question is when is the prime

time to use GP IIb/IIIa receptor inhibitors. Intermediate- and high-risk patients with elevated troponins and/or ST depression, and those undergoing angioplasty and stents early or late after their acute presentation, are good candidates for these receptor inhibitors. Future studies may determine that LMWH, IIb/IIIa receptor inhibitors, and aspirin/clopidogrel in different combinations are first-line drugs, along with IV nitroglycerin and a β-blocker, to stabilize the patient. Both GP IIb/IIIa antagonists and the LMWHs have benefits in a growing array of patients with acute coronary syndromes. Enoxaparin has shown significant reduction in death and myocardial infarction (ESSENCE and TIMI 11b data).

The preliminary experience with combining the IIb/IIIa antagonists abciximab and LMWH enoxaparin (National Investigators Collaborating in Enoxaparin–NICE-4 trial) during percutaneous coronary intervention demonstrates a low incidence of bleeding and infrequent major cardiac events. The combination of tirofiban and enoxaparin (ACUTE-1 pilot trial) produces a greater platelet inhibition than tirofiban plus unfractionated heparin.

Another important question is when invasive strategy or conservative strategy should be considered. In spite of the VANQWISH and TIMI IIIb trials that showed conservative therapy was best, it appears from more recent studies with stents that invasive procedures should be considered, especially in the high-risk group. In the TIMI IIIb study, thrombolytic agents were not effective in unstable angina. Since there is now evidence that inflammatory processes (elevated C-reactive protein) may be involved in the pathogenesis of acute coronary syndrome, anti-inflammatory drugs will be investigated. The benefit of aspirin may stem from its anti-inflammatory effect along with its anti-platelet effect. The Na^+/H^+ exchange inhibitors also are being evaluated, for they reduce severe ventricular arrhythmia, limit necrosis, and reduce contractile dysfunction. In addition, gene-directed therapy may become available in the future.

The present patient was classified in the high-risk group. He received intensive medical therapy and coronary arteriography. Two significant obstructions were found that required stents.

Clinical Pearls

1. Patients with unstable angina should be risk stratified into low-risk, intermediate-risk, and high-risk categories.

2. Low-risk groups can be managed as outpatients.

3. Traditionally, initial therapy is aspirin, IV nitroglycerin, beta-blocker and calcium blocker (diltiazem or verapamil), and IV unfractionated heparin.

4. New agents such as LMWHs and GP IIb/IIIa inhibitors may become first-line drugs. The challenge is to study the combination of these agents to achieve more dramatic effectiveness than with either drug alone.

5. At present, LMWH can be given initially instead of unfractionated heparin—especially by physicians practicing in rural areas, where referral to a medical center may require several hours.

6. Glycoprotein IIb/IIIa receptor blockers can be considered if troponins are elevated, ST depression is present, and angioplasty or stent implantation is planned.

7. Most patients in the intermediate- or high-risk groups should have coronary arteriography. The others, when stable, should be evaluated with noninvasive studies prior to considering coronary arteriography.

REFERENCES

1. Braunwald E, Jones RH, Mark DB, et al: Diagnosis and management of unstable angina. Agency for Health Care Policy and Research. Circulation 1994;90:613–622.
2. Cohen M, Demers C, Gurfinkel EP, et al.: A comparison of low-molecular-weight heparin with unfractionated heparin for unstable coronary artery disease. Efficacy and Safety of Subcutaneous Enoxaparin in Non-Q-Wave Coronary Events Study Group. N Engl J Med 1997;337:447–452.
3. Kereiakes DJ, Fry E, Matthai W, et al: Combination of enoxaparin and abciximab therapy during percutaneous coronary intervention: "Nice Guys Finish First." J Invas Cardiol 2000;12(suppl A):1A–5A.

PATIENT 28

A 59-year-old man with cough, dyspnea, and electrical alternans

A 59-year-old man presents with cough productive of white sputum, dyspnea with exertion, and orthopnea that began 1 week before admission. He denies hemoptysis, fever, chills, and night sweats. For several years, he had exertional chest pain relieved by rest or nitroglycerin, and he was told that he had a myocardial infarction about 10 years ago. The patient denies ethanol use, but has smoked two packs of cigarettes per day for the past several years.

Physical Examination: Vital signs: temperature 100.5°; pulse 125; blood pressure 110/90 (15 mmHg pulsus paradoxus). Neck: jugular venous pulsations up to the angle of the jaw. Chest: decreased breath sounds with dullness over the left upper lobe. Cardiac: normal heart sounds without murmur.

Laboratory Findings: Hct 39%; WBC 8,700/μl. EKG: total electrical alternans. Chest radiograph: large cardiac silhouette; left upper lobe consolidation and bilateral pleural effusions. Echocardiogram: see below.

Question: What is the most probable diagnosis?

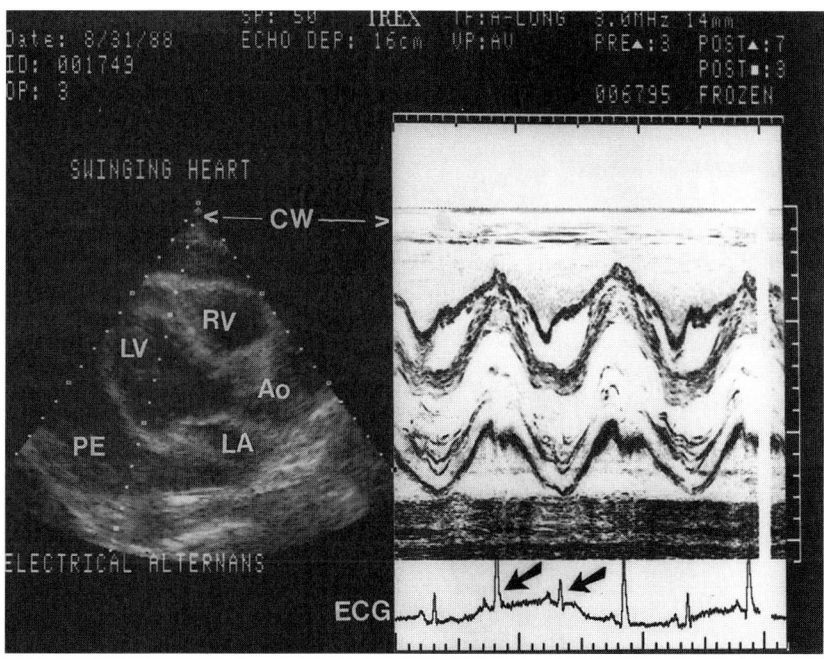

Figure reproduced from Gazes PC: Clinical Cardiology—A Cost-Effective Approach, 4th ed. New York, Chapman and Hall, 1997; with permission.

Diagnosis: Malignant pericardial effusion with cardiac tamponade.

Discussion: Cardiac tamponade develops when a pericardial effusion interferes with diastolic filling of the heart. It is related to the rapidity of fluid accumulation, quantity of fluid, and distensibility of the pericardium. As little as 100 ml or less of fluid accumulating rapidly can produce tamponade, yet a large quantity of fluid developing slowly may not interfere with cardiac function. The most common causes of cardiac tamponade are **trauma with hemopericardium, infectious pericarditis, uremia,** and **neoplastic pericardial effusions.**

Impaired diastolic ventricular filling causes tamponade by reducing stroke volume. The heart rate increases to maintain cardiac output and a narrow pulse pressure subsequently occurs. Increased right-sided pressures distend the jugular veins, and **pulsus paradoxus** can be elicited. Pulsus paradoxus is best detected with a blood pressure cuff by lowering the cuff pressure a few millimeters at a time at the point of the expiratory systolic blood pressure. Pulsus paradoxus is considered to be present if sounds are not heard during the inspiratory phase of respiration for 10 mmHg or more from the systolic blood pressure heard during expiration.

There are many theories to explain the mechanism of the paradoxical pulse. The most plausible explanation is that during inspiration there is an increased venous return to the right side of the heart despite the elevated intrapericardial pressure that resists diastolic filling. The increased venous return distends the right ventricle and shifts the interventricular septum toward the left ventricle, thereby reducing the left ventricular stroke volume and systolic blood pressure. These changes occur normally to a slight degree, but are exaggerated in patients with cardiac tamponade. Pulsus paradoxus can also occur with obstructive emphysema, asthma, pneumothorax, and massive pulmonary embolism. In these conditions, the marked negative intrathoracic pressure with inspiration can produce a decrease in left heart filling.

Pulsus paradoxus may be absent in cardiac tamponade if there is marked elevation of the left ventricular diastolic pressure, as may be noted with aortic regurgitation, left ventricular systolic failure, or hypertrophy. It also may be absent in patients with cardiac tamponade and atrial septal defect, in whom differential ventricular filling cannot occur, or in patients with pulmonary hypertension and right ventricular hypertrophy, in whom inspiration produces little change in right ventricular volume.

The EKG in cardiac tamponade may show total electrical alternans involving the P waves, QRS, and T waves. The diagnosis can be suggested by **echocardiography,** which shows the effusion plus evidence of right ventricular diastolic collapse. Echocardiography can help to make the diagnosis of early tamponade before full-blown hemodynamic compromise occurs. Cardiac tamponade can be confirmed at catheterization of the right heart that shows equalization of right atrial and left atrial pressures. Pericardiocentesis demonstrates a high intrapericardial pressure that is equal to intracardiac filling pressures. Equalization of intracardiac pressures disappears and stroke volume increases after successful pericardiocentesis. Pericardiocentesis or a pericardial window created through a small subxiphoid incision can be lifesaving even when only a small amount of fluid is removed.

Pending pericardial drainage, patients should be treated aggressively with intravenous saline to raise the intracardiac filling pressures and improve cardiac output. Positive inotropic agents are of marginal value in patients with cardiac tamponade. Percutaneous balloon pericardiotomy has been done in patients with tamponade as a part of percutaneous pericardiocentesis. The balloon is dilated to create a tear in the pericardium, and a pericardial catheter is inserted to drain fluid.

In the present patient, M-mode and two-dimensional echocardiogram revealed a large pericardial effusion (PE) with a swinging motion of the heart, and diastolic collapse of the right ventricle and right atrium, and the EKG showed electrical alternans (see figure on previous page). Note in the M-mode tracing that when the cardiac wall swings anteriorly, the QRS voltage is high, and as it swings posteriorly, the voltage is low (*arrows*). The patient's symptoms were relieved when 1900 cc of bloody pericardial fluid was drained. This fluid and a bronchoscopic specimen of the left upper lobe revealed atypical carcinoma, probably adenocarcinoma.

Clinical Pearls

1. Pulsus paradoxus can be diagnostic for cardiac tamponade but is not always present, especially if left ventricular filling pressure is elevated before the tamponade occurred.

2. The EKG often demonstrates total electrical alternans involving the P waves and the T waves, as well as the QRS complexes.

3. Echocardiography can confirm that fluid is present; tamponade is suggested when the study shows diastolic right atrial, right ventricular, and left atrial collapse. The heart may show a pendular swinging motion.

4. Removing a small amount of pericardial fluid by pericardiocentesis can be lifesaving for the person with tamponade.

REFERENCES

1. Shabetai R, Fowler NO, Fenton JC, et al: Pulsus paradoxus. J Clin Invest 1965;44:1882–1898.
2. Leimgruber PP, Kloppenstein, HS, Wann LS: The hemodynamic derangement associated with right ventricular diastolic collapse in tamponade. An experimental echocardiographic study. Circulation 1983;68:612–620.
3. Ziskind AA, Pearce AC, Lemmon CC et al: Percutaneous balloon periocariotomy for the treatment of cardial tamponade and large periocardial effusions: Description of technique and report of the first 50 cases. J Am Coll Cardiol 1993;21:1–5.

PATIENT 29

A 64-year-old man with intermittent chest pain responsive to nitroglycerin

A 64-year-old man has a 10-year history of recurrent midsubsternal chest pain during exercise and at rest. Initially, sublingual nitroglycerin provided some relief. A thallium stress test was nondiagnostic. His chest pain continued intermittently but eventually was controlled with diltiazem and isosorbide dinitrate. Approximately 1 year previously, the patient experienced an episode of upper abdominal pain that seemed different from his usual substernal tightness. An upper gastrointestinal study showed deformity of the duodenal bulb with mild gastritis. One day before admission, he had substernal pressure with radiation down both arms, but no associated dyspnea, nausea, vomiting, or diaphoresis. Three sublingual nitroglycerin tablets provided relief. The following night he was awakened with another attack that required several nitroglycerin tablets to ease the pain. He was admitted for further evaluation.

Physical Examination: Vital signs: normal. Cardiac: normal. Chest: clear.

Laboratory Findings: Serial EKGs and cardiac enzymes: normal. Coronary arteriograms: normal; coronary artery spasm could not be induced with ergonovine, although chest pain occurred. Left ventriculogram: normal.

Question: What further studies are indicated?

Answer: A barium swallow should be performed.

Discussion: Chest pain may have many causes and produces anxiety among patients, their families, and physicians alike. The sudden onset of chest pain must be differentiated from the discomfort caused by anxiety neurosis, organic and functional disturbances of the gastrointestinal tract, costochondritis, musculoskeletal diseases, and other disorders. Four gastrointestinal disorders can mimic myocardial ischemic pain—namely, hiatal hernia with reflux and esophagitis, diffuse esophageal spasm, nutcracker esophagus, and the splenic flexure syndrome. Esophagitis often is relieved by antacids; the splenic flexure syndrome is relieved by passing flatus. A confounding problem is the possibility of so called linked angina. Esophageal acid stimulation can produce anginal attacks by reducing coronary blood flow in patients with coronary artery disease. A neural reflex is possible, since it was not noted in heart transplant patients with heart denervation.

Diffuse esophageal spasm and nutcracker esophagus are the most difficult conditions to differentiate because symptoms more closely resemble those of ischemia and may even respond to coronary vasodilators. At times, the diagnosis is suggested when a cold or carbonated beverage or ice cream precipitates an attack, or when dysphagia is present. As observed in the present patient, however, symptoms can occur at rest while the patient is not swallowing or during periods of exertion or stress, which further confuses the diagnosis with myocardial ischemia. At times, esophageal spasm can even produce electrocardiographic T-wave changes suggestive of myocardial infarction.

To assist in the differential diagnosis, patients with esophageal spasm often undergo **coronary arteriography** to rule out coronary artery disease. Although an **ergonovine challenge** can produce both coronary artery and diffuse esophageal spasm, ST elevation occurs only in patients with a positive challenge due to underlying coronary artery disease. Ergonovine has been safely administered in the coronary care unit setting, but most studies are performed during coronary arteriography. This affords the possibility of intracoronary administration of nitroglycerin, which is occasionally required to reverse ergonovine-induced coronary spasm. Ergonovine testing should be performed when the patient is off all calcium channel antagonists and nitrates, as these agents can render the test falsely negative. **Esophageal manometry** performed during ergonovine challenge may demonstrate an acute increase in pressure indicative of diffuse esophageal spasm. In patients with a nutcracker esophagus, chest pain occurs with distal esophageal peristaltic pressures greater than the upper limit of normal that persist for greater than 6 seconds. The **barium esophagram** in patients with diffuse esophageal spasm shows simultaneous, nonperistaltic contractions throughout the esophagus that cause segmentation of the barium column.

In the present patient, ergonovine was administered during coronary arteriography to exclude Prinzmetal's or variant angina. The patient did not have evidence of coronary spasm but did develop his characteristic chest pain without EKG changes. Because of the persistent pain, a barium swallow was performed. The figure below (*left*) demonstrates **diffuse esophageal spasm** with frank subdivision of the esophageal outline ("rosary bead esophagus"). Subsequently, sublingual nitroglycerin relieved the pain, and a repeat barium swallow (*below right*) demonstrated resolution of the esophageal spasm.

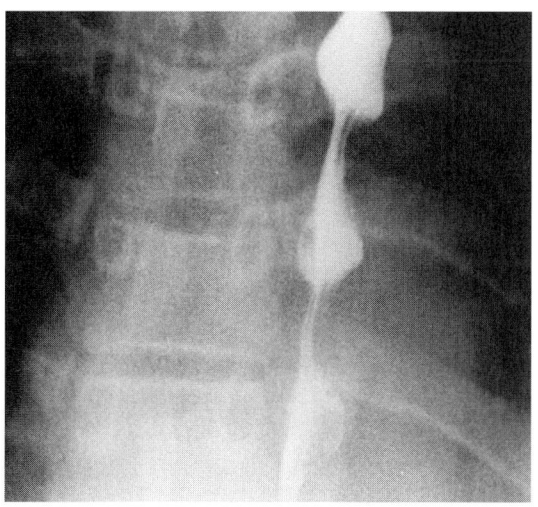 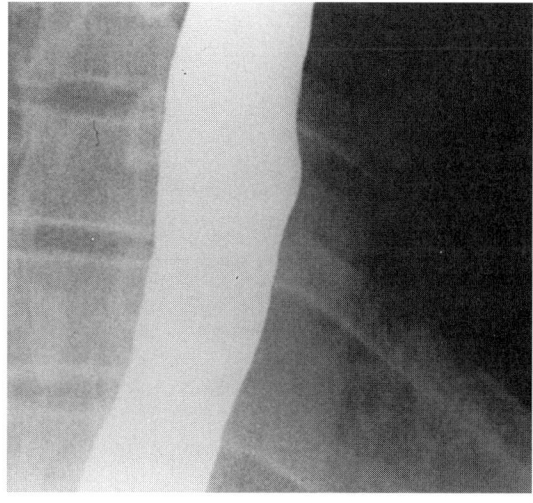

Clinical Pearls

1. Esophageal spasm can mimic chest pain due to coronary artery disease both in the nature of the pain and the associated EKG changes observed.

2. Esophageal spasm may be differentiated from myocardial ischemia by coronary arteriography with an ergonovine challenge and also with a barium swallow.

3. Esophageal spasm responds to coronary vasodilator drugs such as nitrates and calcium blockers.

REFERENCES

1. Brand DL, Martin D, Pope CE: Esophageal manometrics in patients with angina-like chest pain. Am J Diag Dis 1977;22:300–308.
2. Eastwood GL, Weiner BH, Dickerson WJ, et al: Use of ergonovine to identify esophageal spasm in patients with chest pain. Ann Intern Med 1981;94:768–771.
3. Chauhan A, Mullins PA, Taylor G, et al: Cardioephageal reflex: A mechanism for "linked angina" in patients with angiographically proven coronary artery disease. J Am Coll Cardiol 1996;27:1621–1628.

PATIENT 30

A 65-year-old woman with hypertension and chronic atrial fibrillation

A 65-year-old woman with known hypertension experienced atrial fibrillation several months earlier, which converted to regular sinus rhythm upon administration of quinidine, after ventricular rate control with digoxin and a beta-blocking agent. Subsequently, fever and diarrhea developed, both of which disappeared after stopping the quinidine. Regular sinus rhythm could not be maintained with use of beta blockers, disopyramide, or procainamide. The ventricular response to persistent atrial fibrillation was controlled with digoxin and a beta blocker.

Physical Examination: Vital signs: pulse 65–70 (irregular), blood pressure 130/85. Neck: no jugular venous distention. Chest: clear to auscultation and percussion. Cardiac: no murmurs or extra sounds.

Laboratory Findings: CBC, urinalysis, and thyroid profile: normal. EKG: atrial fibrillation with a satisfactory ventricular response at rest and with moderate exercise. Echocardiogram: all chambers normal in size; valves appeared normal; ejection fraction greater than 50%.

Question: Should this patient be on long-term oral anticoagulation?

Answer: The patient has hypertension and chronic atrial fibrillation and should receive long-term anticoagulation.

Discussion: The Framingham study showed that patients with long-term atrial fibrillation have almost a six times higher incidence of stroke. This risk increases to 17-fold if the atrial fibrillation is associated with rheumatic heart disease. In addition, it has been shown that atrial fibrillation can produce left ventricular dysfunction and shorten life. Another study concluded that patients under age 60 with lone atrial fibrillation unassociated with underlying cardiac abnormalities have a low risk of stroke.

Up to 30% of individuals with sustained or recurrent atrial fibrillation have at least one embolic event. Transesophageal echocardiography (TEE) can detect atrial thrombi, but the use of this procedure to guide the need for long-term anticoagulation for chronic atrial fibrillation requires further study. There is clear evidence that patients with rheumatic valvular disease and atrial fibrillation should receive warfarin.

Anticoagulation in nonrheumatic atrial fibrillation had been controversial. Five studies have shown that warfarin reduced the incidence of stroke in such cases. The Copenhagen AFASAK (atrial fibrillation, aspirin, anticoagulation) study showed that warfarin was effective in preventing stroke, but low-dose aspirin (75 mg per day) was ineffective. The Stroke Prevention in Atrial Fibrillation (SPAF) study reported that strokes were significantly higher in patients on placebo compared to warfarin or 325 mg of aspirin. However, aspirin did not benefit patients over 75 years of age. The Boston Anticoagulation Trial, the Canadian Trial, and Veterans Administration studies showed that long-term low-dose warfarin was highly effective in preventing stroke in patients with nonrheumatic atrial fibrillation.

The SPAF II study demonstrated that patients 75 years or less without hypertension, congestive heart failure, or prior thromboembolism are at low risk with aspirin, although they did slightly better with warfarin. The SPAF III study reported that women over 75 years of age and those with hypertension, left ventricular dysfunction, or prior thromboembolism did better with adjusted-dose warfarin than those on fixed doses of aspirin and warfarin. In addition, this study showed that those without these risk factors have a low risk of stroke with aspirin.

At present, warfarin is recommended for all patients over age 75 years with nonvalvular atrial fibrillation, or under age 75 with one or more risk factors (prior thromboembolism, hypertension, heart failure or left ventricular dysfunction). Maintain the INR between 2 and 3. Aspirin is recommended for patients who decline warfarin or are poor candidates and those under age 65 without risk factors. For those between 65 and 75 years without risk factors, aspirin or warfarin can be considered. Patients with atrial fibrillation also may have atherosclerosis of the thoracic aorta, which can produce an embolism. Control ventricular rate in patients with chronic atrial fibrillation with digoxin and a beta-blocker, verapamil or diltiazem.

The present patient was anticoagulated with warfarin, and her INR was maintained between 2 and 3.

Clinical Pearls

1. Overall, approximately 30% of patients with atrial fibrillation have a cerebral embolism during their lifetime.
2. Chronic atrial fibrillation—regardless of the cause—can shorten life.
3. At present, warfarin is recommended for all patients over age 75 years with nonvalvular, chronic atrial fibrillation, or under age 75 with risk factors. Maintain the INR between 2 and 3.
4. Aspirin is recommended for patients who decline warfarin or are poor candidates and those under age 65 without risk factors.
5. For those between 65 and 75 years without risk factors, aspirin or warfarin can be considered.

REFERENCES

1. Kopecky SL, Gersh BJ, McGoon MD, et al: The natural history of lone atrial fibrillation: A population-based study over three decades. N Engl J Med 1987;317:669–674.
2. Stroke Prevention in Atrial Fibrillation Investigators: Warfarin versus aspirin for prevention of thromboembolism in atrial fibrillation: Stroke Prevention in Atrial Fibrillation II Study. Lancet 1994;343:687–691.
3. The SPAF III Writing Committee for the Stroke Prevention in Atrial Fibrillation Investigators: Patients with nonvalvular atrial fibrillation at low risk of stroke during treatment with aspirin. Stroke Prevention in Atrial Fibrillation III Study. JAMA 1998;279:1273–1277.
4. Ezekowitz MD, Levine JA: Preventing stroke in patients with atrial fibrillation. JAMA 1999;281:1830–1835.

PATIENT 31

A 22-year-old man with an abnormal electrocardiogram

A 22-year-old college student was referred for evaluation of a faint systolic murmur and an unusual electrocardiogram. He denies chest pain or exercise limitations. The patient recollects that his brother also might have had an unusual electrocardiogram.

Physical Examination: Vital signs: pulse 65 (regular); blood pressure 120/70. Fundi: normal. Chest: clear. Cardiac: no murmurs or extra sounds on lying, standing, or squatting or after a Valsalva maneuver.

Laboratory Findings: CBC, urinalysis: normal. Chest radiograph: normal. EKG: see below.

Question: What is the likely diagnosis?

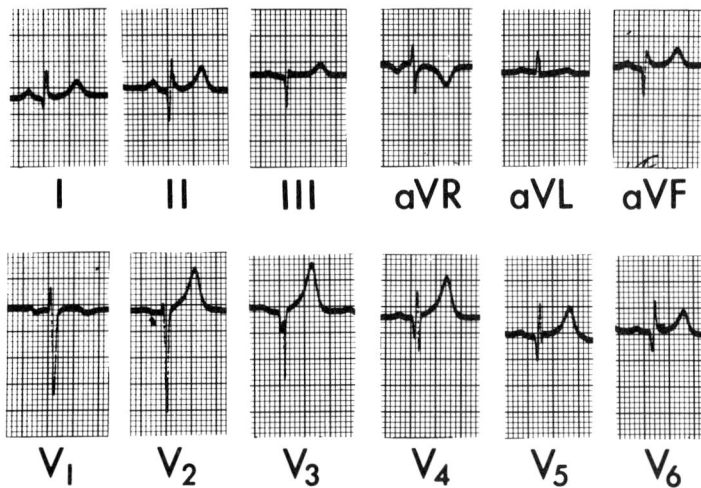

From Gazes PC: Recognition of acute myocardial infarction. In Chest Pain: Problems in Differential Diagnosis, Volume 3. Published by Biomedical Information Corp., New York, for Marion Laboratories, Inc., Kansas City, Missouri, 1977.

Diagnosis: Hypertrophic cardiomyopathy (HCM).

Discussion: HCM is usually inherited in an autosomal dominant pattern. There can be variable types in the same family, such as concentric hypertrophy, asymmetric hypertrophy of the septum with obstruction or without, and rare types involving only the apex as described by the Japanese. In the idiopathic hypertrophic subaortic stenosis (IHSS) type, the degree of obstruction is labile. The obstruction is greater in the standing position or during a Valsalva maneuver, which produces a decrease in left ventricular volume and an increase in the loudness of the murmur. The reverse occurs with squatting, which increases left ventricular volume.

Patients with IHSS may have angina, syncope, or congestive heart failure. When failure occurs, it is due to diastolic dysfunction rather than abnormalities of ventricular systole, as confirmed by a high ejection fraction. The EKG may reveal only left ventricular hypertrophy or unusual narrow Q waves. The Q waves can be due to septal hypertrophy and/or fibrosis. However, myopathic septal muscle has electrophysiologic properties different from those of the remainder of the myocardium and may account for the Q waves.

The apex form of the HCM has giant T-wave inversion in the mid-precordial leads. The EKG in this condition is almost never normal. The diagnosis can be readily made with echo-Doppler studies.

Sudden death is a major risk in patients with HCM. Unfortunately, there is no evidence that beta blockers or antiarrhythmic drugs, such as amiodarone, can prevent sudden death. If the patient with obstructive HCM develops syncope, angina, or ventricular arrhythmias, beta blockers should be given. Verapamil can be effective in ameliorating symptoms, but if the left ventricular filling pressure is very high, it may precipitate pulmonary edema. Disopyramide is another negative inotropic drug that may diminish the obstruction. Digitalis should *not* be given because it can increase contractility and the amount of left ventricular outflow obstruction.

The onset of atrial fibrillation can be catastrophic in patients with HCM, and regular rhythm should be restored pharmacologically or with DC shock. Drugs that reduce the preload, such as nitrates and diuretics, increase the obstruction gradient and should be avoided. If medical therapy fails, myotomy-myomectomy or replacement of the mitral valve relieves the obstruction and improves symptoms. Recently, DDD pacing has been shown to be an effective alternative to surgery in most patients with obstructive HCM with drug-refractory symptoms. Atrioventricular sequential pacing can cause the septum to move away from the left ventricular wall during systole, thus reducing the degree of obstruction. Selective intracoronary alcohol injection to induce localized septal infarction has been done to reduce the extent of obstruction to the left ventricular outflow tract. This technique may provide an alternative to surgical myomectomy in certain patients. Heart block and ventricular arrhythmias may develop.

In the present patient with narrow Q waves, the diagnosis of HCM, rather than infarction, should be considered. Ten years after this EKG was taken, the same cardiologist saw the patient and noted classic findings of IHSS. The carotid pulses were bifid, and at the apex a double pulsation was palpable. In addition, there was a fourth heart sound and a grade III/IV systolic ejection murmur along the left sternal border, which became very loud on standing and decreased with squatting. Echocardiography revealed a thickened ventricular septum and systolic anterior motion of the mitral valve.

Clinical Pearls

1. HCM can present as concentric hypertrophy, asymmetric septal hypertrophy with or without obstruction, or as isolated apical hypertrophy.
2. The electrocardiogram of the IHSS type can simulate infarction.
3. The first clinical manifestation of HCM can be sudden death.
4. Congestive heart failure is due to diastolic dysfunction and can be worsened by digitalis, nitrates, diuretics, and arterial dilators.
5. Prior to surgery, consider a DDD pacemaker for symptomatic patients with obstructive cardiomyopathy refractory to medical therapy.
6. Nonsurgical septal reduction with alcohol injection to produce septal infarction is another alternative to surgery for reducing the obstruction in IHSS.

REFERENCES

1. Cosio FG, Moro C, Alonso M: The Q waves of hypertrophic cardiomyopathy. An electrocardiographic study. N Engl J Med 1980;302:96–99.
2. Maron BJ, Epstein SE: Hypertrophic cardiomyopathy. Recent observations regarding the specificity of three hallmarks of the disease: Asymmetric septal hypertrophy, septal disorganization, and systolic anterior motion of the anterior mitral leaflet. Am J Cardiol 1980;45:141–154.
3. Fananapazir L, Cannan RO III, Tripodi D, et al: Impact of dual-chamber permanent pacing in patients with obstructive hypertropic cardiomyopathy with symptoms refractory to verapamil and β-adrenergic blocker therapy. Circulation 1992;85:2141–2161.
4. Knight C, Kurbaan AS, Seggewiss H, et al: Nonsurgical septal reduction for hypertrophic obstructive cardiomyopathy. Outcome in the first series of patients. Circulation 1997;95:2075–2081.

PATIENT 32

A 55-year-old man with a complication of acute myocardial infarction

A 55-year-old man with known hypertension and diabetes for several years presents with severe substernal chest pain of 8-hour duration. He also is experiencing diaphoresis and nausea.

Physical Examination: Vital signs: pulse 100 (regular); blood pressure 100/60. Neck: jugular venous distention 4 cm above the angle of Louis at 30°. Cardiac: S_3 gallop; no murmurs or rubs. Chest: bibasilar rales up to a quarter of the lung fields posteriorly.

Laboratory Findings: EKG: acute anterior myocardial infarction. Echocardiogram performed several days later: see below.

Question: What complication of myocardial infarction is demonstrated?

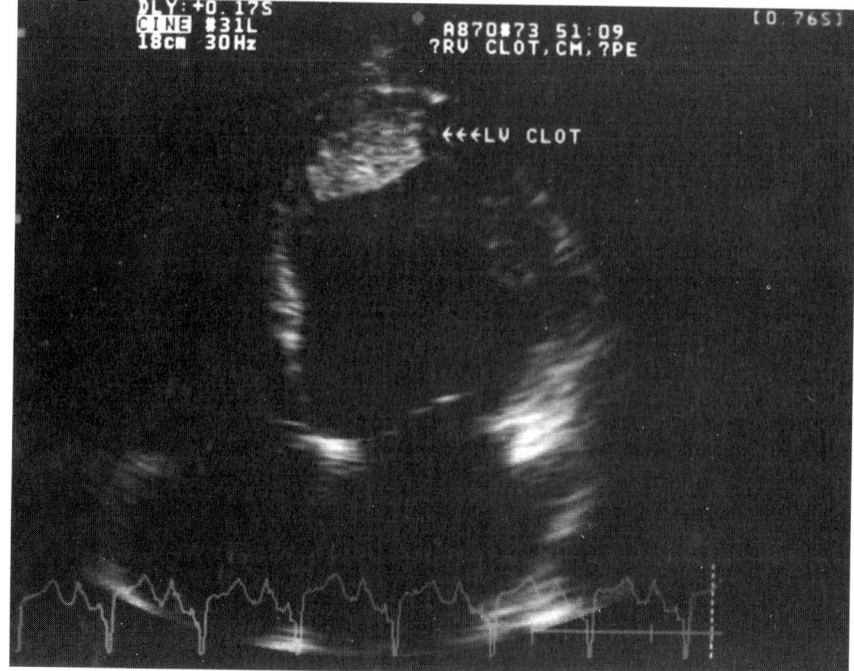

Answer: A large ventricular aneurysm and mural thrombus.

Discussion: A ventricular aneurysm develops most commonly after an anterior infarction, which usually is due to total occlusion of the left anterior descending coronary artery. Often it is the only vessel involved, and there are few or no collaterals present. Only 10% of all aneurysms involve the inferior wall. Patients with anterior ventricular aneurysms have a double left ventricular apical impulse on physical examination. Especially large anterior aneurysms may produce a sustained and diffuse apical impulse that extends medially and upward over two or more interspaces. Patients with inferior aneurysms usually do not have any abnormal physical findings.

About 46% of patients with an acute anterior infarction who have an akinetic or dyskinetic segment develop a mural thrombus 5–21 days after the acute attack. Thrombus formation, however, is rare after an inferior infarction. Embolism can occur in up to 10% of those who have a mural thrombus and usually occurs 1–3 months after the initial onset of the infarction. The mural thrombus can best be detected by two-dimensional echocardiography, which also shows the wall motion abnormalities. Virtually all patients with anterior myocardial infarction (MI) should have at least one echocardiogram several days after the infarction to detect thrombi.

Initially, patients with mural thrombi should receive full heparin dosage, maintaining the partial thromboplastin time 1.5 to 2 times normal. After a few days, warfarin should be added and then heparin stopped when the INR is 3–4. Warfarin should be continued for at least 3 months and, at that time, if an echocardiogram shows no thrombus, the warfarin can be discontinued. If there is a protruding thrombus or if a very large abnormal wall motion abnormality is still present, the warfarin should be continued for a longer time. One study suggested that aspirin was as effective as anticoagulation in causing resolution of thrombi in patients with anterior MI. Further data are needed to confirm this observation. Low-molecular-weight heparin (Dalteparin) significantly reduces left ventricular thrombus formation in acute anterior infarction, but is associated with increased hemorrhagic risk.

Ventricular aneurysms rarely rupture. They can cause ventricular tachycardia, intractable congestive heart failure, and angina and may be the source for thromboembolic events. Surgical resection is indicated if the complications cannot be controlled. Prior to surgery, the amount of mechanical dysfunction and the extent of reversible ischemia should be determined by hemodynamic and radionuclide studies at rest and during exercise. If exercise testing reveals reversible ischemia, revascularization should be performed at the time of aneurysmectomy. Outcome is enhanced if the ejection fraction of the nonaneurysmal portion of the heart is normal or supernormal. Ventricular aneurysm and left ventricular thrombi may be prevented by early reperfusion with thrombolytic agents and/or angioplasty with stents and the use of ACE inhibitors to attenuate the remodeling process in patients with anterior MI.

The present patient's EKG showed persistent ST segment elevation over several weeks, which suggested a ventricular aneurysm. Echocardiogram after several days revealed a large anterior infarction with apical dyskinesis and a protruding apical thrombus.

Clinical Pearls

1. Ventricular aneurysms occur almost exclusively secondary to anterior MI. Perform an echocardiogram to detect mural thrombi in all patients suffering an anterior MI.

2. Mural thrombi occur frequently in patients with ventricular aneurysm, and resolve with anticoagulation.

3. Consider resection for a ventricular aneurysm if complications such as intractable heart failure, ventricular arrhythmias, and thromboembolic events cannot be controlled medically.

REFERENCES

1. Asinger RW, Mikell FL, Elsperger J, et al: Incidence of left ventricular thrombosis after acute transmural myocardial infarction: Serial evaluation by two-dimensional echocardiography. N Engl J Med 1981;305:297–302.
2. Kouvaras G, Chronopoulos G, Soufras G, et al: The effects of long-term antithrombotic treatment on left ventricular thrombi in patients after an acute myocardial infarction. Am Heart J 1990;119:73–78.
3. Kontny F, Dale J, Abildgaard U, et al: Randomized trial of low molecular weight heparin (Dalteparin) in prevention of left ventricular thrombus formation and arterial embolism after acute myocardial infarction: The Fragmin in Acute Myocardial Infarction (FRAMI) Study. J Am Coll Cardiol 1997;30:962–969.
4. Ileri M, Tandğan I, Koşar F: Influence of thrombolytic therapy on the incidence of left ventricular thrombi after acute anterior myocardial infarction: Role of successful reperfusion. Clin Cardiol 1999;22:477–480.

PATIENT 33

A 18-year-old man with frequent premature ventricular beats

An 18-year-old man was noted to have an irregular heart rhythm while donating blood. After an EKG showed premature ventricular beats (PVBs), he was referred to a cardiologist. Except for influenza several years earlier, he has no past illnesses and denies a history of rheumatic fever. His mother states that his birth was normal and no cardiac murmur was noted during infancy. The patient is unaware of the premature beats.

Physical Examination: Vital signs: regular rhythm with intermittent premature beats; blood pressure 140/70. Cardiac: no murmurs or extra sounds.

Laboratory Findings: CBC and urinalysis: normal. EKG (see below): PVBs with a vertical axis; left bundle branch block (LBBB) appearance; and slurred R wave in V_1 and V_2. With exercise, the premature beats cleared. 24-hour Holter monitor: frequent unifocal PVBs. Echo/Doppler: normal.

Question: How would you manage this patient?

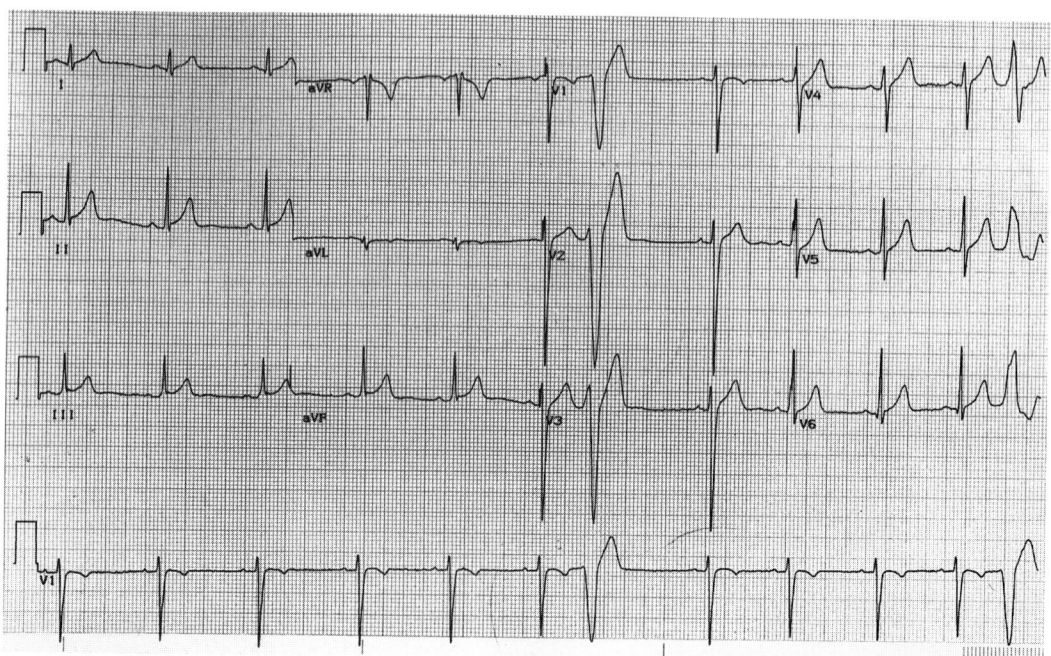

Answer: Offer reassurance plus dietary and exercise advice.

Discussion: Unifocal PVBs often are noted in healthy persons. Numerous studies have shown that PVBs are present in about one-third of healthy persons between the ages of 20 and 59 years, and in 69–100% of patients over 60. Complex forms (salvos, multifocal, greater than 30/hr) are present in less than 10% of healthy subjects between the ages of 20 and 60 years and in about 36–50% of patients between 60 and 85 years.

In one study, cardiac magnetic imaging was performed in patients with idiopathic right ventricular outflow tract PVBs (monomorphic LBBB and inferior axis morphology) and without evidence of structural heart disease. These patients had a higher rate of morphologic and functional abnormalities of the right ventricular outflow tract as compared to the controls without PVBs. Large-scale studies with long-term followup are needed to determine if these findings could identify a localized form of arrhythmogenic cardiomyopathy and its clinical significance.

The following configuration of PVBs is typical of persons with no evidence of cardiac disease: (1) left bundle branch block configuration; (2) slowly inscribed R waves in the PVBs in V_1 and V_2 positions; and (3) inferior direction of the main forces of the PVBs in the limb leads, producing an axis between +60° and +120°. It is believed that these PVBs arise from the anterior wall of the right ventricle, and because the initial part of the QRS in V_1 and V_2 is inscribed slowly, these originate from the general myocardium rather than from the Purkinje tissues. It is postulated that stretching of the anterior papillary muscle of the right ventricle during mechanical activity could trigger these extrasystoles. The present patient's PVBs had this type of configuration. For years it was thought that PVBs produced by exercise were associated with a cardiac abnormality; however, exercise-induced PVBs frequently are found in normal subjects during exercise.

Antiarrhythmic drugs are not recommended for PVBs of any type in patients without cardiac disease, unless PVBs cause symptoms. If patients are symptomatic, a beta-blocker can be effective. Beta-blockers are helpful for arrhythmias due to excessive cardiac adrenergic stimulation, such as those initiated by exercise or emotion. At times, PVB frequency may be diminished by reduction or elimination of the following: smoking; excessive coffee, tea, alcohol, and drugs such as thyroid hormone; amphetamines; and medications containing caffeine. In patients taking diuretics, hypokalemia and hypomagnesemia, which can precipitate PVBs, should be ruled out. Avoiding stress and exercising regularly should be encouraged. If all general measures fail and the patient is emotionally disturbed by the PVBs, a short course of mild tranquilizers can be helpful in addition to reassurance that the PVBs are benign. The long-term prognosis of healthy patients with PVBs compares favorably to those without PVBs.

The present patient was reassured that the PVBs noted during blood donation were benign and did not require therapy or further evaluation. He was advised to limit his consumption of dietary cardiac stimulants and to exercise regularly.

Clinical Pearls

1. PVBs are common in healthy persons, and their incidence increases with age.
2. In the absence of other findings, PVBs occurring with exercise do not indicate that cardiac disease is present.
3. Do not give antiarrhythmic drugs for PVBs unless the patient is symptomatic.
4. Reassure healthy persons with PVBs, and encourage them to avoid stimulants and exercise regularly.

REFERENCES

1. Rosenbaum MB: Classification of ventricular extrasystoles according to form. J Electrocardiogr 1969;2:289–298.
2. Kennedy HL, Whitlock JA, Sprague MK, et al: Long-term follow-up of asymptomatic healthy subjects with frequent and complex ventricular ectopy. N Engl J Med 1985;312:193–197.
3. Drory Y, Pines A, Fisman EZ, Kellerman JJ: Persistence of arrhythmia exercise response in healthy young men. Am J Cardiol 1990;66:1092–1098.
4. Alpert MA, Mukerji V, Bikkina M, et al: Pathogenesis, recognition, and management of common cardiac arrhythmias. Part I: Ventricular premature beats and tachyarrhythmias. South Med J 1995;88:1–21.
5. Proclemer A, Basadonna PT, Slavich GA, et al: Cardiac magnetic resonance imaging findings in patients with right ventricular outflow tract premature contractions. Eur Heart J 1997;18:2002–2010.

PATIENT 34

An 18-year-old man with palpitations, lightheadedness, and an abnormal electrocardiogram

An 18-year-old man presents to the emergency department with complaints of palpitations and lightheadedness. He has experienced no prior symptoms and has no significant past medical history. The patient is taking no medications and denies illicit drug use.

Physical Examination: Vital signs: pulse 270 and regular; blood pressure 100/60. General: mild respiratory distress. No jugular vein distention. Chest: clear. PMI in normal position; tachycardia present, but no murmurs. No hepatomegaly and no peripheral edema.

Laboratory Findings: CBC and SMA-7: normal. Chest radiograph: normal. EKG: see below.

Question: What is your diagnosis?

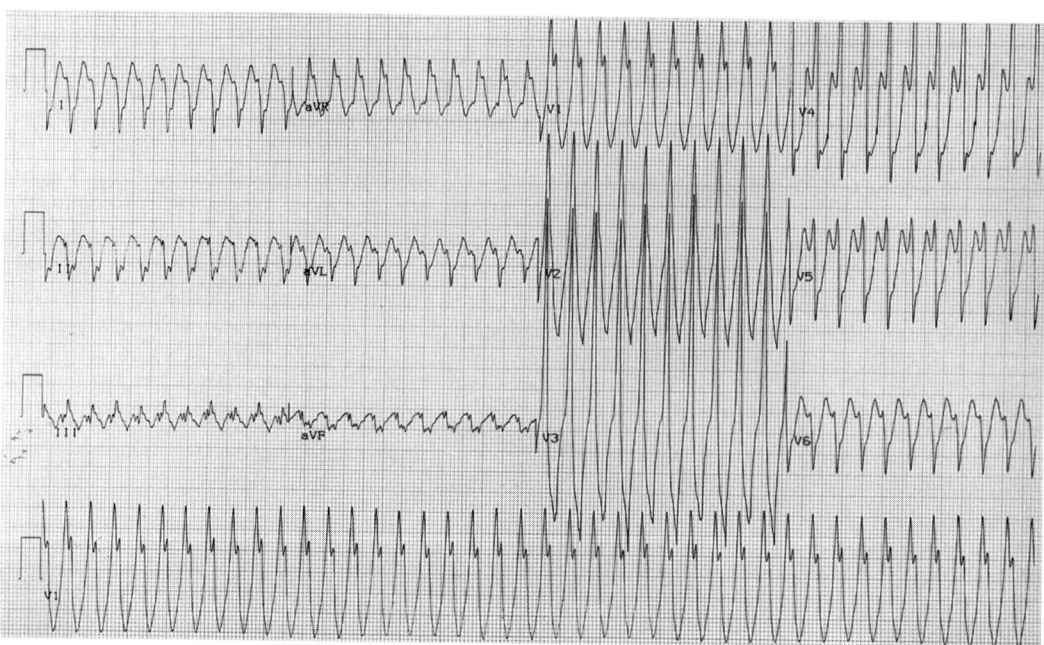

Diagnosis: Wolff-Parkinson-White syndrome (WPW).

Discussion: The true incidence of WPW syndrome is unknown, but varies in different reports from 0.1 to 3 per 1000 EKGs. In the most common manifestation of this syndrome, an accessory pathway connects the atria and ventricles. When conduction is through the accessory pathway, the EKG shows a short PR interval (0.1 second or less) and slurring of the initial portion of the QRS (delta wave). Activation of the ventricle over two pathways (normal pathway and accessory pathway) produces a fusion QRS configuration that depends on the contribution of the two activation pathways.

Traditionally, three types of QRS configuration are described, depending on the direction of the accessory pathway. **Type A** (left-sided or septal connection) has upright QRS complexes in all precordial leads. **Type B** (right-sided connection) has negative QRS complexes in V_1 and a positive complex in V_6. **Type C** (left lateral wall connection) has a positive QRS complex in V_1 and a negative QRS complex in V_6, and occurs infrequently. A patient may have more than one accessory pathway.

The European Study Group has standardized the nomenclature by using "tract" for pathways that insert into specialized conducting tissue and "connection" when pathways enter the general myocardium. Other preexcitation syndromes, besides that involving the atrioventricular (AV) connection (Kent bundle), involve bypass tracts from the atria to the His bundle (L-G-L syndrome or atriofascicular tract); the Mahaim fibers that connect the lower AV node, bundle of His, or upper bundle branches to the ventricular myocardium (nodoventricular or fasciculoventricular connections); and the James fibers that connect the atrium to the AV node (internodal bypass tract).

About 20–30% of all supraventricular tachycardias are associated with WPW syndrome. In at least 90% of patients, conduction proceeds down the AV node and returns retrograde through the accessory pathway to the atrium (orthodromic). In this situation the QRS is normal. In less than 10% of patients, conduction is in the reverse direction (antidromic) and, in such cases, the QRS complex is widened, demonstrating WPW syndrome. Regular orthodromic tachycardias usually are quite rapid in WPW, 190–250 beats min, and respond to vagal maneuvers, adenosine, or verapamil, just as AV nodal reentry tachycardia responds to such therapy. If the attacks are symptomatic or frequent, and do not respond to medical therapy, perform electrophysiologic studies and consider radiofrequency ablation of the pathway. In this procedure, alternating current is converted into radio waves, which causes thermal destruction of the accessory pathway. Success of radiofrequency ablation ranges from 65–95%, depending on operator experience and the site of the pathway.

Antidromic atrioventricular tachycardias (conducting down the accessory pathway) are usually due to atrial flutter or atrial fibrillation; the QRSs have the WPW configuration. Such cases (as in the present patient; see figure) respond best to **procainamide,** which prolongs the refractory period of the accessory pathway, or to **DC shock.** Digitalis and verapamil may shorten the refractory period of the accessory pathway, further increasing the ventricular rate, and may precipitate ventricular fibrillation.

The present patient received one 6-mg dose of adenosine without effect. Adenosine does not effect conduction in normal accessory pathways, and it may predispose to the development of atrial fibrillation. A rapid procainamide infusion converted his rhythm to atrial fibrillation with a ventricular response of 130 beats/min, then to sinus rhythm. His echocardiogram was normal. An electrophysiologic study revealed a left lateral accessory pathway with inducible atrial flutter with 1:1 conduction at a rate of 286 beats/min. Both antidromic and orthodromic tachycardias were inducible. Subsequently this patient underwent radiofrequency ablation of the accessory pathway.

Clinical Pearls

1. When an arrhythmia is conducted downward by the accessory pathway, it is easily confused with ventricular tachycardia.

2. Atrial flutter or fibrillation in the presence of WPW syndrome responds best to intravenous procainamide. Do *not* give digitalis and verapamil, especially if antidromic conduction has been demonstrated.

3. Catheter ablation of WPW pathways is highly successful and obviates the need for chronic drug administration.

REFERENCES

1. Anderson RH, Becker AE, Brechenmacher C, et al: Ventricular preexcitation: A proposed nomenclature for its substrate. Eur J Cardiol 1975;3:27.
2. Prystowsky EN: Diagnosis and management of the preexcitation syndromes. Curr Probl Cardiol 1988;13:225–310.
3. Capucci A, Villani GQ, Aschieri D: Risk of complications of atrial fibrillation. Pacing Clin Electrophysiol 1997;20:2684–2691.
4. Iesaka Y, Yamane T, Takahashi A, et al.: Retrograde multiple and multifiber accessory pathway conduction in the Wolff-Parkinson-White syndrome: Potential precipitating factor of atrial fibrillation. J Cardiovasc Electrophysiol 1998;9:141–151.

PATIENT 35

A 72-year-old woman on quinidine with presyncopal episodes

A 72-year-old woman has experienced recurrent palpitations since menopause. The episodes are frequent, but not associated with dizziness, syncope, or changes in mental status. Frequent premature ventricular beats (PVBs) have been noted, and she has become increasingly aware of them. She has been started on quinidine, 200 mg every 6 hours, because she is symptomatic. The patient returns 3 weeks later because of three episodes of dizziness and near syncope.

Physical Examination: Vital signs: normal. Cardiac: normal, with occasional premature beats.

Laboratory Findings: CBC: normal. Serum electrolytes: normal. Quinidine blood level: normal range. EKG: rare unifocal premature ventricular beats; QT interval 560 msec (corrected QT 490 msec). 24-hour Holter monitor: rhythm strip recorded during an episode of near-syncope (see below).

Question: What is the diagnosis of this arrhythmia?

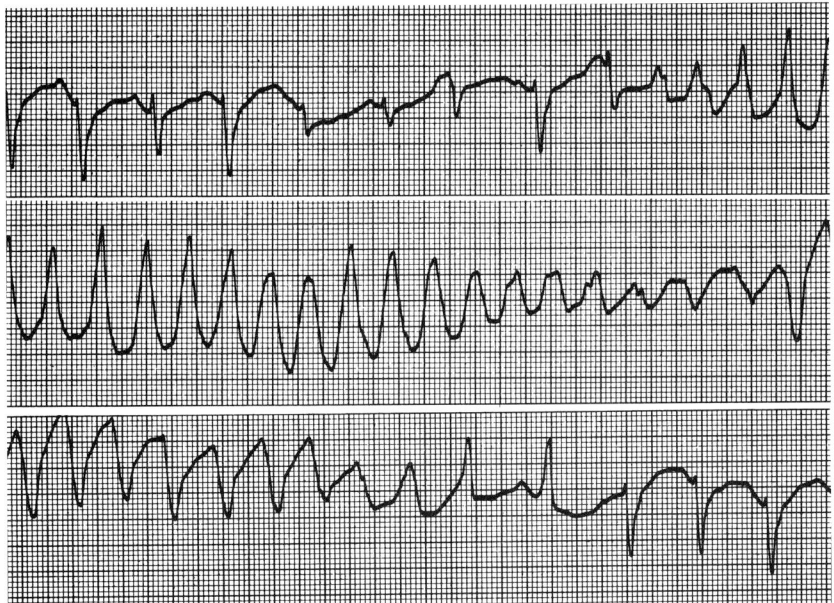

Figure reproduced from Gazes PC: Clinical Cardiology—A Cost-Effective Approach, 4th ed. New York, Chapman and Hall, 1997; with permission.

Diagnosis: Polymorphic ventricular tachycardia—torsade de pointes.

Discussion: Polymorphic ventricular tachycardia appears to be a transition between conventional ventricular tachycardia and ventricular fibrillation. The EKG shows cycles of changing electrical polarity, so that the peaks of the QRS twist about the isoelectric baseline (see figure). When it is associated with a long QT interval, it is referred to as torsade de pointes. Type 1A drugs such as quinidine, procainamide, and disopyramide and class III drugs such as amiodarone, sotalol, ibutilide, all of which prolong the QT interval, can produce such attacks despite blood levels that are not considered toxic. Approximately 50% of patients who experience torsade do so within the first few days of therapy with these drugs. The remainder manifest the arrhythmias weeks or years later.

Torsade de pointes also occurs soon after conversion of atrial fibrillation to sinus rhythm. Other causes of QT prolongation, such as hypomagnesemia, hypokalemia, congenital long QT interval syndromes, central nervous system lesions, high-grade AV block, and the use of psychotropic drugs (tricyclics, tetracyclics, phenothiazines) also can produce this arrhythmia. Five cases of torsade have been reported after administration of erythromycin. Erythromycin prolongs ventricular repolarization, which could explain the arrhythymia, but the drug often is given to ill patients with other predisposing factors that contribute to prolonging the QT interval. Terfenadine can lead to a prolonged QT interval and torsade if it is given to patients with hepatic dysfunction, in doses greater than 60 mg b.i.d., or in conjunction with ketoconazole, itraconazole, or erythromycin.

The QTc interval (corrected for heart rate) is generally considered prolonged if it is greater than 440 msec seconds. Torsade de pointes occurs in about 50% of those with a QT interval of 600 msec seconds or greater. Marked "U" wave—accentuation in the beat following a premature ventricular contraction (postpause beat)—or a new bigeminal pattern often precedes torsade. Episodes of torsade de pointes usually terminate spontaneously, but continue to recur, and may lead to ventricular fibrillation.

Therapy is directed at removing the predisposing cause of the QT interval prolongation. Overdrive suppression with atrial or ventricular pacing or isoproterenol has been successful in emergency situations. Magnesium sulfate as a 1–2-gm bolus given intravenously, followed by continuous infusion of 2–7 mg/min for several hours, is now the therapy of choice. Those with congenital long QT intervals may require left-sided cervical thoracic sympathetic ganglionectomy for control of the arrhythmia. In some congenital types, beta blockers may be effective. If the QT interval is normal, the polymorphic ventricular tachycardia should be treated with standard antiarrhythmic therapy.

The present patient recovered after the quinidine was discontinued. In fact, this elderly patient with PVBs and good ventricular function probably should not have been treated with antiarrhythmic therapy.

Clinical Pearls

1. Torsade de pointes is a form of polymorphic ventricular tachycardia associated with drugs or conditions that prolong the QT interval.
2. Torsade de pointes most often occurs when the QT interval is 600 msec seconds or greater, when the postpause "U" wave amplitude is accentuated, or when new ventricular bigeminy occurs.
3. The predisposing causes of the prolonged QT intervals should be removed. Until this can be accomplished, manage torsade de pointes with intravenous magnesium sulfate or overdrive suppression pacing.
4. Avoid giving antiarrhythmic drugs to patients with PVBs and good ventricular function, because these drugs can cause proarrhythmias.

REFERENCES

1. Smith WM, Gallagher JJ: "Les torsades de pointes." An unusual ventricular arrhythmia. Ann Intern Med 1980;93:578–584.
2. Jackman WM, Friday KJ, Anderson JL, et al: The long QT syndromes: A critical review, new clinical observations and a unifying hypothesis. Prog Cardiovasc Dis 1988;31:115–172.
3. Locati EH, Maison-Blanche P, Dejode P, et al.: Spontaneous sequences of onset of torsade de pointes in patients with acquired prolonged repolarization: Quantitative analysis of Holter recordings. J Am Coll Cardiol 1995;25:1564–1575.
4. Roden DM: A practical approach to torsade de pointes. Clin Cardiol 1997;20:285–290.

PATIENT 36

A 60-year-old man with an acute inferior myocardial infarction and pulmonary edema

A 60-year-old man presents with an acute inferior myocardial infarction (MI) and no significant prior history. Within 2 hours of presentation, he develops pulmonary edema, which responds to intravenous nitroglycerin and diuretics. The patient is given thrombolytic therapy, and the chest pain resolves within 3 hours of onset. An echocardiogram reveals inferior akinesis, overall ejection fraction of 50%, and trivial mitral regurgitation. Twelve hours later, recurrent chest pain develops, and the manifestations of acute pulmonary edema return. He again responds to diuretics and an increased dosage of nitroglycerin.

Physical Examination: Vital signs: pulse 100; respirations 30; blood pressure 110/60. General: moderate respiratory distress. Neck: no jugular venous distention. Chest: rales over lower one-third of lung fields. Cardiac: III/VI holosystolic murmur at the apex radiating to the axilla. Extremities: no edema.

Question: Why did episodic pulmonary edema develop in this patient?

Answer: The episodic pulmonary edema is due to left atrial overload in ischemic mitral regurgitation.

Discussion: Mitral regurgitation is the only valvular lesion commonly caused by ischemic heart disease. The papillary muscles to which the mitral valve leaflets are attached through the chordae tendineae are extensions of the endocardium—the layer of the myocardium most susceptible to ischemia. The ischemic or infarcted papillary muscle fails to contract during systole, allowing the mitral valve leaflets to prolapse into the left atrium, producing mitral regurgitation. As observed in the present patient, intermittent ischemia of a papillary muscle can cause episodic mitral regurgitation.

A severe manifestation of ischemic papillary muscle dysfunction is necrotic rupture of one of the papillary muscle heads. This causes partial flail of a mitral valve leaflet and consequent severe mitral regurgitation. Either the anterior or posterior papillary muscle may be involved, but posterior involvement during inferior infarction is more common than anterior involvement during anterior infarction. In extreme cases, infarction can result in complete transection of a papillary muscle, which produces overwhelming mitral regurgitation that is incompatible with life. The likelihood of papillary muscle dysfunction does not depend on the size of the infarct; severe mitral regurgitation often is found in relatively small infarcts isolated to the area contiguous with the papillary muscles.

The new onset of a **holosystolic murmur** following an MI raises the suspicion that either acute mitral regurgitation or a ventricular septal defect has developed. Both conditions may be associated with shock and pulmonary edema. The left atrial overload observed in mitral regurgitation, however, makes pulmonary edema a more prominent finding in that condition than in acute ventricular septal defect. The murmur in mitral regurgitation is apical in location, whereas the murmur of a ventricular septal defect is heard loudest along the sternum and frequently radiates to the right of the sternum. If septal rupture occurs near the apex, however, the murmur may be best heard apically, thus mimicking mitral regurgitation. The diagnosis of acute mitral regurgitation is usually confirmed at **echocardiography with color flow mapping,** which demonstrates systolic flow across the mitral valve.

Initial management of acute severe mitral regurgitation should be monitored by the insertion of a Swan-Ganz catheter. The pulmonary capillary wedge pressure tracing usually demonstrates an accentuated V wave and no oxygen step-up. Large V waves also can be seen in the presence of an acute ventricular septal defect, which also overloads the left atrium. Further, the absence of a large V wave does not rule out the diagnosis of severe mitral regurgitation.

The mainstay of medical therapy is **afterload reduction.** Nitroprusside is the drug of choice because it causes both venodilatation, which reduces left atrial filling pressure directly, and arterial vasodilatation, which permits increased flow into the aorta and differentially less flow into the left atrium. However, note that many patients with acute mitral regurgitation already are severely hypotensive, which may preclude the use of a vasodilator. In such patients, intra-aortic balloon counterpulsation reduces afterload and also augments systemic blood pressure.

The definitive therapy for mitral regurgitation is surgery. Unfortunately, despite advances in surgery for nonischemic mitral regurgitation, the operative mortality for ischemic mitral regurgitation is still high, approximately 25%. Although in some instances simple revascularization may improve ischemic papillary muscle function, valve repair usually is required. Valve repair may be difficult, however, because the valve itself is typically normal, reducing the options for repair available to the surgeon. A Carpentier annuloplasty may help to restore valvular competence.

In the present patient, echocardiogram revealed moderate mitral regurgitation, and cardiac catheterization revealed three-vessel coronary disease. He underwent revascularization without mitral valve surgery. Postoperatively, his intermittent mitral regurgitation disappeared because revascularization improved the ischemic papillary muscle function.

Clinical Pearls

1. Ischemic mitral regurgitation has a much higher mortality than does mitral regurgitation from any other cause.
2. Either inferior or anterior MI can produce ischemic mitral regurgitation. The condition occurs more frequently, however, in patients with inferior MI.
3. Large V waves in the pulmonary capillary wedge tracing can be seen both in acute mitral regurgitation and acute ventricular septal defect—two conditions that produce a new holosystolic murmur.

REFERENCES

1. Rankin JS, Feneley MP, Hickey MSJ, et al: A clinical comparison of miral valve repair versus valve replacement in ischemic mitral regurgitation. J Thora Cardiovasc Surg 1988;95:165–177.
2. Himelman RB, Kusumoto F, Oken K, et al: The flail mitral valve: Echocardiographic findings by precordial and transeosophageal imaging and Doppler color flow mapping. J Am Coll Cardiol 1991;17:272–279.
3. Kishon Y, Oh JK, Mullany CJ, et al: Mitral valve operation in post-infarction rupture of papillary muscle: immediate results and long-term followup of 22 patients. Mayo Clin Proc 1992;67:1023–1030.
4. Ryan TJ, Antman EM, Brooks NH, et al: 1999 update: ACC/AHA guidelines for the management of patients with acute myocardial infarction. A report of the American College of Cardiology/American Heart Association Task Force on Practice Guidelines (Committee on Management of Acute Myocardial Infarction). J Am Coll Cardiol 1999;34:890–911.

PATIENT 37

A 60-year-old man with acute interscapular pain and a cold right hand

A 60-year-old man is admitted to the hospital 3 hours after the onset of sudden, severe interscapular pain. His pain reached full intensity almost immediately. Presently he notes that his right hand is cold. He has had hypertension for many years and is a heavy cigarette smoker.

Physical Examination: Vital signs: pulse 80; blood pressure left arm 220/140—after receiving nitroprusside IV 220/110, right arm 90/80. General: diaphoretic. Cardiac: faint diastolic murmur left sternal border. Extremities: right hand cold; right radial pulse absent; pulses present in the lower extremities; systolic bruits heard over the femoral arteries.

Laboratory Findings: Hct: 40%. Chest radiograph: see below. EKG: left ventricular hypertrophy.

Questions: What is the most likely diagnosis? Which diagnostic test should be performed next?

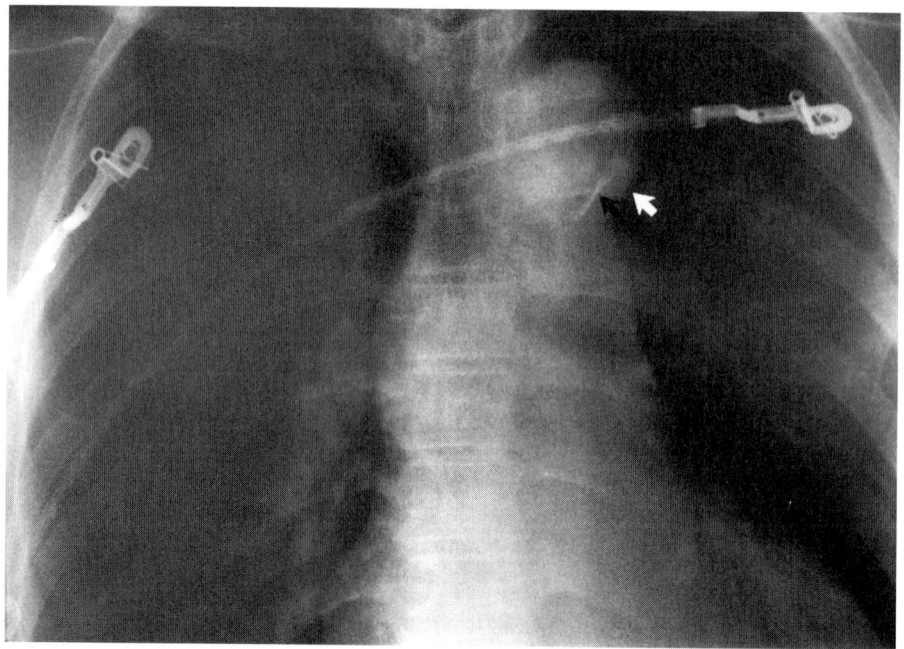

Answer: The most likely diagnosis is type I aortic dissection producing aortic insufficiency. Confirmatory imaging is the next test.

Discussion: The incidence of aortic dissection is approximately 1 per 10,000 hospital admissions and 1 per 360 autopsies. Most patients are between the ages of 40 and 70. Dissection usually is due to Marfan syndrome or a congenital anomaly if dissection occurs before age 40. Predisposing factors in older patients are hypertension and degeneration of the aortic media (cystic medial necrosis). Cystic medial necrosis occurs normally with aging, suggesting that dissections occur when this "normal" process is accelerated. An entrance tear is noted in 90% of dissections. If an exit intimal tear also is present, it produces a double-barreled appearance of the aorta.

Aortic dissection has been classified by Debakey as type I, which begins in the ascending aorta just above the aortic valve; type II, which is limited to the ascending aorta; and type III, which begins at or just distal to the origin of the left subclavian artery. If dissection is limited to the descending thoracic aorta, it is classified as type IIIA; type IIIb extends to the abdominal aortic bifurcation and lower. Another and simpler classification system that works well prognostically categorizes dissection as proximal (type A) when the ascending aorta is involved, and distal (type B) when the ascending aorta is spared. Type A includes Debakey types I and II, and type B is analogous to Debakey type III.

Patients with dissection have severe pain that reaches maximum intensity immediately. Pain may be located in the anterior or posterior chest, back, or abdomen. Pulses can become absent or diminished as the dissection advances to involve major arteries. If the aortic root is involved, aortic insufficiency may occur. The aorta also may rupture into the pericardial cavity, producing tamponade and cardiovascular collapse. Rarely, the right sternal clavicular joint pulsates. The patient may appear to be in shock despite elevated blood pressure. Partial occlusion of the branches of the aorta, as in the present patient, can produce differences in blood pressure between the two upper extremities. Chest pain may lead to the misdiagnosis of an acute myocardial infarction. However, the lack of Q waves on the EKG, the lack of serum enzyme elevation, and the persistence of pain associated with hypertension should lead to the presumptive diagnosis of dissection. Rarely, the dissection involves the ostium of a coronary vessel and causes a Q wave infarction. Such patients usually have associated aortic insufficiency.

Widening of the aorta on chest radiograph with intimal calcification separated from the outer edge of the aortic shadow (see figure on previous page) should increase suspicion of dissection. The best imaging modality for confirming the diagnosis currently is under debate. **Transesophageal echocardiography, MRI, CT scanning,** and **aortography** all have high sensitivity and specificity.

Drug therapy to reduce the propulsive stress on the aortic wall is the initial treatment for all patients with dissection. Agents are given to reduce the velocity of left ventricular ejection (DV/DT) and systolic blood pressure. Reduction in pulse pressure may be more important than the reduction in absolute blood pressure. Sodium nitroprusside combined with a beta blocker has become standard therapy to reduce both blood pressure and left ventricular propulsive force. Once the patient is stable, imaging should be performed to establish the diagnosis. Serious complications such as severe aortic insufficiency, aortic rupture, cardiac tamponade, or compromise of vital organs may require immediate surgery.

The standard treatment for acute aortic dissection is either surgical or medical, depending on the features of the lesion and any associated complications. Stent-graft coverage of the primary entry tear is a very promising new treatment for selected patients with acute aortic dissection. Transluminal endovascular stent-grafts appear particularly useful in covering the primary intimal tear in the descending aorta (type B) in the treatment of peripheral arterial complications. Initial studies showed a lower mortality rate and no instance of paraplegia, stroke, embolization, side-branch occlusions, or infection in the stent-graft. Post-implantation syndrome can occur with transient C-reactive protein levels rising, mild temperature rise, and leukocytosis.

In the present patient, the diagnosis of aortic dissection was confirmed by aortography, which showed a dissection beginning in the aortic root and extending beyond the great vessels (see figure below). The patient underwent successful surgery.

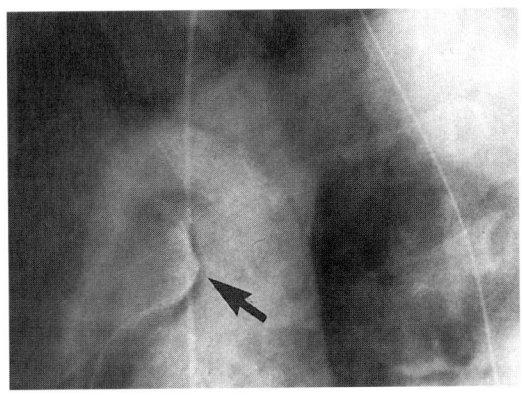

Clinical Pearls

1. Suspect aortic dissection if the patient has chest, back, or abdominal pain that reaches maximum intensity immediately. Hypertension, despite an appearance of shock, and a relatively normal EKG should increase your suspicion.
2. Evaluate for aortic dissection in any patient with chest pain who develops aortic insufficiency.
3. Marfan syndrome is likely if the dissection occurs under age 40.
4. Drug therapy with nitroprusside and a beta blocker is the initial treatment in almost all cases of dissection; surgery should be performed if the ascending aorta is involved.
5. Transluminal endovascular stent-grafts can be used in selected cases.

REFERENCES

1. Schlatmann TJM, Becker AE: Histologic changes in the normal aging aorta: Implications for dissecting aortic aneurysm. Am J Cardiol 1977;39:31–20.
2. Wheat MW Jr: Acute dissecting aneurysms of the aorta: Diagnosis and treatment—1979. Am Heart J 1980;99:373–387.
3. Debakey ME, McCollum CH, Crawford ES, et al: Dissection and dissecting aneurysms of the aorta: Twenty-year follow-up of 527 patients treated surgically. Surgery 1982;92:1118–1134.
4. Nienaber CA, Von Kodolitsch Y, Nicolas V, et al: The diagnosis of thoracic aortic dissection by noninvasive imaging procedures. N Engl J Med 1993;328:1–9.
5. Dake MD, Kato N, Mitchell RS, et al: Endovascular stent-graft placement for the treatment of acute aortic dissection. N Engl J Med 1999;340:1546–1552.

PATIENT 38

A 35-year-old man who received thrombolytic therapy for chest pain and ST elevation

A 35-year-old African-American man developed substernal chest tightness and a fullness in his throat—without nausea, vomiting, or diaphoresis—while moving beds. He has never experienced a similar pain previously, and denies hypertension, diabetes, and a smoking history. He recently experienced a stressful divorce. Family history is negative for coronary artery disease. The patient presents with stable vital signs, but an EKG showing ST elevation. After sublingual nitroglycerin fails to relieve the chest pain or resolve the ST elevation, tissue plasminogen activator (tPA) and heparin are administered in the emergency department. His pain subsides after 45 minutes of tPA infusion.

Physical Examination: Vital signs: pulse 80 (regular); blood pressure 118/70. Neck: no jugular venous distention. Cardiac: no murmurs.

Laboratory Findings: CBC, urinalysis, and cardiac enzymes: normal. EKG: see below.

Question: What etiologies for the EKG abnormalities, other than myocardial infarction, should be considered?

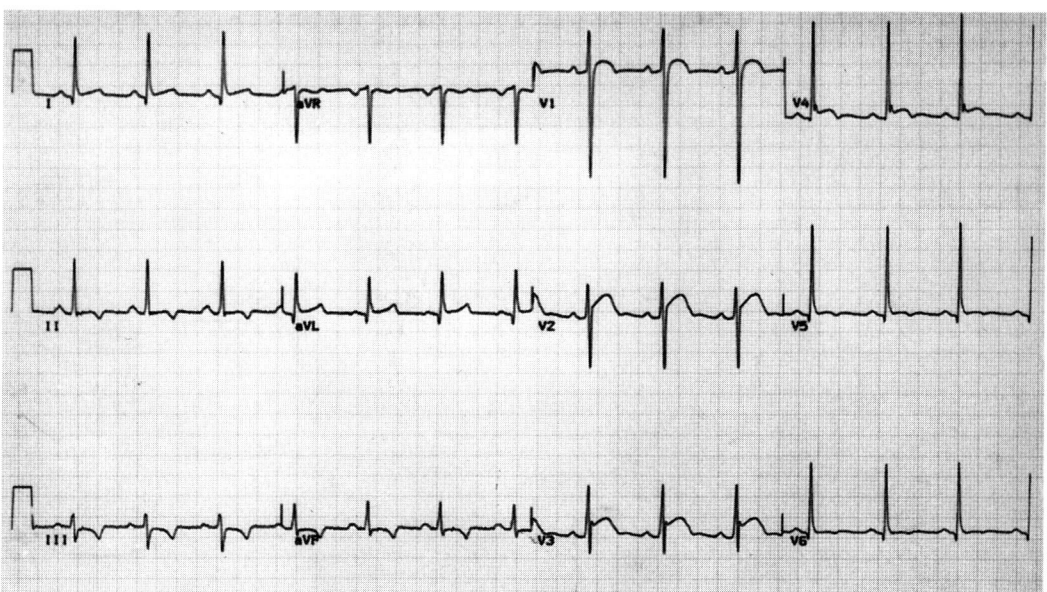

Answer: Early repolarization.

Discussion: It is estimated that only 30% of patients who suffer an acute myocardial infarction receive thrombolytic therapy—despite unequivocal evidence that this therapy is effective. There is an understandable impetus, therefore, to broaden the application of this form of treatment. On the other hand, because thrombolytic therapy has a clear risk, every effort should be made to avoid its use in patients with chest pain *unrelated* to myocardial infarction.

Criteria have been formulated to assist patient selection for thrombolytic therapy and identify patients with a high likelihood of clinical benefit. The usual **indications for thrombolysis** are: onset of pain within 12 hours of presentation; pain not relieved by nitroglycerin; 1 mm or more of ST elevation in two inferior leads, in two contiguous precordial leads, or in both leads I and aVL; new or presumably new left bundle branch block with a history suggesting acute myocardial infarction; ST-segment depression equal or greater than 2 mm in V_1, V_2 (true posterior infarction); and no contraindications to anticoagulation. **Absolute contraindications** include active internal bleeding, active cerebrovascular disease, and uncontrolled severe hypertension. **Relative contraindications** are hemostatic disorders, major surgery (less than 10 days previously), gastrointestinal or genitourinary tract bleeding (in the previous 6 months), prolonged CPR, recent trauma, diabetic hemorrhagic retinopathy, and pregnancy. There is no age limit to thrombolytic therapy. The earlier therapy begins, the better the outcome. The greatest benefit occurs when thrombolytic therapy is given within the first 2 hours.

In using these selection criteria, conditions unassociated with myocardial ischemia that may cause ST-segment elevation must be carefully excluded. Early repolarization is a normal variant of unknown etiology that often is noted in African-American patients. It can simulate the injury pattern of acute pericarditis or myocardial infarction. In early repolarization, however, the ST-segment elevation usually is concave *upward* without reciprocal changes, and the ratio of ST-segment elevation to T-wave height is less than 0.25 in lead V_6. Also, early repolarization frequently is associated with increased R-wave amplitude, especially in the left precordial leads. Additionally, the T waves often are inverted above the baseline and commonly variable in daily tracings.

When EKG abnormalities cannot be clearly contributed to early repolarization in patients with acute chest pain, an emergency echocardiogram may reveal abnormal segmental wall motion consistent with myocardial ischemia. The ST elevation of pericarditis may also be a source of diagnostic error in patients with acute chest pain. An echocardiogram is helpful in this condition by showing normal wall motion and the presence of a pericardial effusion.

The present patient had ST-segment elevation without reciprocal ST depression, consistent with early repolarization. The ST-segment elevation in V_1–V_3 was concave *downward*, however, suggesting a current of injury—but no evolution of the EKGs occurred, and serial cardiac enzymes studies were negative. Coronary arteriorgrams revealed normal arteries. The diagnosis was nonspecific chest pain, and the patient was discharged with reassurance.

Clinical Pearls

1. In early repolarization, ST elevation usually is concave upward and is not associated with ST depression in other leads.

2. When the diagnosis of myocardial infarction is in doubt, employ echocardiography to examine for regional left ventricular functional abnormalities.

3. In early repolarization, the ratio of ST-segment elevation to T-wave height ratio is less than 0.25 in lead V_6, R-wave amplitudes may be increased especially in the left precordial leads, and T waves often are inverted above the baseline and commonly vary in daily tracings.

REFERENCES

1. Goldman MJ: RS-T segment elevation in mid and left precordial leads as a normal variant. Am Heart J 1953;46:817–820.
2. Gazes PC: Pericarditis. Cardiovasc Dis Chest Pain 1985;1:28.
3. Spodick DH: Early repolarization: An underinvestigated misnoner. Clin Cardiol 1997;20:913–914.
4. Ryan TJ, Antman EM, Brooks NH, et al: 1999 update: ACC/AHA guidelines for the management of patients with acute myocardial infarction. A report of the American College of Cardiology/American Heart Association Task Force on Practice Guidelines (Committee on Management of Acute Myocardial Infarction). J Am Coll Cardiol 1999;34:890–911.

PATIENT 39

A 26-year-old woman with headache, nausea, blurred vision, and an abnormal electrocardiogram

A 26-year-old woman with no significant past medical history presents with a severe acute headache. She also reports blurred vision and nausea, with one episode of vomiting.

Physical Examination: Vital signs: temperature 98.5°; pulse 80; respirations 18; blood pressure 100/60. Neurologic: nuchal rigidity.

Laboratory Findings: Lumbar puncture: grossly bloody. Head CT: subarachnoid hemorrhage. EKG: see below.

Question: What is the cause of these EKG abnormalities?

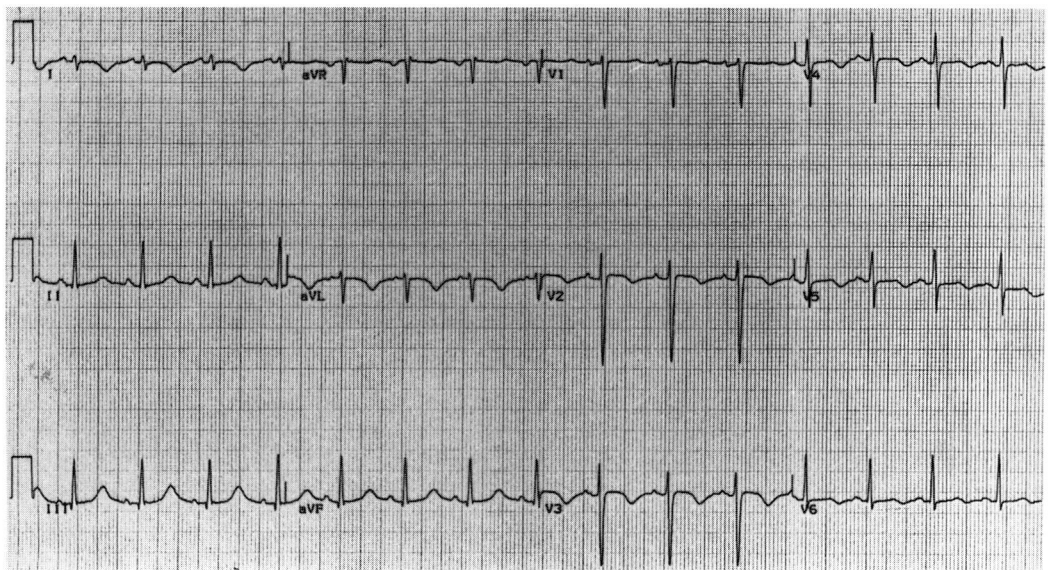

Answer: The exact mechanism is unknown.

Discussion: Symmetrically inverted T waves, prominent "U" waves, and prolonged QT intervals frequently are observed following a cerebrovascular accident (CVA). They may be misinterpreted as myocardial ischemia, infarction, or electrolyte imbalance. The exact mechanism by which a CVA causes these EKG changes is unknown. It is clear, however, that the heart receives a high level of nerve traffic from the brain, which may exert profound physiologic effects on the heart. Both circulating and myocardial catecholamines are increased following a CVA. The **high levels of catecholamines** may directly damage the myocardium. Such damage is indicated by an increase in the MB fraction of serum creatine kinase and the development of wall motion abnormalities. This damage might be the genesis of the EKG abnormalities.

Pulmonary edema also may occur in the setting of a CVA and may be related to increased catecholamines. The hypertension that results from the rise in catecholamines increases afterload, forcing the use of preload reserve to compensate, in turn increasing pulmonary capillary wedge pressure. Heightened sympathetic tone also may decrease vascular capacity and increase hydrostatic pressure at any given vascular volume, which leads to alveolar transudation of fluid. Vascular permeability also may increase, contributing to the syndrome.

Treatment is primarily supportive and includes oxygenation, diuresis, and control of hypertension. Significant cardiac arrhythmias can develop and should be monitored and treated when they become life-threatening.

The present patient suffered repolarization changes due to a cerebrovascular accident. Her EKG showed symmetrically inverted T waves throughout the tracing and a long QT interval. She developed progressive neurologic deficits and died as a result of subarachnoid hemorrhage.

Clinical Pearls

1. Profound EKG changes mimicking myocardial ischemia may occur following intracranial catastrophes.
2. The constellation of acute pulmonary edema and EKG changes due to increased intracranial pressure can be confused with a primary cardiac disorder.
3. Circulating and myocardial catecholamines increase following a cerebrovascular accident and may directly damage the myocardium, causing wall motion abnormalities and the observed EKG abnormalities.

REFERENCES

1. Yamour BJ, Sridharan MR, Rice JF, et al: Electrocardiographic changes in cerebrovascular hemorrhage. Am Heart J 1980;99:294–300.
2. Samuels MA: Electrocardiographic manifestations of neurologic disease. Semin Neurol 1984;4:453–461.
3. Malik AB: Mechanisms of neurogenic pulmonary edema. Cir Res 1985;57:1–18.
4. Maron MB: Pulmonary vasoconstriction in a canine model of neurogenic pulmonary edema. J Appl Physiol 1990;68:912–918.
5. Oppenheimer SM, Hachinski VC: The cardiac consequences of stroke. Neurol Clin 1992;10:167.

PATIENT 40

A 56-year-old man on digoxin with supraventricular tachycardia

A 56-year-old man with ischemic heart disease and a history of congestive heart failure presents with increasing dyspnea on exertion and palpitation. His heart failure had been compensated until approximately 12 hours before admission when he noted the onset of palpitations. There is no lightheadedness or syncope. Although he complains of a "funny feeling in his chest," there is no angina. His regimen for congestive heart failure prior to admission was digoxin 0.25 mg q.d., furosemide 40 mg p.o. q.d., and enalapril 10 mg b.i.d.

Physical Examination: Vital signs: pulse 150 (regular); blood pressure 110/60. Chest: clear. Cardiac: summation gallop; I/VI systolic ejection murmur. Extremities: no peripheral edema.

Laboratory Findings: Na^+ 140 mEq/L; K^+ 3.7 mEq/L; Cl 102 mEq/L; HCO_3 26 mEq/L; calcium 9.0 mEq/L; phosphate 3.0 mEq/L; magnesium 0.9 mEq/L. Digoxin level: 0.9 ng/ml. EKG: see below.

Question: What is the likely cause of the patient's arrhythmia?

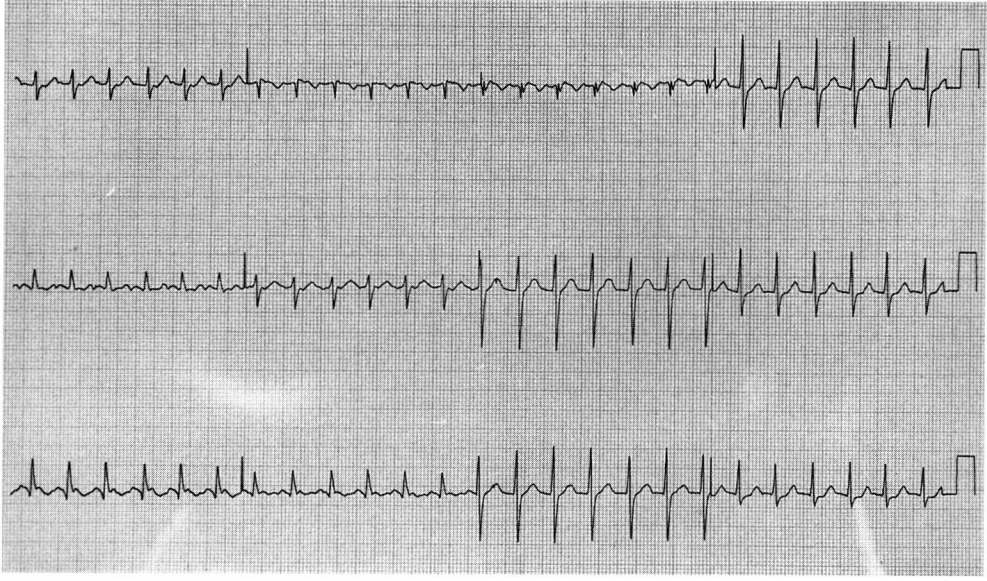

Diagnosis: Atrial flutter associated with hypomagnesemia.

Discussion: Loop diuretics such as furosemide, thiazide diuretics, and digitalis enhance the renal excretion of magnesium. Although diuretics typically also increase the excretion of potassium (the typical hypomagnesemic patient is also hypokalemic) and most physicians provide potassium replacement when needed, magnesium replacement is frequently overlooked. Although in the present patient the serum magnesium level is low, it may not reflect hypomagnesemia in skeletal or cardiac muscle.

Hypomagnesemia leads to increased sinus node discharge and may produce atrial and ventricular ectopy, potentially leading to sustained atrial or ventricular arrhythmias. Hypomagnesemia also may prolong the QT interval and lead to torsade de pointes. Thus, magnesium administration is an important therapy in torsade de pointes caused by hypomagnesemia or by type IA antiarrhythmic agents. Other consequences of magnesium depletion are increased sensitivity to digitalis and coronary spasm. A recent controlled study of magnesium used in patients with acute myocardial infarction demonstrated reduced mortality following administration of magnesium. This reduction might have occurred because magnesium reduces peri-infarction arrhythmias and also may reduce infarct size.

The present patient clearly requires repletion of magnesium. In acute circumstances, 1 g of magnesium can be given in the sulfate form over 20 minutes. Chronically, magnesium chloride may be administered orally in doses of as much as 3 g a day in divided doses. Because serum magnesium levels do not correlate well with overall magnesium depletion, many advocate daily magnesium therapy for patients receiving chronic diuretics.

The present patient returned to sinus rhythm with a normal QT interval after repletion of magnesium and administration of sotalol.

Clinical Pearls

1. Serum magnesium levels frequently do not reflect magnesium depletion in cardiac and skeletal muscle.
2. Consider chronic magnesium replacement in patients receiving chronic diuretics.
3. Magnesium excretion is enhanced by digitalis.
4. Hypomagnesemia can produce atrial and ventricular arrhythmias.

REFERENCES

1. Gottlieb SS, Baruch L, Kukin ML, et al: Prognostic importance of the serum magnesium concentration in patients with congestive heart failure. J Am Coll Cardiol 1990;16:827–831.
2. Perticone F, Borelli D, Ceravolo R, et al: Antiarrhythmic short-term protective magnesium treatment in ischemic dilated cardiomyopathy. J Am Coll Nutr 1990;9:492–499.
3. Rosenberger K: Management of electrolyte abnormalities: Hypocalcemia, hypomagnesemia, and hypokalemia. J Am Acad Nurse Pract 1998;10:209–217.
4. Liao F, Folson AR, Brancati FL: Is low magnesium concentration a risk factor for coronary heart disease? The Atherosclerosis Risk in Communities (ARIC) Study. Am Heart J 1998;136:480–490.
5. Agus ZS: Hypomagnesemia. J Am Soc Nephrol 1999;10:1616–1622.

PATIENT 41

A 42-year-old man with stable angina referred for a thallium stress test

A 42-year-old man presents with a 3-month history of exertional substernal chest pain. He describes the pain as a squeezing sensation across his chest, radiating down the inner aspect of his left arm. The pain occurs primarily when he walks fast; at a slow pace, the patient can go two miles without symptoms. An EKG stress test becomes positive at 8 minutes (1.5-mm ST-segment depression) of a Bruce protocol, with a heart rate of 150 beats/min. He is started on a beta blocker and calcium channel blocker and has no further symptoms. Subsequently, a thallium stress test is performed (see below). The patient denies hypertension or diabetes, but admits smoking two packs of cigarettes per day for many years. His father had a myocardial infarction at age 40 and died at age 51.

Physical Examination: Vital signs: pulse 80; blood pressure 118/80. Cardiac: normal.
Laboratory Findings: CBC and electrolytes: normal. Cholesterol: 230 mg/dl.

Question: Considering the thallium stress test result, should the patient undergo coronary arteriography?

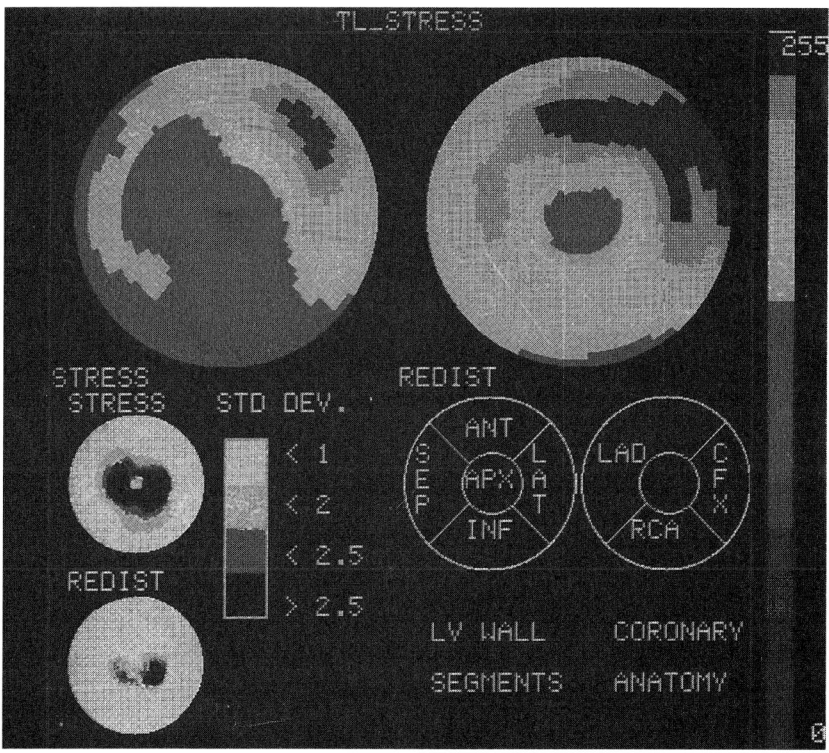

Answer: Yes. The thallium study demonstrated a large area of myocardium at risk in the distribution of the left anterior descending artery.

Discussion: Thallium stress testing has contributed significantly to the management of patients with coronary artery disease (CAD). In addition to **planar thallium imaging,** the use of **single photon emission computed tomography** (SPECT) has become popular because results are displayed as a polar map, or "bullseye," in color, which better demonstrates the location and extent of perfusion abnormalities. Thallium, which is taken up by myocytes like a potassium derivative, distributes only in viable and perfused areas of the myocardium. Increased thalium uptake in the lung indicates exercise-induced left ventricular dysfunction and portends a poor prognosis.

The following clinical conditions are considered the major indications for a thallium stress test:
- Diagnosis of CAD in the patient with atypical chest pain, positive EKG stress test without symptoms, or negative EKG stress test with chest pain suggestive of ischemia.
- Exercise testing in patients with resting EKG abnormalities such as left bundle branch block (LBBB), use of digitalis and other drugs that alter the EKG, or left ventricular hypertrophy
- Determination of the physiologic significance of borderline coronary stenoses detected by coronary arteriorgraphy
- Evaluation of coronary bypass graft patency
- Determination of the efficacy of angioplasty and stents
- Determination of whether the myocardium is at risk in patients with angina.

Although of value for the diagnosis of CAD, thallium scanning is used more often for predicting the risk of cardiovascular morbidity and mortality. Thallium scintigraphy is not cost effective in screening for silent CAD in asymptomatic patients. Asymptomatic patients at high risk for coronary disease should have an **EKG stress test** as the first step. The sensitivity for the EKG stress test (1.0 mm or greater ST depression) is about 60% and the specificity 80%. The sensitivity and specificity of thallium imaging are in the range of 90%. Thus, ≤10% of patients with a normal thallium stress test will have significant coronary disease. This level of probability is sufficient for many physicians to manage low-risk patients. When coronary disease is suspected on clinical grounds, coronary arteriography may be required for a definitive diagnosis.

Individuals unable to walk on a treadmill can be tested for ischemia by combining thallium scintigraphy with the infusion of **dipyridamole, adenosine, or dobutamine.** Dobutamine is a selective beta$_1$ agonist that has inotropic and chronotropic effects on the heart. Its infusion selectively stresses the heart, whereas dipyridamole and adenosine vasodilate the coronary vessels. Adenosine, which has a 10-second half-life, can be used instead of dipyridamole since dipyridamole actually achieves vasodilation by increasing endogenous adenosine release.

All three agents increase coronary blood flow. In areas of the myocardium supplied by diseased coronaries, flow does not increase normally during infusion of these agents, and the abnormal flow is detected by the thallium images. If scanning at 4 hours after stress has not demonstrated a return to normal, scanning is repeated at 24 hours, looking for late redistribution. Alternatively, reinjection of thallium 3–4 hours after the initial administration of the radioisotope helps differentiate viable but severely ischemic myocardium from scar. Thallium injected at rest, followed by rest tomographic imaging and then immediate treadmill or pharmacologic stress with sestamibi injected at peak exercise, has become very popular, and it takes only 1½ hours. **Rest thallium** is best for viability, and a delayed image can be done if necessary. **Stress sestamibi** gives functional data with an ejection fraction and is gated to give wall motion images.

Stress echocardiography can be performed with treadmill exercise or with dobutamine, dipyridamole, or adenosine in those who cannot exercise. It detects development of regional systolic dysfunction indicating ischemia, whereas nuclear perfusion detects regional differences in perfusion and does not not necessarily reflect ischemia. Stress echo is highly specific (up to 100%) as a marker for CAD, but has a sensitivity of 78%. Dipyridamole (Persantine) is the drug of choice for patients with significant hypertension, abdominal aneurysms, or LBBB (false positive occurs with exercise or dobutamine). Dobutamine is best if there is congestive heart failure, hypotension, or reactive airway disease.

Patients with minimal CAD rarely have a positive **noninvasive test,** whereas those with high-grade stenosis rarely have a negative test. The non-invasive stress test is best for those who have inbetween lesions at 40–60%. Unfortunately, these noninvasive tests and coronary arteriography do not elevate the arterial wall and cannot predict if a plaque will rupture and produce an unstable coronary syndrome.

The present patient had stable angina that responded well to medical therapy. In view of the history, exercise EKG, and response to medical therapy, continued observation with medical management would have been justified. The thallium stress test, however, showed a large area of anterior, septal, apical, and inferior ischemia. The extent of this area led to the performance of coronary arteriography, which revealed a long, left anterior, descending coronary artery that coursed around the apex to the inferior wall. It had a 95% lesion proximal to the first septal perforator and proximal to a large diagonal branch. Angioplasty reduced the lesion to about 20%. A thallium stress test 6 weeks later showed no ischemia.

Clinical Pearls

1. Employ thallium stress testing preferentially to EKG stress testing in patients with left ventricular hypertrophy or left bundle branch block and in those receiving digitalis.

2. The sensitivity and specificity of thallium stress testing for detecting coronary artery disease are in the range of 90% when SPECT is employed.

3. If the patient cannot use a treadmill, use of dipyridamole, adenosine, or dobutamine is an alternative method for increasing coronary blood flow.

4. Lung thallium uptake results from increased left ventricular filling pressure due to ventricular dysfunction during exercise. Its presence worsens prognosis significantly.

REFERENCES

1. Iskandrian AS, Heo J, Askenase A, et al: Thallium imaging with single photon emission computed tomography. Am Heart J 1987;114:852–865.
2. Zellner JL, Elliott BM, Robinson JG, et al: Preoperative evaluation of cardiac risk using dobutamine-thallium imaging in vascular surgery. Ann Vasc Surg 1990;4:238–243.
3. Pohost GM, Henzolva MJ: The value of thallium-201 imaging. N Engl J Med 1990;323:190–192.
4. Beller GA: Current status of nuclear cardiology techniques. Curr Probl Cardiol 1991;16:451–535.
5. Cheitlin MD, Alpert JS, Armstrong WF, et al.: ACC/AHA guidelines for the clinical application of echocardiography: Executive summary. A report of the American College of Cardiology/American Heart Association Task Force on practice guidelines (Committee on Clinical Application of Echocardiography). Developed in collaboration with the American Society of Echocardiography. J Am Coll Cardiol 1997;29:862–879.
6. Pingitore A, Picano E, Varga A, et al.: Prognostic value of pharmacological stress echocardiography in patients with known or suspected coronary artery disease: A prospective, large-scale, multicenter, head-to-head comparison between dipyridamole and dobutamine test. Echo-Persantine International Cooperative and Echo-Dobutamine International Cooperative Study Groups. J Am Coll Cardiol 1999;34:1769–1777.

PATIENT 42

A 62-year-old man with nausea and an arrhythmia

A 62-year-old man with ischemic cardiomyopathy is admitted because of nausea and a rapid heart rate. He has had several prior myocardial infarctions, resulting in left ventricular dysfunction and an ejection fraction of about 20%. The patient has been admitted repeatedly to the hospital because of congestive heart failure. During the most recent previous admission, cardiomegaly, an S_3 gallop, and multifocal premature ventricular beats (PVBs) were detected. He was receiving maintenance digoxin 0.25 mg daily and diuretics. Quinidine was added for control of PVBs.

Physical Examination: Vital signs: pulse 120; blood pressure 110/60. Cardiac: neck veins not distended; cardiomegaly; S_3 gallop at the apex. Abdomen: no hepatomegaly. Extremities: no peripheral edema.

Laboratory Findings: Digoxin level 3.5 ng/ml, quinidine level 3.1 μg/ml, potassium 3.5 mEq/L, creatinine 2.0 mg/dl. EKG: see below.

Question: What is the arrhythmia and the patient's diagnosis?

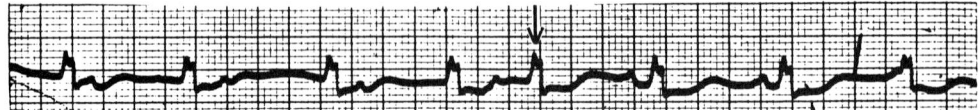

Diagnosis: Nonparaoxysmal junctional tachycardia with atrioventricular (AV) dissociation and occasional captured beats, indicating digitalis toxicity.

Discussion: Digitalis toxicity is a major problem in hospitalized patients. The reported incidence is 15–20% and is even higher in elderly hospitalized patients. Several factors promote the onset of digitalis toxicity. **Digoxin** is excreted by the kidneys and accumulates in patients with renal dysfunction. Coadministration of **quinidine** causes a decrease in renal glycoside clearance and increases serum digoxin concentration, even when the digoxin is given at a constant dose. After the addition of quinidine, the serum digoxin level can double within 48 hours. Even with previously well-tolerated blood digitalis levels, the onset of hypokalemia or hypomagnesemia can initiate manifestations of cardiac digitalis toxicity.

Digitalis toxicity may present with vomiting, visual spots (yellow objects), dizziness, and facial pain. These clinical manifestations were prominent when digitalis leaf was administered and do not occur with the purified crystalline glycosides presently available. Today, the initial toxic effect of digoxin is usually a **cardiac arrhythmia.** The toxic arrhythmias associated with digitalis toxicity usually result from conduction block or increased pacemaker cell automaticity and include PVBs, ventricular bigeminy, multifocal PVBs, ventricular tachycardia, bidirectional tachycardia, sinoatrial (SA) block or sinus pauses with or without escape rhythms, atrial tachycardia with block, AV heart block, and nonparoxysmal junctional tachycardia with AV dissociation.

The presence of **nonparoxysmal junctional tachycardia with AV dissociation** often is noted with digitalis toxicity, but is mistaken at the bedside for sinus rhythm. This arrhythmia occurs from enhanced automaticity of the AV junction and has a rate of 70–130 beats/min. The presence of AV dissociation causes the sinus P waves to occur at a slower rate with no relationship to the QRS complexes. At times, however, the P wave may conduct downward (see figure, *arrow*) and capture the ventricle, producing an irregular rhythm easily mistaken for atrial fibrillation.

Occasionally, nonparoxysmal junctional tachycardia may be associated with **atrial fibrillation** or flutter, in which case P waves are not present. At the bedside this tachycardia may be misinterpreted to mean that the atrial fibrillation has converted to regular sinus rhythm. Further confusion may occur when digitalis toxicity produces a Wenckebach exit block in patients with nonparoxysmal junctional tachycardia. In the presence of atrial fibrillation, the exit block causes the nonparoxysmal junctional tachycardia to be irregular and simulate conducted atrial fibrillation with a controlled ventricular response.

Ventricular arrhythmias are one of the more dangerous manifestations of digitalis toxicity. Studies now suggest that digitalis-induced ventricular arrhythmias may be due to triggered activity (delayed afterdepolarizations) and may respond to verapamil, which decreases the magnitude of the oscillating delayed afterdepolarization. Life-threatening digoxin-induced arrhythmias may also be treated with digoxin-immune Fab fragments. This digoxin-specific antibody is most often used for massive intoxication, as in a suicide attempt. Usually, however, digitalis toxic arrhythmias cease when the drug is discontinued.

The present patient had his digoxin dose held and his hypokalemia corrected. When the digoxin blood level was reduced, digoxin was restarted at half the previous dose. The arrhythmias resolved.

Clinical Pearls

1. Digitalis intoxication can produce many tachyarrhythmias or bradyarrhythmias. Nonparosyxmal junctional tachycardia with AV dissociation often is overlooked because at the bedside it is misinterpreted as sinus rhythm (if regular) or as atrial fibrillation when sporadic P-wave capture makes the rhythm irregular.
2. Massive intoxication requires treatment with digoxin-specific antibodies.
3. Digitalis toxicity may occur within 48 hours of the addition of quinidine.
4. If quinidine is added, the maintenance digoxin dose should be reduced by half.

REFERENCES

1. Beller GA, Smith TW, Abelmann WH, et al: Digitalis intoxication: A prospective clinical study with serum level correlations. N Engl J Med 1971;284:989–997.
2. Smith TW, Butler VP Jr, Haber E, et al: Treatment of life-threatening digitalis intoxication with digoxin-specific Fab fragments: Experience in 26 cases. N Engl J Med 1982;307:1357–1362.
3. Hickey AR, Wenger TL, Carpenter VP, et al: Digoxin immune Fab therapy in the management of digitalis intoxication: Safety and efficacy results of an observational surveillance study. J Am Coll Cardiol 1991;17:590–598.
4. Hauptman PJ, Kelly RA: Digitalis. Circulation 1999;99:1265–1270.

PATIENT 43

A 55-year-old woman with episodes of wide QRS tachycardia

A 55-year-old woman is admitted for management of metastatic breast cancer. She has had episodes of tachycardia for about 30 years, which, on occasion, have been stopped with right carotid pressure. Soon after admission, she has an attack associated with dizziness and lightheadedness, but no chest pain or dyspnea.

Physical Examination: Vital signs: pulse 214; blood pressure 80/50. Cardiac: no murmurs or extra sounds.

Laboratory Findings: Hct 26%; WBC 3500/μl. EKG: see below.

Question: What type of tachycardia is present?

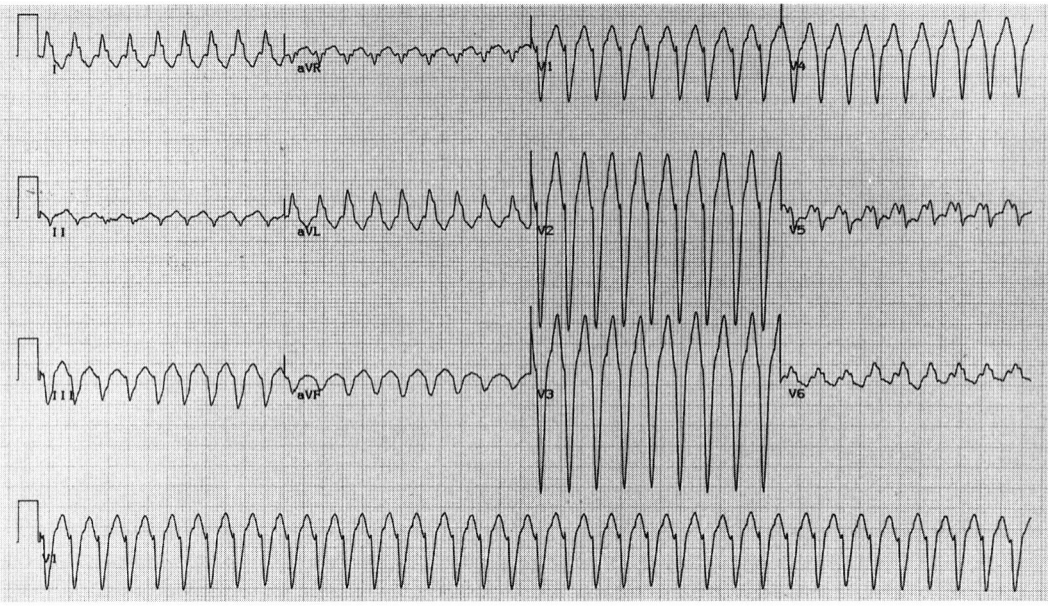

Diagnosis: Supraventricular tachycardia with left bundle branch block.

Discussion: Atrioventricular (AV) nodal reentrant tachycardia is the most common form of paroxysmal supraventricular tachycardia. In this condition, the reentry pathway is within the AV nodal or perinodal atrium. Before this mechanism was clarified, **AV nodal reentrant tachycardia** was known as **paroxysmal atrial tachycardia.**

The AV node in patients with AV nodal reentrant tachycardia manifests electrophysiologic features of longitudinal dissociation with two pathways (alpha and beta). The alpha pathway conducts slowly and has a short refractory period. In contrast, the beta pathway conducts rapidly and has a long refractory period. A premature atrial beat arriving at the AV node is blocked from the beta pathway because of its long refractory period. The atrial beat is therefore conducted down the alpha pathway, which conducts slowly. The slow conduction allows for the impulse to exit the alpha pathway and travel retrograde through the beta pathway, which now has recovered its excitability. Subsequent antegrade conduction down the alpha pathway establishes a reentrant tachycardia.

The retrograde P resulting from this reentry wave may be buried in the QRS or may occur less than 70 msec after the R wave (short RP type). Rarely, conduction occurs initially down the beta pathway (10% or less) and retrograde through the alpha pathway. In this instance, the P waves are noted later after the QRS (long RP type) and appear to be associated with the next QRS. As such, this type of AV nodal reentrant tachycardia can be difficult to differentiate from intra-atrial reentrant or automatic types of tachycardia without performing electrophysiologic studies.

Evaluation of tachycardias is further complicated when **left bundle branch block** is present. Careful evaluation of the EKG assists in diagnosis of this arrhythmia. Clues to the diagnosis of supraventricular tachycardia with left bundle branch block are that the R-wave duration is less than 30 msec in V_1 and V_2, no notch is present on the downstroke of the S wave, and there is less than 70 msec from the R wave to the nadir of the S wave. The present patient had these findings, which all suggest that the tachycardia is the AV nodal reentrant type, with left bundle branch block rather than ventricular tachycardia. Other features that suggest an AV nodal reentrant tachycardia are (1) the tachycardia is initiated and terminated by a premature atrial beat and (2) the rate is usually greater than 150/min and very regular.

Any vagal maneuver or block of the slow calcium channels in the AV node can restore sinus rhythm. The drugs of choice are **adenosine** first and **verapamil** second. Various other antiarrhythmic drugs have been used to prevent the arrhythmia, but often are unsuccessful. Selective radiofrequency catheter ablation of the atrial insertion of the alpha pathway has been successful in eliminating this arrhythmia without affecting normal atrioventricular nodal conduction.

In the present patient, the arrhythmia was terminated by infusion of 6 mg of adenosine, another point in favor of an AV nodal origin of the arrhythmia.

Clinical Pearls

1. AV nodal reentrant tachycardia is the most common supraventricular tachycardia.

2. AV nodal reentrant tachycardia may be present in patients with bundle branch block or aberrant conduction, imitating ventricular tachycardia.

3. The main features of AV nodal reentrant tachycardia are: rate greater than 150 beats/min and very regular; tachycardia may be initiated by an ectopic beat and terminated by an ectopic beat; tachycardia depends on critical conduction delay within some part of the circuit.

4. AV nodal reentrant tachycardia responds to vagal maneuvers, digitalis, verapamil, or adenosine. The drug of choice is now adenosine.

5. Symptomatic refractory AV nodal reentrant tachycardia is successfully treated by radiofrequency perinodal ablation.

REFERENCES

1. Manolis AS, Estes NA III: Supraventricular tachycardia. Mechanisms and therapy. Arch Intern Med 1987;147:1706–1716.
2. Mitrani RD, Klein LS, Hackett FK, et al: Radiofrequency ablation for atrioventricular nodal reentrant tachycardia: Comparison between fast (anterior) and slow (posterior) pathway ablation. J Am Coll Cardiol 1993;21:432–441.
3. Patterson E, Scherlag BJ: Longitudinal dissociation within the posterior AV nodal input of the rabbit. A substrate for AV nodal reentry. Circulation 1999;99:143–155.
4. Glatter KA, Cheng J, Dorostkar P: Electrophysiologic effects of adenosine in patients with supraventricular tachycardia. Circulation 1999;99:1034–1040.

PATIENT 44

A 60-year-old man with severe chronic obstructive lung disease and edema

A 60-year-old man is admitted to the hospital for chronic obstructive lung disease, which has been present for many years, and for evaluation of a recent increase in abdominal girth and peripheral edema. He is a heavy cigarette smoker and has had dyspnea on exertion for several years. The patient denies a history of coronary disease, hypertension, or diabetes.

Physical Examination: Vital signs: pulse 90 (regular); blood pressure 110/70. Cardiac: jugular veins pulsated to 5 cm above the angle of Louis at 45°; loud P2 in the pulmonic area; S_3 gallop with inspiration along lower left sternal border; grade III/VI systolic high-pitched murmur audible with inspiration near the xiphoid; palpable downward thrust under the xiphoid. Chest: distant diffuse rales and increased AP diameter of chest. Abdomen: distended with ascites. Extremities: 2+ peripheral edema noted almost to the knees.

Laboratory Findings: CBC and urinalysis: normal. P_{aCO_2}: elevated. P_{aO_2}: low. EKG: see below. Chest radiograph: normal heart size and pulmonary emphysema.

Question: What is your diagnosis?

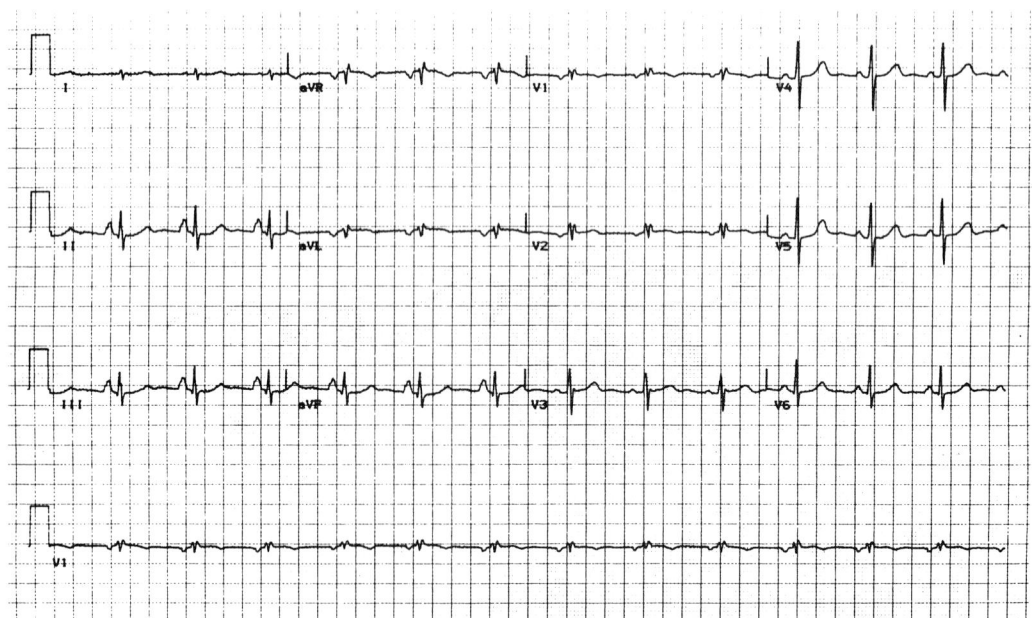

Diagnosis: Chronic obstructive lung disease with cor pulmonale.

Discussion: It is difficult to diagnose cor pulmonale by physical examination in a patient with chronic obstructive lung disease in the absence of overt congestive heart failure, because right ventricular enlargement is difficult to detect. Lung distention increases thoracic AP diameter, which may obscure a right ventricular lift. In some patients, however, the right ventricular enlargement may be palpable as a downward thrust under the xiphoid in the epigastric area. Additional confusion results because **chronic obstructive pulmonary disease** (COPD) without cor pulmonale may result in adventitious chest sounds, a palpable liver because of a low diaphragm, and peripheral edema due to inactivity and venous stasis, all of which could be misinterpreted as signs of right-sided congestive heart failure. The variation in intrapleural pressure due to respiratory effort makes it difficult to evaluate the level of neck vein pulsations, obscuring another finding of right-sided heart failure.

In patients with cor pulmonale, the heart often appears normal in size on chest radiography due to lung hyperinflation; however, the lateral projection may suggest right ventricular enlargement. EKG abnormalities may be due to chest configurational changes associated with COPD producing large P waves in the inferior leads and clockwise rotation. The tall R waves of right ventricular hypertrophy seldom develop in the right ventricular leads of patients with increased AP diameter. Thus, the diagnosis of cor pulmonale often must be made by hemodynamic measurements, radionuclide studies, or echo-Doppler findings. Electrocardiographic signs of chronic cor pulmonale and very low P_{aO_2} indicate patients with severe short-term prognosis.

Therapy for cor pulmonale in patients with emphysema is directed at the underlying lung disease and relieving hypoxemia if present. Digitalis is not given unless there is associated left heart failure or a supraventricular tachycardia such as atrial fibrillation and flutter. **Multifocal atrial tachycardia** (MAT), frequently present in chronic obstructive lung disease, responds best to treatment of the underlying pulmonary disease. MAT may be precipitated or aggravated by theophylline. If direct medical therapy is required to treat MAT, verapamil is the drug of choice.

Diuretics should be used cautiously in cor pulmonale because excessive volume depletion can decrease cardiac output and produce hypokalemic, metabolic alkalosis that may further reduce ventilatory response to carbon dioxide. On the other hand, treatment of right-sided volume overload may improve pulmonary function by reducing left ventricular filling pressure. While it is well appreciated that left ventricular failure may lead to right-sided failure, it is not well recognized that right-sided failure may cause left-sided failure. The latter condition occurs as the failing right-sided chambers enlarge, compressing the left-sided chambers through septal and pericardial interaction. Left-sided compression increases left-sided filling pressure, in turn increasing lung water and worsening pulmonary function. Diuresis may reverse this process by reducing right-sided chamber size.

The present patient's EKG showed right axis, right atrial enlargement (P pulmonale) and right ventricular enlargement (late R in V_1). His echocardiogram was compatible with cor pulmonale. Right atrial and right ventricular enlargement were present. Tricuspid insufficiency was noted by Doppler, and the peak right ventricular systolic pressure was 90 mmHg. The patient initially responded to diuresis, but eventually died of respiratory failure.

Clinical Pearls

1. It may be difficult to diagnose cor pulmonale by physical examination in patients with chronic obstructive pulmonary disease unless there is overt congestive heart failure.

2. Therapy for cor pulmonale should concentrate on treating the lung disease rather than treating the heart failure directly. Digitalis should be avoided unless there is concomitant left ventricular systolic dysfunction or a supraventricular tachycardia.

3. Although it is well known that left-sided failure may cause right-sided failure, it is also true that right-sided failure may cause diastolic left-sided failure.

4. Electrocardiographic signs of chronic cor pulmonale and very low P_{aO_2} indicate patients with severe short-term prognosis.

REFERENCES

1. Scott RC: The electrocardiogram in pulmonary emphysema chronic cor pulmonale. Am Heart J 1961;61:843–845.
2. Palevsky HI, Fishman AP: Chronic cor pulmonale: Etiology and management. JAMA 1990;263:2347–2353.
3. Incalzi RA, Ruso L, De Rosa M, et al.: Electrocardiographic signs of chronic cor pulmonale: A negative prognostic finding in chronic obstructive pulmonary disease. Circulation 1999;99:1600–1605.
4. Tutar E, Kaya A, Gulec S, et al.: Echocardiographic evaluation of left ventricular diastolic function in chronic cor pulmonale. Am J Cardiol 1999;83:1414–1417.

PATIENT 45

A 52-year-old man with chest pain and a normal coronary arteriogram

A 52-year-old man presents with typical exertional angina. He describes his chest discomfort as substernal squeezing with radiation to the neck and down his left arm. It occurs during exertion, and is relieved by rest and/or nitroglycerin. His only risk factor is smoking, which he discontinued several months previously.

Physical Examination: Pulse 80; blood pressure 130/80. Chest: clear. Cardiac: normal heart sounds. Extremities: normal pulses without bruits.

Laboratory Findings: Complete blood count and chemistry: normal. Cholesterol 240 mg/dl; HDL 42 mg/dl. EKG: see below. Echocardiogram: normal. Coronary arteriography: normal except for slow filling of the coronary vessels; no spasm provoked with ergonovine. 24-hour Holter monitor: intermittent left bundle branch block; normally conducted betas showed ST segment depression that occurred with and without angina. Thallium stress test: normal. Radionuclide (MUGA) stress test: normal wall motion but a flat response to exercise; the ejection fraction remained at 68% at rest and with exercise.

Question: What is this patient's diagnosis?

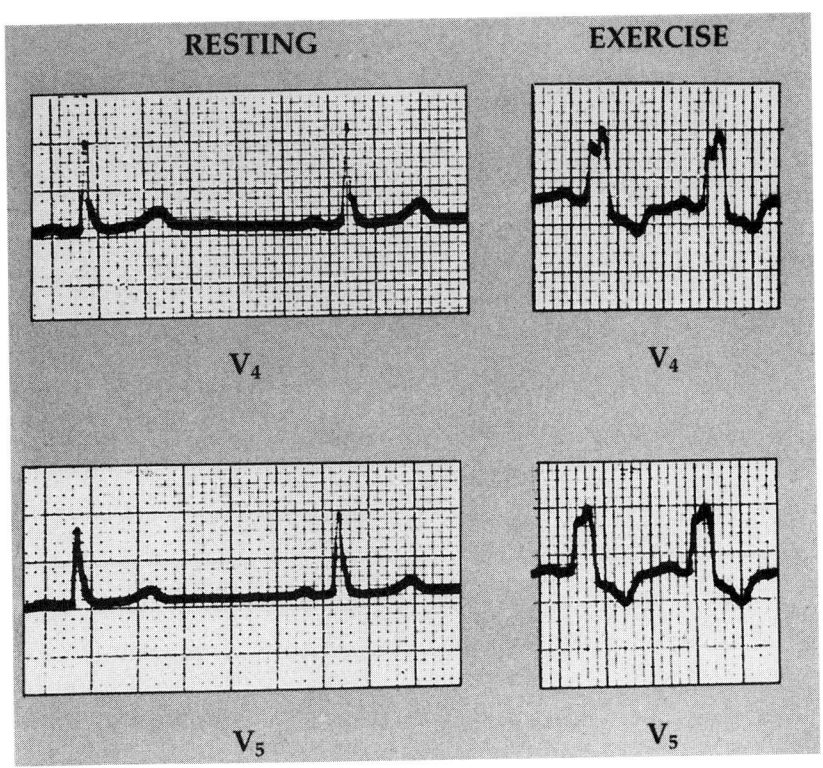

From Gazes PC: Syndrome X in 1988. Cardiovasc Dis Chest Pain 1988;4:3–8.

Diagnosis: Syndrome X—angina with normal coronary arteriograms.

Discussion: The terms "syndrome X" and "microvascular angina" have been used to describe patients who have angina, normal coronary arteriograms, and no other conditions, such as coronary artery spasm or ventricular hypertrophy, that could account for the pain. It has been conjectured that such patients have inappropriate coronary arteriolar or small coronary artery constriction with deficient vasodilator reserve in response to atrial pacing. Attenuated epicardial coronary dilation response to **adenosine** may be a marker of microvascular dysfunction. Other factors considered in the metabolic and vascular alterations found in syndrome X are enhanced exercise-induced hyperkalemia, enhanced activity of sodium-lithium countertransport, stimulated hyperinsulinemia, and abnormal perception of chest pain. Pathologically, myofibrillar hypertrophy with patchy fibrosis and hyperplastic fibromuscular thickening of the intramural coronary arteries have been described.

The anginal pain in this condition often continues for more than 30 minutes beyond the precipitating effort. The prolonged nature of the pain may result from release of adenosine, which causes arteriolar vasodilatation and a resultant drop in coronary artery distending pressure. Compensatory constriction of the distal end of the prearteriole diminishes myocardial perfusion and stimulates additional release of adenosine, thereby perpetuating the process. A study with acetylcholine suggested that endothelium-dependent dilatation of the smaller coronary resistance vessels (microvascular) is defective, which may contribute to the altered regulation of myocardial perfusion in these patients.

Patients with syndrome X demonstrate an interesting constellation of clinical and laboratory findings. They often have a positive stress EKG, and the ejection fraction may decrease during exercise. They may occasionally experience left bundle branch block, as noted in the present patient. Some have shown reversible perfusion defects, mainly in the septal segment, and reduced or delayed thallium washout. In contrast to patients with epicardial coronary artery stenosis or spasm, signs of left ventricular dysfunction during pain are usually mild or nonexistent in patients with syndrome X. Atrial pacing can produce increased lactate production, and myocardial biopsy may show nonspecific changes and narrowing of capillaries.

Other conditions that can cause angina in the presence of normal coronary artery anatomy should be excluded. These conditions include myocardial bridging, disorders of coronary blood flow associated with left ventricular hypertrophy, and coronary vasospasm. Once diagnosed, patients should be treated with **nitrates, calcium blockers,** and **beta blockers** in a similar fashion to patients with epicardial coronary artery stenosis. Variation in response to treatment may be related to the potential existence of multiple mechanisms of the prearteriolar vasoconstriction. The prognosis for patients with syndrome X is very good, although they may continue to have pain. Those who have left bundle branch block at rest or heart rate–independent pain have a worse prognosis and may experience deterioration of left ventricular function. Some clinicians consider such patients to have a form of cardiomyopathy.

The present patient was treated with a calcium channel–blocking agent, with improvement of pain. He will be followed very closely because of the presence of intermittent left bundle branch block, which carries a less favorable prognosis.

Clinical Pearls

1. Consider syndrome X in patients with typical angina and normal coronary arteriograms.

2. Reduced coronary dilatory capacity and ultrastructural changes have been noted in such patients.

3. The prognosis is very good except in patients who have left bundle branch block at rest or with exertion.

4. Medical management is the same as that for epicardial coronary artery disease.

REFERENCES

1. Romeo F, Rosano GMC, Martuscelli E, et al.: Long-term follow-up of patients initially diagnosed with syndrome X. Am J Cardiol 1993;71:669–673.
2. Chauhan A, Mullins PA, Thuraisingham SI, et al.: Abnormal cardiac pain perception in syndrome X. J Am Coll Cardiol 1994;24:329.
3. Gaspardone A, Ferri C, Crea F, et al.: Enhanced activity of sodium-lithium countertransport in patients with cardiac syndrome X. A potential link between cardiac and metabolic syndrome X. J Am Coll Cardiol 1998;32:2031–2034.
4. Botker HE, Sonne HS, Frobert O, et al.: Enhanced exercise-induced hyperkalemia in patients with syndrome X. J Am Coll Cardiol 1999;33:1056–1061.
5. Reis SE, Holubkov R, Lee JS, et al.: Coronary flow velocity response to adenosine characterizes coronary microvascular function in women with chest pain and no obstructive coronary disease. Results from the Pilot Phase of the Women's Ischemia Syndrome Evaluation (WISE) Study. J Am Coll Cardiol 1999;33:1469–1475.

PATIENT 46

A 63-year-old man with sudden cardiac death

A 63-year-old man without any previous cardiac history is referred for outpatient stress testing after resuscitation from an episode of sudden death (ventricular fibrillation) that occurred while dancing. During hospitalization, a CT scan of his head, electroencephalogram, and 24-hour Holter monitoring were normal. A myocardial infarction was ruled out by negative enzymes and EKGs.

Physical Examination: Vital signs: pulse 60 (regular); blood pressure 127/79. Neck: right carotid bruit with an overlying well-healed surgical scar. Cardiac: no murmurs or gallops. Chest: clear. Abdomen: liver not enlarged. Extremities: no peripheral edema.

Laboratory Findings: EKG: sinus bradycardia. Stress test: 1.5-mm horizontal ST-segment depression in leads I, II, aVF, V_5, V_6 during stage II of a Bruce protocol; heart rate increased from 75 beats/min to 130 beats/min; blood pressure increased from 160/70 to 180/90; no arrhythmias noted.

Question: What would you recommend?

Answer: The patient should be evaluated with coronary arteriography and electrophysiologic studies.

Discussion: About 25% of patients with sudden death have had no known prior cardiac disease. Once such patients are identified following resuscitation, the mortality is 30% during the first year unless effective antiarrhythmic therapy is instituted. The prognosis is even worse if left ventricular dysfunction is present. To ameliorate this poor prognosis, such patients should be fully evaluated in an effort to find correctable causes. Evaluation should include coronary arteriography because the most common underlying cardiac disorder in patients with sudden death is coronary artery disease (about 75%). In fact, autopsy studies of patients dying suddenly have shown that most patients have multivessel disease and evidence of one or more prior infarctions.

All patients who have had cardiac arrest or hypotensive ventricular tachycardia not associated with an acute event such as myocardial infarction should also have electrophysiologic studies. Programmed electrical stimulation is used to initiate ventricular tachyarrhythmias and to test the efficacy of pharmacologic, electrical, or surgical therapy. If ventricular tachyarrhythmia is inducible on antiarrhythmic drugs or after surgery, then an implantable cardioverter defibrillator (ICD) should be inserted. The Multicenter Automatic Implantation Trial (MADIT) randomized high-risk coronary patients to ICD versus best conventional treatment, namely, amiodarone. These patients had a previous myocardial infarction; ejection fraction ≤35%; and nonsustained ventricular tachycardia, inducible ventricular tachycardia, or fibrillation. The ICD cohort showed significantly fewer deaths during a followup period of 3 years. The Antiarrhythmics Versus Implantable Defibrillators (AVID) trial also reported less arrhythmic cardiac death with ICDs than antiarrhythmic drugs. Based in part on the Coronary Artery Surgical Study, which showed that bypass surgery reduced the 5-year sudden death rate to 2% in patients with coronary disease compared with 6% in the medically treated group, revascularization should probably be performed when significant correctable coronary disease is found.

In the present patient, because of his episode of sudden death and the results of his exercise test, coronary arteriograms were performed. They revealed a 90% proximal left anterior descending lesion at the level of a second large diagonal vessel. The left anterior descending coronary artery was a long vessel going around the apex. The ventriculogram was normal, with an ejection fraction of 61%. Subsequently, he had a 10-run beat of ventricular tachycardia at a rate of 150 beats/min. The patient underwent two-vessel coronary bypass grafting with a left internal mammary artery to the left anterior descending artery and a saphenous vein graft to the diagonal. Postoperatively, ventricular tachycardia could not be induced during electrophysiologic studies. A signal-averaged electrocardiogram was normal.

Clinical Pearls

1. Sudden cardiac death frequently is due to asymptomatic coronary artery disease, but most often occurs in the absence of an acute myocardial infarction.

2. Patients who have suffered ventricular fibrillation in the absence of an acute myocardial infarction have a mortality rate of up to 30% during the first year following resuscitation unless effective antiarrhythmic therapy is instituted.

3. Nearly all patients who experience sudden cardiac death should undergo coronary arteriography and electrophysiologic studies.

4. Studies are now showing that devices are superior to drugs in most patients with coronary artery disease and sudden death in the absence of acute myocardial infarction.

REFERENCES

1. Nalos PC, Gang ES, Mandel WJ, et al: The signal-averaged electrocardiogram as a screening test for inducibility of sustained ventricular tachycardia in high risk patients: A prospective study. J Am Coll Cardiol 1987;9:539–548.
2. Moss A, Hall J, Cannon D, et al (for the MADIT investigators): Improved survival with an implanted defibrillator in patients with coronary disease at high risk of ventricular arrhythmias. N Engl J Med 1996;335:1933–1940.
3. Gregoratos G, Cheitlin MD, Conill A, et al: ACC/AHA guidelines for implantation of cardiac pacemakers and antiarrhythmia devices. J Am Coll Cardiol 1998;31:1175–1209.
4. Sra J, Dhala A, Blanck Z, et al: Sudden cardiac death. Curr Probl Cardiol 1999;24:468–538.
5. The AVID investigators: Cause of death in the antiarrhythmics versus implantable defibrillators (AVID) trial. J Am Coll Cardiol 1999;34:1552–1559.

PATIENT 47

A 54-year-old woman with coma and ST-segment electrocardiographic abnormalities

A 54-year-old woman was found unconscious at home and brought to the emergency department by her family. She has a history of metastatic breast carcinoma and long-term hypertension. The patient had gradually become obtunded over the 2 days before admission and was unarousable that morning.

Physical Examination: Vital signs: pulse 72 (regular); respirations 20; blood pressure 160/90. General: responsive only to deep pain. Fundi: normal optic disk. Chest: clear. Cardiac: normal except for a fourth heart sound.

Laboratory Findings: EKG: see below.

Question: What underlying diagnosis requires urgent consideration?

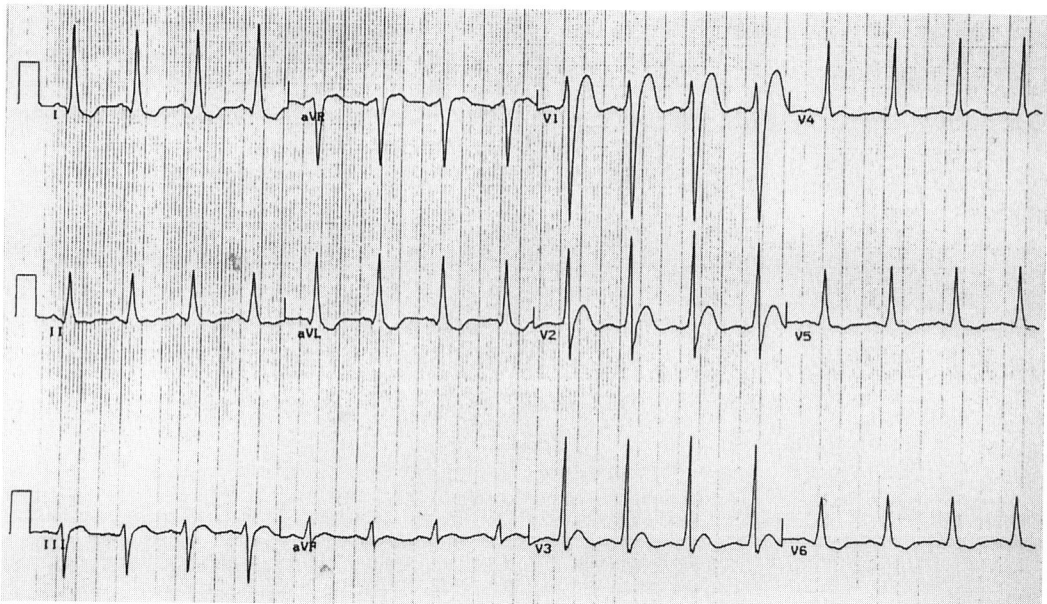

Diagnosis: Hypercalcemia with secondary EKG manifestations.

Discussion: The EKG can assist in the diagnosis of hypercalcemia by demonstrating characteristic findings before blood chemistry results return from the lab. Severe hypercalcemia may produce virtual absence of the ST segment in the right anterior precordial leads, with resultant extreme shortening of the QT interval. ST-segment shortening also may be seen in patients with hypermagnesemia and secondary to digitalis. However, extreme ST-segment shortening, as seen on the present patient's EKG, almost always is due to hypercalcemia. The clinical conditions most commonly associated with hypercalcemia are **malignancy, hyperparathyroidism, sarcoidosis, thiazide-induced hypercalcemia,** and **hypervitaminosis D.**

Severe hypercalcemia (>16 mg/dl) constitutes a medical emergency. Initial therapy includes aggressive hydration and forced diuresis with intravenous furosemide, 10–20 mg every 2–3 hours, which increases urinary calcium excretion. Normal saline is infused at a rate of 500 cc/hr in the absence of underlying cardiovascular disease that might predispose the patient to congestive heart failure. In patients at risk for congestive heart failure, a Swan-Ganz catheter should be placed to monitor therapy. If hypercalcemia appears to be life-threatening, calcitonin may be indicated, because it is the most rapidly acting inhibitor of osteoclastic function. Other adjunctive agents, such as corticosteroids, bisphosphonates, or plicamycin (mithramycin) may be used, depending on the etiology of the hypercalcemia and the patient's underlying condition.

Once serum concentration of calcium has decreased to less than 13 mg/dl, oral hydration and oral furosemide may be used to maintain serum calcium levels in an acceptable range. During diuresis, serum sodium, potassium, and magnesium levels also may fall and should be monitored carefully and repleted as necessary. During hypercalcemia, the dose of digitalis should be reduced or the drug should be discontinued, because hypercalcemia increases the risk of digitalis intoxication.

After initial therapy, the cause of the hypercalcemia should be sought and reversed when possible. If hyperparathyroidism is the primary cause, removal of the parathyroid adenoma should be definitive therapy. In the case of malignancy, chronic therapy with hydration and furosemide may be adequate to maintain serum calcium. If this measure fails, addition of oral phosphate to the diet or IV and oral bisphosphonate therapy may be effective. Plicamycin (mithramycin), which reduces osteoclastic activity and calcium mobilization from bone, also may be used to maintain normal serum calcium concentrations. However, this cytotoxic agent can cause severe marrow, renal, and hepatic toxicity, limiting its long-term usefulness.

The present patient's serum calcium was 17.2 mg/dl. She improved with aggressive hydration and diuresis. Further evaluation revealed metastatic breast cancer.

Clinical Pearls

1. A short or absent ST segment that produces a very short QT interval almost invariably is due to hypercalcemia. Hypermagnesemia or digitalis also causes a short ST interval, but not to the degree observed with severe hypercalcemia.

2. Decrease a patient's digitalis dose during intervals of hypercalcemia.

3. During diuretic therapy for hypercalcemia, serum concentrations of sodium, potassium, and magnesium also may fall and should be monitored carefully and repleted as necessary.

REFERENCES

1. Suki WN, Yium JJ, Von Minden M, et al: Acute treatment of hypercalcemia with furosemide. N Engl J Med 1970;283:836–840.
2. Rodman JS, Sherwood LM: Disorders of mineral metabolism in malignancy. In Avioli LV, Krane SM (eds): Metabolic Bone Disease, Vol 2. New York, Academic Press, 1978, pp 577–631.
3. Bilezikian JP: Management of acute hypercalcemia. N Engl J Med 1992;326:1196–1203.
4. Mosseri M, Porath A, Ovsyshcher I, et al: Electrocardiographic manifestations of combined hypercalcemia and hypermagnesemia. J Electrocardiol 1990;23:235–241.

PATIENT 48

A 35-year-old apparently healthy man with profound T-wave abnormalities

A 35-year-old patient is referred for evaluation when an abnormal EKG is obtained as part of a routine physical examination. The patient denies any symptoms. He regularly participates in athletic activities, including calisthenics and rowing, but denies dyspena, chest pain, palpitation, or syncope.

Physical Examination: Unremarkable.

Laboratory Findings: EKG: see below.

Question: What is the most likely diagnosis?

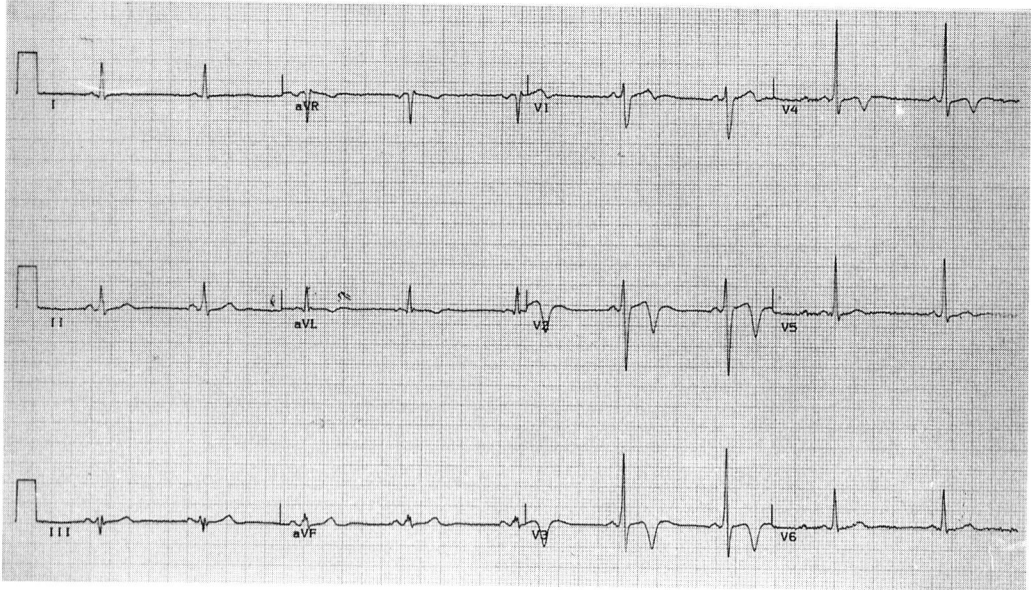

Diagnosis: Apical ("Japanese") hypertrophic cardiomyopathy.

Discussion: Hypertrophic cardiomyopathy (HCM) presents with several variations in the location of the hypertrophy. When the septum is hypertrophied out of proportion to the free wall, the term **asymmetric septal hypertrophy** is used. This variation usually produces left ventricular outflow obstruction, in which case it is called **idiopathic hypertrophic subaortic stenosis** (IHSS). There also may be **concentric symmetric hypertrophy** or hypertrophy confined to the distal septum and sometimes the apex (Japanese variety). In this variety, because the hypertrophic bulge does not lie in close proximity to the mitral valve, most of the usual features of IHSS are absent. Thus, systolic anterior motion of the mitral valve, the murmur, and other findings of outflow tract obstruction usually are not found.

The giant T waves seen in the precordial leads of the EKG are typical of the Japanese variety of HCM and almost diagnostic in a young, otherwise healthy patient. However, many patients with this form of disease fail to show giant negative T waves. As in the present patient, the diagnosis is confirmed echocardiographically.

In the United States, only approximately 2% of patients with HCM have the distal septal form of the disease, whereas in Japan the incidence may be as high as 25%. These data may, in fact, reflect two entirely different diseases, because in Japan, the hypertrophy involves not only the septum but the apex of the heart, producing a spade-like configuration of the left ventriculographic silhouette.

Although the features of obstruction on physical examination usually are absent, and catheterization usually fails to detect an outflow tract gradient, the hypertrophic process alone can produce symptoms. Many patients report dyspnea on exertion and fatigue. Beta blockers are probably the therapy of choice, but experience with this form of the disease is too limited to provide controlled studies of efficacy.

The prognosis for this form of HCM appears favorable compared with that of the classic disease. In most patients, the disease has remained stable during followup observation. It is, however, *not* totally benign. Atrial fibrillation, life-threatening arrhythmias, and myocardial infarction with normal coronaries have been reported. Because this type of HCM has been recognized as a discrete entity for only 20 years, its natural history has yet to be completely delineated.

The present patient had negative thallium and Holter studies. He enjoys moderate activity and does not experience symptoms.

Clinical Pearls

1. Giant precordial T-wave inversion is the classic EKG sign of apical idiopathic hypertrophic cardiomyopathy.
2. The true apical form, which occurs in Japan, may differ from that seen in the United States, where typically the distal septum alone is affected.
3. Outflow tract obstruction is rare in the Japanese variety of HCM.
4. In general, prognosis seems to be more favorable than that of typical IHSS.

REFERENCES

1. Epstein SE, Henry WL, Clark CE, et al: Asymmetric septal hypertrophy. Ann Intern Med 1974;81:650–680.
2. Yamaguchi H, Ishimura T, Nishiyama S, et al: Hypertrophic nonobstructive cardiomyopathy with giant T-waves (apical hypertrophy): Ventriculographic and echocardiographic features in 30 patients. Am J Cardiol 1979;44:401.
3. Maron BJ: Apical hypertrophic cardiomyopathy: The continuing saga. J Am Coll Cardiol 1990;15:91–93.
4. Koga Y, Katoh A, Matsuyama K, et al: Disappearance of giant negative T waves in patients with the Japanese form of apical hypertrophy. J Am Coll Cardiol 1995;26:1672–1678.
5. Wang Y, Takigawa O, Handa S, et al: The mechanism of giant negative T wave in electrocardiogram in patients with apical hypertrophic cardiomyopathy: Evaluation with thallium-201 and iodine-123 metaiodobenzylguanidine myocardial scintigraphy. Kaku Igaku 1996;33:999–1004.

PATIENT 49

A 34-year-old woman with a wide QRS tachycardia

A 34-year-old woman is admitted to the hospital because of an episode of tachycardia associated with weakness. During the 3 months before admission, she had several similar episodes. She has no history of heart disease and denies hypertension, diabetes, a recent viral infection, and drug use.

Physical Examination: Vital signs: regular rhythm at 150 beats/min; blood pressure 100/60. General: obese. Cardiac: no jugular venous distention.

Laboratory Findings: CBC, urinalysis, electrolytes: normal. EKG: see below.

Question: What is the arrhythmia?

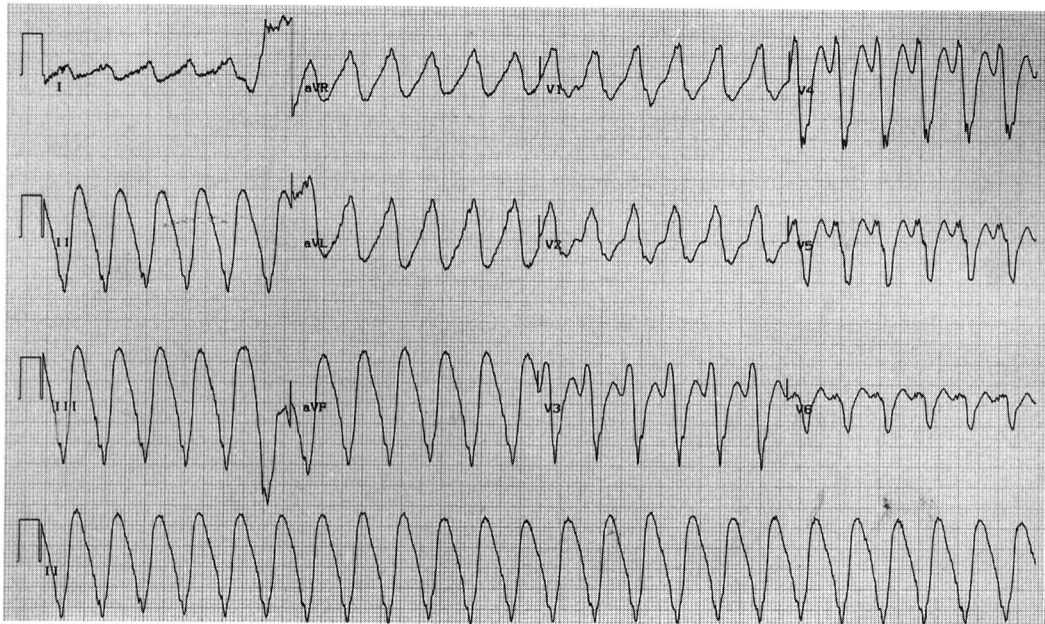

Diagnosis: Ventricular tachycardia.

Discussion: Wide QRS tachycardia (usual rate 140–250) may be ventricular tachycardia or a supraventricular tachycardia with bundle branch block or aberrant conduction. Ventricular tachycardia should be suspected if atrioventricular (AV) dissociation is noted and P waves are seen at a slower rate than the ventricular rate. Occasionally, a P wave may be conducted, producing capture or fusion beats that have a normal QRS configuration or are at least different from those that predominate in the tachycardia. The sensitivity for AV dissociation is ±25%, and specificity is ±90%. Capture and fusion beats have a sensitivity of ±5% and specificity of ±100% for diagnosing ventricular tachycardia.

The application of **Wellens' criteria** to the configuration of the QRS complexes of the tachycardia increases diagnostic accuracy to 90%. A QRS width of more than 140 msec, a monophasic QRS in V_1, a biphasic QRS in V_1 with R greater than R' (or qR configuration), positive or negative QRS complexes in all the precordial leads, a frontal axis between $-90°$ and $-180°$, and an R:S ratio in $V_6 <$ 1 all suggest ventricular tachycardia. Brugada has added another criterion: an RS greater than 100 msec in at least one precordial lead. A right bundle branch block configuration of the QRS complex in V_1 (rsR') suggests a supraventricular tachycardia with aberration. If the QRS complexes have a left bundle branch block morphology, ventricular tachycardia should be suspected if: the R wave duration in V_1 and V_2 is greater than 30 msec; there is any Q wave in V_6; there is greater than 70 msec to the S wave nadir in V_1 or V_2; a notch is present on the downstroke of the S wave in V_1 or V_2; or the QRS duration is greater than 160 msec.

Ventricular tachycardia may have retrograde conduction to the atria, with QRS complexes followed by P waves. This is difficult to differentiate from reentrant supraventricular tachycardia with aberration and P waves after the QRS complexes. If uncertain, the diagnosis of ventricular tachycardia can be made with the use of an esophageal lead or an intra-atrial electrode, which will demonstrate P waves clearly dissociated from the QRS.

Clinically, during an episode of ventricular tachycardia, intermittent **Cannon A waves** may be noted in the jugular venous pulse. Cannon A waves occur during ventricular tachycardia when AV dissociation causes P waves to occur after the QRS, producing atrial contraction against a closed tricuspid valve. On auscultation of the patient with ventricular tachycardia, there is variability in intensity of the first heart sound.

When in doubt as to the diagnosis of a wide QRS tachycardia, treatment should be DC cardioversion if the patient is unstable, or lidocaine infusion if the patient is stable. Adenosine can be used to differentiate wide QRS tachycardias in the stable patient. It has a short half-life, and if hypotension occurs, it is transient. Adenosine may terminate many supraventricular tachycardias with bundle branch block or aberrancy, or slow them and allow P waves to be noted. Rarely, it terminates some monomorphic ventricular tachycardias that occur in those without structural heart disease (EKG shows left bundle branch block with an inferior axis). In such cases, the origin of the ventricular tachycardia most often is located in or near the right ventricular outflow tract.

The EKG in the present patient had the following features that suggest ventricular tachycardia: a QRS complex wider than 140 msec, an axis between $-90°$ and $-180°$, a biphasic R in V_1, and an R:S ratio in $V_6 < 1$. The diagnosis of ventricular tachycardia was confirmed in the present patient with electrophysiologic studies.

Clinical Pearls

1. The EKG diagnosis of ventricular tachycardia should be suspected if AV dissociation or fusion beats are present. The use of Wellens' criteria further aids in making the diagnosis.

2. Intermittent Cannon A waves in the jugular venous pulse in a person with rapid heart rate suggests ventricular tachycardia, as does variability in the intensity of the first heart sound.

3. If there is hemodynamic instability, perform immediate countershock regardless of the type of tachycardia.

4. Adenosine can be used to differentiate wide QRS tachycardias in the stable patient.

5. The diagnosis can be confirmed by an esophageal or intra-atrial EKG or by electrophysiologic studies.

REFERENCES

1. Wellens HJJ, Bar FWHM, Lie KI: The value of the electrocardiogram in the differential diagnosis of a tachycardia with a widened QRS complex. Am J Med 1978;65:27–33.
2. Akhtar M: Clinical spectrum of ventricular tachycardia. Circulation 1990;82:1561–1573.
3. Brugada P, Brugada J, Mont L, et al: A new approach to the differential diagnosis of a regular tachycardia with a wide QRS complex. Circulation 1991;83:1649–1659.

PATIENT 50

A 40-year-old man with cyanosis and palpitations

A 40-year-old man presents with a lifelong history of cyanosis. Although he experiences easy fatigue and moderate dyspnea on exertion, he has been able to maintain a job as a file clerk. He denies orthopnea and paroxysmal nocturnal dyspnea, but has peripheral edema. Recently, he noted the onset of palpitations and rapid heart beat. During the episodes of palpitations, he felt lightheaded, but did not experience syncope. The episodes lasted as long as a half hour and resolved spontaneously.

Physical Examination: Vital signs: pulse 80 (regular); blood pressure 100/60. Skin: cyanosis. Chest: clear. Cardiac: neck veins elevated with large V waves; quintuple cadence and a III/VI holosystolic murmur heart beat along the left sternal border. Extremities: trace peripheral edema; no clubbing.

Laboratory Findings: EKG: see below.

Question: What condition explains the physical examination and EKG findings?

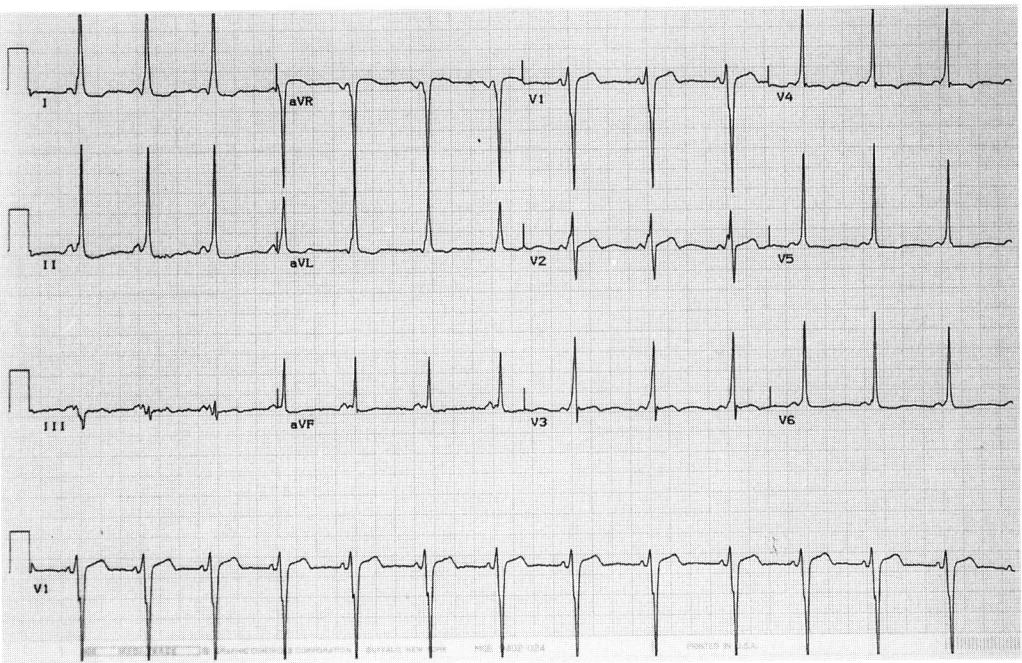

Diagnosis: Ebstein's anomaly with preexcitation syndrome.

Discussion: Ebstein's anomaly of the tricuspid valve is a downward displacement of the tricuspid valve into the right ventricle. Thus, a portion of the right ventricle lies above the tricuspid valve and is "atrialized." One portion of the tricuspid valve is attached to the tricuspid annulus, whereas other portions are attached directly to the right ventricular wall by anomalous connections. In some cases, the posterior leaflet is small or absent. These abnormalities result in a small, frequently ineffective right ventricle and often severe tricuspid regurgitation.

Cyanosis occurs when increased right atrial pressure from the tricuspid regurgitation causes right-to-left shunting through a patent foramen ovale or through an atrial septal defect, which coexists in 75% of cases. In some patients, the cyanosis disappears shortly after birth when pulmonary vascular resistance falls, but then reappears when tricuspid regurgitation leads to right ventricular volume overload, failure, and increased right atrial pressure. The disease also may be associated with **pulmonary stenosis,** which further contributes to right ventricular failure, and increased right atrial pressure, which increases the right-to-left shunt. As in the present patient, preexcitation syndrome (usually type B Wolff-Parkinson-White [WPW] syndrome) is present in approximately one-quarter of patients with Ebstein's anomaly of the tricuspid valve.

The diagnosis is suspected on the basis of history and physical examination. This is one of the few uncorrected cyanotic congenital heart diseases that allows survival into adult life. A history of bipolar disorder—a condition often treated with lithium—in the patient's mother is a predisposing factor. On physical examination, differential closure of the tricuspid and mitral valves causes a wide splitting of the first heart sound; the addition of right ventricular third and fourth heart sounds to S_2 and a split S_1 produce the characteristic **quintuple auscultatory cadence.** The tricuspid component of the first sound may be clicking and loud ("sail sound").

The EKG shows prominent P waves and right bundle branch block with low voltage when conduction is not down the WPW accessory pathway. Deep Q waves may be present in the inferior leads and precordial leads.

An adequate echocardiogram almost always makes the diagnosis. Echocardiography demonstrates the inferior displacement of the tricuspid valve and its abnormal alignment with the mitral valve. In the apical four-chamber view, the displacement of the septal tricuspid leaflet can be demonstrated.

If for technical reasons an adequate echocardiogram cannot be obtained, the diagnosis can be made by cardiac catheterization. During cardiac catheterization, a pacing electrode catheter with a lumen is advanced across the tricuspid valve, and the right ventricular electrogram and right ventricular pressure tracing are recorded. The catheter is then gradually withdrawn across the tricuspid valve until a position is reached where a right *atrial* pressure tracing is recorded simultaneously with a right *ventricular* electrogram, reflecting that portion of the right ventricle that has been "atrialized" by the downward displacement of the tricuspid valve.

If medical management fails to control the symptoms, tricuspid valve replacement may relieve cyanosis by restoring tricuspid competence, thereby lowering right atrial pressure. If the right ventricle is extremely small, employ the Glenn procedure (anastomosis of the superior vena cava to the pulmonary artery) to increase pulmonary blood flow. If the preexcitation syndrome cannot be controlled medically, perform surgical or catheter ablation of the accessory pathway.

The present patient underwent catheter ablation of the preexcitation pathway, with resolution of palpitations. He remains cyanotic but in New York Heart Association functional Class II.

Clinical Pearls

1. Suspect Epstein's anomaly of the tricuspid valve in any patient with cyanotic congential heart disease who has survived without correction into adulthood.
2. Disappearance of the cyanosis shortly after birth with reappearance later in life is typical of the syndrome.
3. A quintuple cadence upon auscultation strongly suggests the diagnosis.
4. Preexcitation is a common coexisting anomaly in this disease.

REFERENCES

1. Kastor JA, Goldreyer BN, Josephson ME, et al: Electrophysiologic characteristics of Ebstein's anomaly of the tricuspid valve. Circulation 1975;52:987–995.
2. Giuliani ER, Fuster V, Brandenberg RO, et al: Ebstein's anomaly: The clinical features and natural history of Ebstein's anomaly of the tricuspid valve. Mayo Clin Proc 1979;54:163–173.
3. Roberson DA, Silverman NH: Ebstein's anomaly: Echocardiographic and clinical features in the fetus and neonate. J Am Coll Cardiol 1989;14:1300–1307.
4. Khan IA, Cohen RA: Ebstein's anomaly of the tricuspid valve associated with congenital deaf-mustism. Int J Cardiol 1999;70(3):219–221.

PATIENT 51

A 68-year-old woman with lower-extremity weakness

A 68-year-old woman with long-standing hypertension, treated with a potassium-sparing diuretic, recently was prescribed an angiotension-converting enzyme (ACE) inhibitor for additional blood pressure control. On presentation, she complains of lower-extremity weakness.

Physical Examination: Vital signs: temperature 98.6°; pulse 120 and regular; respirations 16; blood pressure 150/85. Neck: no jugular vein distention. Chest: clear. Cardiac: S_4; no murmurs. Neurologic: general muscle weakness.

Laboratory Findings: EKG: see below.

Question: What is the cause of the patient's lower-extremity weakness?

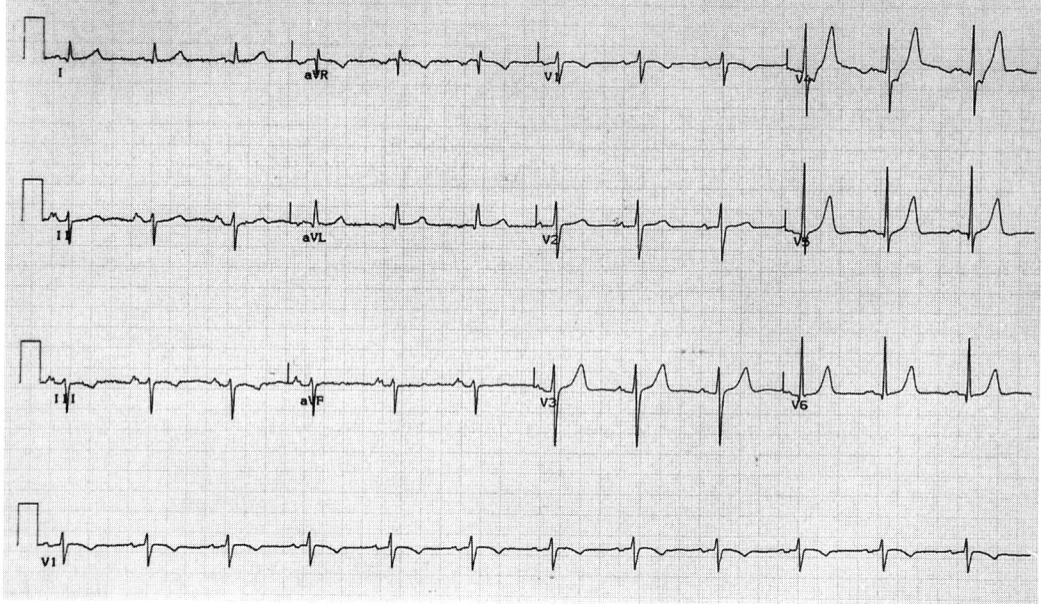

Diagnosis: Hyperkalemia.

Discussion: Potassium ion is critical in determining cardiac cellular resting potential. The higher the serum potassium, the more electronegative the myocyte becomes, moving further away from its ability to generate an action potential. Hyperkalemia, therefore, reduces the excitability of cardiac tissue.

The EKG manifestations of hyperkalemia are manifold. As the serum potassium level increases, the EKG progresses through four stages: (1) peaking of the T waves with a narrow base (as shown in EKG on the previous page) and QT-interval shortening; (2) sinus node dysfunction with exit block; (3) widening of the QRS complex; and (4) a sine wave pattern or ventricular fibrillation. While this typical progression may be seen in some patients, in others the first EKG manifestation may be one of the more advanced patterns indicating severe hyperkalemia. The earliest EKG abnormality is peaking of the T waves with symmetry and a narrow base. These features help to differentiate the effect of hyperkalemia from other causes of tall T waves, such as ischemia, which may normalize the T waves and have a tall, broad base. There is a correlation between the serum potassium level and specific EKG findings, but variation exists among patients. For instance, if the patient has had a prior myocardial infarction, the previously inverted T waves may become more inverted and do not normalize. At times, ST elevation (dialyzable current of injury) can occur, and it may be mistaken for acute ischemia.

Hyperkalemia occurs either when there is failure of appropriate renal excretion of potassium or when excess potassium is introduced either endogenously or exogenously. Renal causes of hyperkalemia include renal failure, type IV renal tubular acidosis, which usually is associated with hypoaldosteronism, and drugs that interfere with renal potassium handling. The most common drugs causing hyperkalemia include the ACE inhibitors, spironolactone, triamterene, and amiloride. ACE inhibitors decrease angiotension II, so that less aldosterone is secreted by the adrenal glands. Since aldosterone enhances potassium excretion, reduced aldosterone secretion leads to potassium retention. Hyperkalemia also may occur when extracellular potassium has been added to the system either from oversupplementation or mobilization of potassium from body tissues. Mobilization occurs from severe muscle injury, hemolysis, lack of insulin, digitalis poisoning, and massive hematomas.

The therapy for hyperkalemia is to lower the potassium acutely while at the same time discover and remove the etiologic agent responsible. The administration of glucose and insulin or sodium bicarbonate effectively transfers potassium into the cell, acutely lowering serum potassium. These maneuvers are the most effective in life-threatening hyperkalemia. Administration of calcium, which does not lower serum potassium, helps to restore myocardial excitability and also may be lifesaving. Once the potassium level has been lowered to a safe range, potassium must then be removed from the body. Potassium exchange resins or vigorous hydration (if there is adequate renal function) will accomplish this goal. If these measures are ineffective, dialysis will restore normal extracellular potassium levels.

The present patient had a serum potassium of 7 mEq/L and serum creatinine of 2 mg/dl. She was treated initially with an insulin and glucose infusion that reduced her potassium to 5.9 mEq/L; her potassium-sparing diuretic and ACE inhibitor were discontinued.

Clinical Pearls

1. ACE inhibitors, potassium-sparing diuretics, or potassium supplements can cause hyperkalemia, especially in patients with renal insufficiency, by impairing renal excretion of potassium.

2. Hyperkalemia must be included in the differential diagnosis of sinus node failure and conduction system block.

3. Abnormalities in sinus impulse formation and intracardiac conduction worsen rapidly if the serum potassium level continues to increase. Hyperkalemia of this magnitude is a medical emergency.

4. Severe hyperkalemia must be treated acutely with agents that rapidly lower potassium, such as insulin and glucose. Exchange resins should not be employed for the acute control of severe hyperkalemia, but are useful once serum potassium levels have decreased from life-threatening levels.

REFERENCES

1. Ponce SP, Jennings AE, Madias NE, et al: Drug-induced hyperkalemia. Medicine 1985;64:357–370.
2. Tannen RL: Potassium disorders. In Kokko JP, Tannen RL (eds): Fluids and Electrolytes. Philadelphia, W. B. Saunders, 1986.
3. Fisch C: Electrocardiography and vectorcardiography. In Braunwald E (ed): Heart Disease, 4th ed. Philadelphia, W. B. Saunders, 1992, pp 150–151.
4. Martinez-Vea A, Bardaji A, Garcia C, et al: Severe hyperkalemia with minimal electrocardiographic manifestations: A report of seven cases. J Electrocardiol 1999;32(1):45–49.

PATIENT 52

A 66-year-old man with a heart rate of 38 bpm

A 66-year-old man with angina and peripheral vascular disease for several years is noted to have a slow heart rate. He had been clinically stable on nifedipine and nitrates. He denies presyncope and syncope, and continues to work as a farmer.

Physical Examination: Vital signs: pulse 38; blood pressure 150/60. General: moderately obese. Cardiac: intermittent Cannon A waves in the jugular pulse; no murmurs.

Laboratory Findings: CBC, urinalysis, electrolytes: normal. EKG: see below.

Question: Should a pacemaker be recommended for this patient? If so, what type?

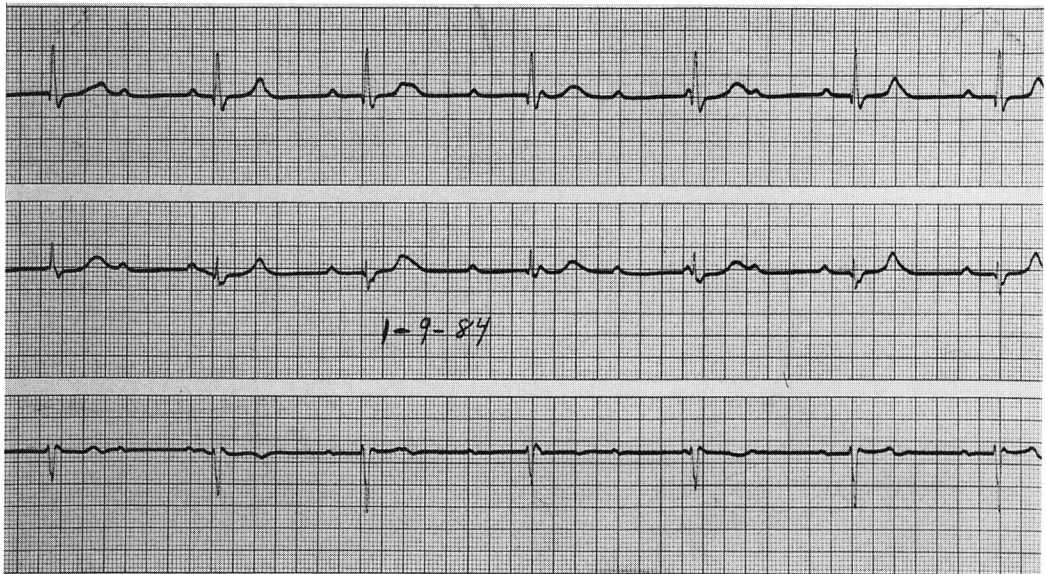

Answer: A pacemaker is indicated for the management of third-degree atrioventricular (AV) block with a heart rate < 40 beats per minute.

Discussion: Patients with lightheadedness or syncope or both should be evaluated for a bradyarrhythmia. Permanent pacing is indicated for patients with symptoms of reduced cerebral perfusion due to bradycardia, regardless of its type, unless it is associated with an acute, transient event such as drug use, infarction, or electrolyte imbalance. The most common causes of symptomatic bradyarrhythmias are the **sick sinus syndrome** (with a maximum R-R interval of more than three seconds or a minimum heart rate below 40 beats/min, sometimes associated with intermittent tachycardia) and **high-grade AV block.** Permanent pacing also is indicated if the patient has: third-degree AV block and congestive heart failure; confusional states that clear with temporary pacing; or arrhythmias and other medical conditions which require drugs that result in symptomatic bradycardia.

In an asymptomatic patient, such as the present one, the decision for pacemaker insertion is more difficult. Generally, in an asymptomatic patient, a permanent pacemaker is indicated if there is: **(1)** a persistent bradycardia with a maximum R-R interval of more than 3 seconds or with a minimum rate of 40 beats/min, or **(2)** bifascicular and trifascicular block with intermittent type II AV block. Asymptomatic patients with right bundle branch block and left anterior or posterior fascicular block, or those with left bundle branch block, are not candidates for pacemakers even if the H-V interval is prolonged, since the incidence of progression to complete heart block in this group is low.

Many types of pacemakers are available today. A three-letter pacemaker code is used to describe them. The first letter is the chamber that is paced, the second represents the chamber that is sensed, and the third letter indicates the pacemaker's response to a sensed event. The letter V refers to the ventricle, A to the atrium, and D to both. The letter I refers to inhibited response and T to a triggered response. A fourth letter R has been added to indicate that the device is rate responsive. If the patient has sinus node disease and normal AV conduction, an AAI pacemaker can be used. These letters indicate that the pacemaker will pace the atrium and become inhibited if it senses atrial depolarization. If AV block is present, a VVI or DDD can be used, depending on the patient's needs. A DDD pacer is implanted to maintain the physiologic sequence of activation if there is abnormal AV conduction. Physiologic pacing provides higher cardiac output than does ventricular pacing and is better suited to active lifestyles. A VVI is used if atrial fibrillation is present, because it is then impossible to pace the atria. Rate-adaptive VVIR and DDDR pacemakers also are available.

A review of the patient's EKGs from 1981, when the tracing was normal, showed a progression of changes. In 1982, the initial septal vector disappeared without chest pain, indicating either a silent infarction or an incomplete left bundle branch block. Such tracings in the absence of a history of infarction often precede a higher grade left bundle branch block. In 1983, the patient's EKG began to show a typical left bundle branch block with a QRS width of 0.12 seconds. In late 1983, right bundle branch block with left anterior fascicular block was noted, with occasional Mobitz II second-degree block. A few months later his tracing was noted to have third-degree AV block.

The present patient had an active lifestyle; therefore, a DDDR pacemaker with rate responsiveness was selected.

Clinical Pearls

1. In an asymptomatic person, a pacemaker usually is indicated if there is persistent bradycardia with a maximum R-R interval of more than 3 seconds or with a minimum rate of 40 beats/min, or bifascicular or trifascicular block is present with intermittent type II second-degree AV block.
2. Patients with symptomatic bradyarrhythmias should receive a permanent pacemaker unless the bradyarrhythmia is caused by acute temporary pathology.
3. The type of pacemaker implanted depends on the patient's lifestyle and needs.

REFERENCES

1. Parsonnet V, Furman S, Smyth NPD: Implantable cardiac pacemakers: Status report and resource guideline. Am J Cardiol 1974;34:487–500.
2. Greenspan AM, Kay HR, Berger BC, et al: Incidence of unwarranted implantation of permanent cardiac pacemakers in a large medical population. N Engl J Med 1988;318:158–163.
3. Gregoratos G, Cheitlin D, Conill A et al: ACC/AHA guidelines for implantation of cardiac pacemakers and antiarrhythmia devices. J Am Coll Cardiol 1998;31:1175–209.
4. Mitrani RD, Simmons JD, Interian A, et al: Cardial pacemakers current and future status. Curr Probl Cardiol 1999;24:348–420.

PATIENT 53

A 40-year-old man with chronic malaise and sudden numbness in the right arm

A 40-year-old man is well until 2 months prior to admission, when he notes the onset of weakness, malaise, and fatigue. He has two episodes of hives on his trunk and arms. He also has two-block dyspnea on exertion, but denies orthopnea, paroxysmal nocturnal dyspnea, edema, and chest pain. On the morning of admission, he notes that his right forearm and hand are cold, pale, and numb. His other extremities are normal, and there are no other neurologic symptoms. There is no chest pain.

Physical Examination: Vital signs: temperature 98.6°; pulse 100 and regular; blood pressure 110/70. Chest: clear. Cardiac: S_4; no S_3; no murmurs. Extremities: right arm cold and pale; brachial pulse present but radial and ulnar pulses absent; other pulses normal.

Laboratory Findings: Hgb 13.5 g/dl; Hct 38%; WBC 14,400/µl with 45% neutrophils, 15% lymphocytes, 37% eosinophils, and 3% monocytes. EKG: normal sinus rhythm; nonspecific ST- and T-wave abnormalities. Echocardiogram: mild global hypokinesis with a suggestion of an apical thrombus.

Question: What diagnosis best explains the clinical presentation?

Diagnosis: Hypereosinophilic syndrome.

Discussion: Tropical endomyocardial fibrosis and nontropical Löffler's syndrome (hypereosinophilic syndrome) are considered by some to be the same entity. However, tropical endomyocardial fibrosis has less eosinophilia, and these two diseases have some different clinical presentations. Tropical endomyocardial fibrosis affects the right ventricle, the left ventricle, or both ventricles, whereas Löffler's disease often is biventricular.

The usual causes of extreme blood eosinophilia are allergy, connective tissue disease, neoplasm, and parasitic infection. In the absence of the aforementioned illnesses and in the presence of organ damage, the diagnosis of idiopathic hypereosinophilic syndrome can be made. It is a **primary myeloproliferative disorder** in which persistently elevated numbers of eosinophils cause organ damage. Organ infiltration with eosinophils followed by release of toxic proteins (eosinophil basic protein and eosinophilic cationic protein) directly damages the tissues.

As in the present patient, the heart is an important target and a major source of morbidity in hypereosinophilic syndrome. Eosinophils cause damage and scarring of the endocardium, producing ventricular diastolic dysfunction and heart failure. Endocardial damage also leads to valvular regurgitation and mural thrombi that can become emboli. Left ventricular wall thickness is usually increased. Because of the predisposition toward mural thrombi and embolization, lifelong anticoagulation is advisable once the diagnosis is established. The skin also may be involved, manifesting angioedema, dermatographia, and other rashes. Nonembolic neurologic involvement is common, presenting as altered behavior, psychosis, or peripheral neuropathy. Pulmonary and hepatic dysfunction also may occur.

The heart failure of hypereosinophilic syndrome is best treated with **diuretics,** since its restrictive physiology causes preload dependence unlikely to respond favorably to vasodilators. Treatment of the hypereosinophilia includes **corticosteroid therapy** and, in some cases, **hydroxyurea.** Earlier studies suggested a very poor prognosis, with over half the patients dying within 1 year after organ system involvement was diagnosed. A recent study from the National Institutes of Health suggests a much better outcome, however, with only a 20% 10-year mortality. Still, the presence of heart disease combined with any other organ system involvement worsens prognosis, with a 40% mortality after 10 years.

Although no EKG or echocardiographic findings are specific for hypereosinophilic heart disease, the presence of mural thrombi in the absence of myocardial infarction or severe left ventricular dysfunction should raise clinical suspicion. Autopsy demonstrates increased cardiac collagen and fibrotic thickening of the endocardium, thrombosis, and infiltration of eosinophils.

The present patient responded to prednisone with a decrease in his eosinophilia. He also was begun on warfarin. Surgical resection of the thickened fibrotic endocardium with repair of the mitral and tricuspid valves has given some palliation of symptoms. (Valve replacement would have been necessary if significant regurgitation was present.)

Clinical Pearls

1. Persistent hypereosinophilia damages the myocardium directly by release of toxic eosinophil products.
2. Unexplained or unexpected thromboembolism in the presence of an increased eosinophil count and good systolic ventricular function strongly suggests the hypereosinophilic syndrome.
3. The heart failure of hypereosinophilic syndrome is best treated with diuretics alone.

REFERENCES

1. Parrillo JE, Borer JS, Henry WL, et al: The cardiovascular manifestations of the hypereosinophilic syndrome. Am J Med 1979;67:572–582.
2. Fauci AS, Harley JB, Roberts WC, et al: The idiopathic hypereosinophilic syndrome. Ann Intern Med 1982;97:78–92.
3. Weller PF, Bubley GJ: The idiopathic hypereosinophilic syndrome. Blood 1994;83:2759.
4. Touze JE, Fourcade L, Heno P, et al: The heart and the eosinophil. Med Trop (Mars) 1998;58:459–464.
5. Corssmit EP, Trip MD, Durrer JD: Löffler's endomyocarditis in the idiopathic hypereosinophilic syndrome. Cardiology 1999;91:272–276.
6. Imoto Y, Tominaga R, Morita S, et al: Surgical treatment of tricuspid regurgitation caused by Löffler's endocarditis. Jpn J Thorac Cardiovasc Surg 1999;47:570–573.

PATIENT 54

A 52-year-old man with a right bundle branch block

A 52-year-old asymptomatic man is noted on a routine electrocardiogram to have a right bundle branch block. He has no cardiovascular risk factors other than his age and gender.

Physical Examination: Vital signs: pulse 70; blood pressure 120/80. Cardiac: normal.

Laboratory Findings: CBC, SMA 12, electrolytes, and urinalysis: normal. EKG: right bundle branch block. Chest radiograph: normal.

Question: What further studies would you recommend?

Diagnosis: The patient should have an echocardiogram and stress test to evaluate right bundle branch block of unknown etiology.

Discussion: Right bundle branch block (RBBB) may occur as a **congenital abnormality** or present in an acquired fashion due to **conduction system fibrosis, myocardial disease,** or **myocardial infarction.** It is not unusual to detect RBBB in patients with no other clinical evidence of cardiac disease.

Some studies indicate that the new development of RBBB in the absence of myocardial infarction is a benign condition—at least as defined by these studies, which had short-term patient followup. The Baltimore Longitudinal Study, for instance, tracked 24 men with RBBB for 8 years. The incidence of cardiovascular events in this patient population was similar to that in the general population. The Manitoba Study identified 59 patients who developed RBBB over a 28-year followup period. Only one of the patients developed ischemic heart disease, and no sudden deaths occurred. Data from the Framingham Study on RBBB, however, was less favorable. Over an 18-year period, approximately half of the 70 patients who developed RBBB subsequently experienced clinically apparent heart disease.

A more recent study, including a 30-year followup, shows that bundle branch block is **a marker of a slowly progressive, degenerative disease** that affects the myocardium. No correlation to risk factors for coronary artery disease at age 50 years, incidence of infarction in the followup, or cardiovascular deaths was found. However, the numbers were small, and no mention was made of whether LBBB had a worse prognosis.

Based on the Framingham data, many cardiologists recommend cardiac evaluation with an echocardiogram and a stress test in patients with coronary risk factors and new-onset RBBB. The stress EKG can be interpreted in the presence of RBBB, but not in the presence of LBBB. The right precordial leads with the RBBB morphology on exercise can show depressed ST segment, which is not significant. The ST changes must be over the left ventricular leads, V_4 to V_6, to be significant. There are a variety of forms with an RBBB, such as noted in the "Brugada" syndrome. In these cases, there is a distinct EKG pattern consisting of RBBB with ST elevation in the right precordial lead (V_1–V_3) in the absence of any structural heart disease. These patients are prone to sudden ventricular fibrillation.

The new appearance of LBBB is decidedly more ominous. In virtually all of the available studies that examine the clinical courses of patients with new-onset LBBB, the morbidity and mortality are significant—especially if coronary artery disease is present. In the Framingham Study, for instance, only 15% of patients with new LBBB were free of heart disease 10 years after initial detection.

The present patient's echocardiogram was normal, but his electrocardiographic stress test showed 2-mm ST-segment depression in the anterolateral leads after 5 minutes of a Bruce protocol. His heart rate increased from 77 to 140 beats/min, but no symptoms occurred. A thallium stress test several days later revealed reversible ischemia in the septum, apical, and inferior areas. The patient was advised to return for coronary arteriography, but on the morning before the planned study, he experienced substernal chest pain that lasted 1 hour and was relieved by nitroglycerin. Coronary arteriography demonstrated a 99% proximal left anterior descending lesion that was dilated by angioplasty, leaving a 20% residual lesion.

Clinical Pearls

1. Although most patients with new-onset RBBB follow a benign course during short-term followup, up to 50% may develop significant heart disease over the ensuing 20 years.

2. Due to the high incidence of cardiac disease during long-term followup, patients with new RBBB should undergo echocardiography and EKG stress testing.

3. An EKG stress test is interpretable in the presence of RBBB, but not in the presence of LBBB.

REFERENCES

1. Schneider JF, Thomas HE, Kregar BF, et al: Newly acquired right bundle-branch block: The Framingham study. Ann Intern Med 1980;92:37–44.
2. Fleg JL, Das DN, Lakatta EG: Right bundle branch block: Long-term prognosis in apparently healthy men. J Am Coll Cardiol 1983;1:887–892.
3. Gibbons RJ, Beasley JW, Duvernoy WFC, et al: ACC/AHA Guidelines for exercise testing: Executive summary. Circulation 1997;96:345–354.
4. Eriksson P, Hansson P-O, Eriksson H, et al.: Bundle-branch block in a general male population. The study of men born 1913. Circulation 1998; 98:2494-2500.
5. Agarwal AK, Venugopalan P: Right bundle branch block: Varying electrocardiography patterns. Aetiological correlation, mechanisms, and electrophysiology. Int J Cardiol 1999;71:33–99.
6. Alings M, Wilde A: "Brugada" syndrome. Clinical data and suggested parthophysiology mechanism. Circulation 1999;99:666–673.

PATIENT 55

A 45-year-old man with hypotension following an acute inferior myocardial infarction

A 45-year-old man is admitted for alcohol detoxification. One week after admission, the patient begins complaining of recurrent episodes of substernal chest pain at rest. These episodes are relieved by sublingual nitroglycerin. He has no prior cardiac history, but is a heavy cigarette smoker and has a strong family history of cardiac disease. He also has a history of alcoholic gastritis, and 1 year prior to this admission he experienced some hematemesis.

Physical Examination: Vital signs: pulse 125 (regular); blood pressure 105/60. General: anxious, in obvious discomfort, pale, and diaphoretic. Neck: no jugular vein distention. Cardiac: no murmurs, rubs, or gallops. Chest: clear to auscultation. Abdomen: normal. Extremities: cool, moist, without peripheral edema.

Laboratory Findings: CBC and electrolytes: normal. Chest radiograph: normal. 12-lead EKG (during pain): see below. Right-sided chest leads reveal ST elevation in V_4R.

Hospital Course: After no improvement with nitroglycerin and morphine, streptokinase provides almost immediate relief of his chest pain. The patient then develops jugular vein distention and hypotension (85/60) that responds partially to fluid challenge. A Swan-Ganz catheter reveals the following data:

	Pressure (mmHg)
Right atrium	20
Right ventricle	35/18
Pulmonary artery	35/20
Pulmonary capillary wedge	17

Question: What is this patient's diagnosis?

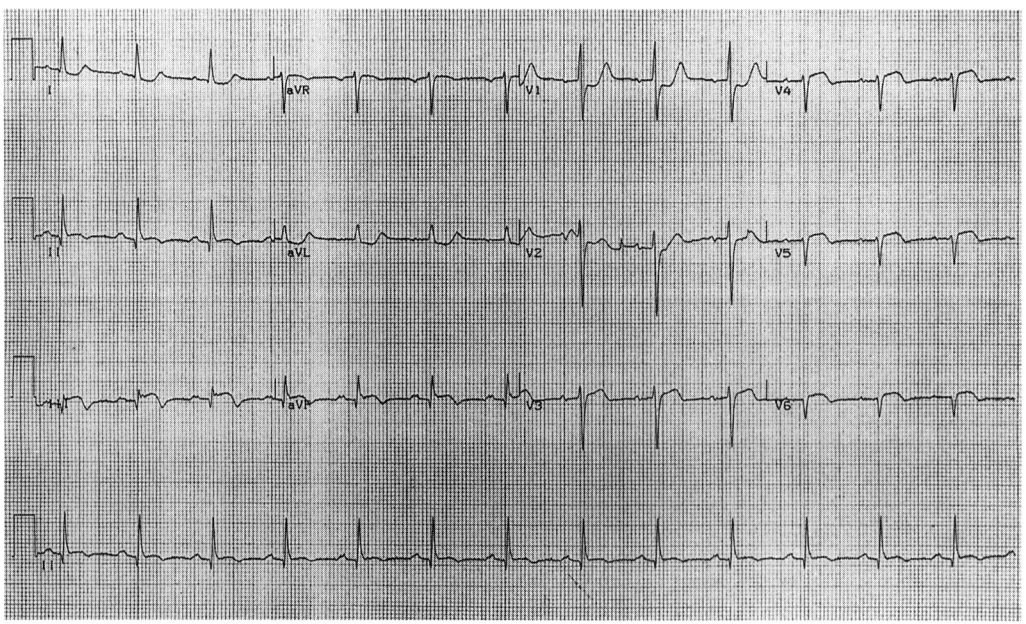

Diagnosis: Inferior posterior myocardial infarction with infarction of the right ventricle.

Discussion: In approximately 35% of patients with inferior myocardial infarctions, EKG evidence of concomitant right ventricular infarction exists. However, most of these patients do not experience clinical manifestations of right ventricular dysfunction. When ventricular dysfunction does occur, the right ventricle loses its ability to fill the left ventricle, resulting in a decrease in cardiac output and systemic hypotension. The right ventricle then becomes dilated and displaces the interventricular septum to the left, further reducing left ventricular filling and cardiac output. Clinically, such patients tend to have evidence of right-sided heart failure with distended neck veins during inspiration (Kussmaul's sign), clear lung fields, and hepatomegaly. These findings can **mimic pericardial tamponade** in the setting of the acute myocardial infarction. Hypotension, shock, and bradyarrhythmias also can occur.

Suspect the diagnosis of right ventricular infarction when the EKG shows ST elevation in the right-sided chest leads, especially in the V_4R position. As shown in the present patient, the prominent R waves in V_1 and V_2 and ST depression indicate that the posterobasal area also is involved. The diagnosis can be confirmed by echocardiography, radionuclide studies, or right heart catheterization. Echocardiography or radionuclide studies will show the decrease in right ventricular contraction, and right heart catheterization will show elevated right atrial pressure that is sometimes greater than the pulmonary capillary wedge pressure, as in the present patient. Note that patients with preinfarction angina have less incidence of right ventricular infarction. This may be due to adequately formed collateral vessels.

Volume expansion is the primary treatment for patients with right ventricular failure and hypotension. However, at times, an **inotropic agent** such as dobutamine is necessary because in the presence of significant left ventricular infarction, a volume load may increase left ventricular filling pressure, resulting in an increase in pulmonary vascular resistance and right ventricular afterload, which may further impair right ventricular systolic function. In addition, volume loading may increase intracardiac pressure but not transmural pressure because of pericardial restraint. On the other hand, diuretics or nitroglycerin may cause right and left ventricular underfilling and therefore produce hypotension. If bradyarrhythmia necessitates pacing, employ **sequential pacing** to retain the atrial "kick," which helps improve cardiac output.

The echocardiogram in the present patient revealed akinesis of the left ventricular inferoposterior wall from the base to the apex, with an ejection fraction of approximately 35%. The right ventricle was dilated with an aneurysm at its mid portion. He was treated with dobutamine with marked hemodynamic improvement. Three days later the dobutamine was discontinued without deterioration in the patient's condition.

Clinical Pearls

1. Right ventricular infarction is a reversible cause of shock in the patient with an inferior infarction.

2. Suspect the diagnosis in a patient with an inferior infarction who has findings of right-sided failure simulating pericardial tamponade.

3. Right-sided precordial leads showing ST elevation is very suggestive of the diagnosis, which can be confirmed by echocardiography or right heart catheterization.

4. Patients with right ventricular infarction respond to volume expansion, but they also may require dobutamine.

5. Patients with right ventricular infarction may receive nitroglycerin, but great caution should be exercised because this agent can reduce the preload and further drop the cardiac output.

REFERENCES
1. Williams JF Jr: Right ventricular infarction. Clin Cardiol 1990;13:309–315.
2. Bowers TR, O'Neill WW, Grines C: Effect of reperfusion on biventricular function and survival after right ventricular infarction. N Engl J Med 1998;338:933–940.
3. Shiraki H, Yoshikawa T, Anzai T: Association between preinfarction angina and a lower risk of right ventricular infarction. N Engl J Med 1998;338:941–947.
4. Horan LG, Flowers NC: Right ventricular infarction: Specific requirements of management. Am Family Physician 1999;60:1727–1734.

PATIENT 56

An 84-year-old man with chest pain and a left bundle branch block

An 84-year-old man with hypertension is admitted because of severe substernal chest pain with radiation to his left arm. The pain is of 1-hour duration. He noted mild episodes of such discomfort at rest several times during the preceding week.

Physical Examination: Vital signs: pulse 90 (regular); blood pressure 140/70. Cardiac: S_2 split with expiration; no murmurs.

Laboratory Findings: Total CPK and MB fractions: pending. Echocardiogram: ordered. EKG: see below.

Question: What is the cause of the patient's chest pain?

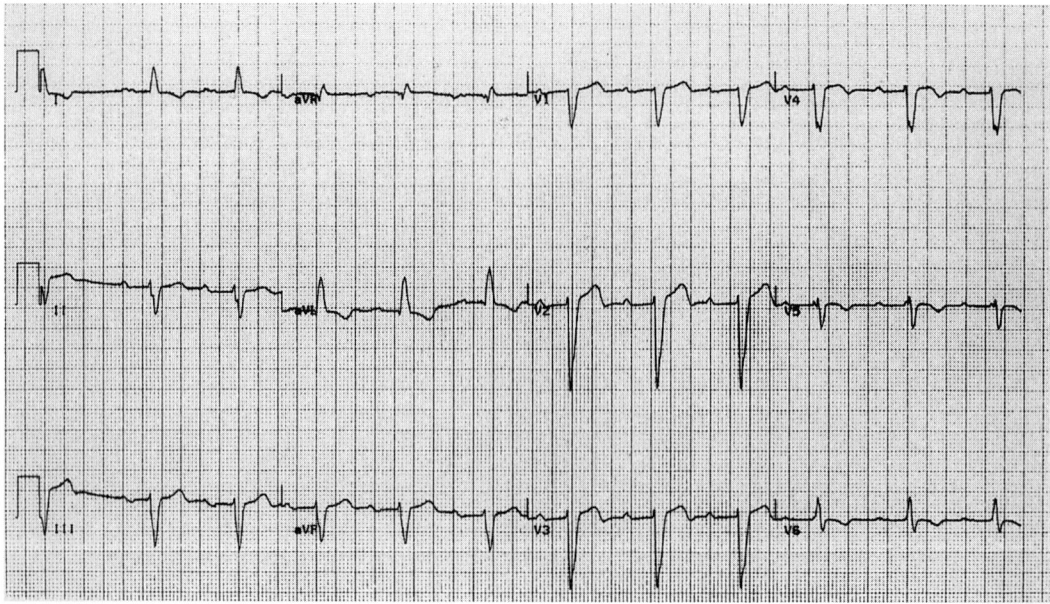

Diagnosis: Anterior myocardial infarction in the setting of left bundle branch block.

Discussion: Because the direction of septal activation is reversed, it is problematic to make the diagnosis of myocardial infarction in the presence of left bundle branch block, especially the diagnosis of infarction of the free left ventricular wall. The abnormal right-to-left septal activation in left bundle branch block produces R waves in the precordial leads instead of the expected Q waves and, thus, the changes of infarction are obscured. In addition, uncomplicated left bundle branch block has Q waves in V_1 and V_2, and ST elevation in these leads that can resemble an anteroseptal infarction. There also are secondary ST-T changes in the left precordial leads that may obscure the findings of a nontransmural infarction.

In some instances, however, myocardial infarction can be diagnosed in the face of left bundle branch block. If there is ST elevation in the *left* chest leads or in the inferior leads, infarction should be suspected. Frequently with such changes, serial tracings show an evolutionary pattern, i.e., the ST segments return toward the baseline and the T waves become coved (symmetrically inverted). If the interventricular septum is infarcted, then there is transmission of right ventricular cavity negativity to the left ventricular cavity, and Q waves may appear in leads I, aVL, V_5 or V_6, as noted in the present patient's tracing. Progressive, diffuse T wave inversion also can indicate infarction in the presence of left bundle branch block.

In addition, an abnormal S wave in the left chest leads (V_5 or V_6) is suggestive of infarction of the anterior free wall in this setting. In the presence of left bundle branch block, a free wall left ventricular infarction allows the left precordial leads to record the left ventricular cavity, which shows an RS complex. Although left precordial lead S waves may be due to the transitional zone being more to the left than normal, in such instances the R wave usually is not slurred, and the T waves are upright. When the R waves are slurred and the T waves are inverted, left precordial S waves often indicate infarction of the free wall, as in the present patient's tracing.

In the present patient, the Q wave in aVL and the S wave in V_6 suggested anterior myocardial infarction, which was confirmed by an anterioapical wall motion abnormality detected by echocardiography and by elevated total CPK and MB fractions.

Clinical Pearls

1. Although left bundle branch block usually obscures the findings of an acute myocardial infarction, there are several instances in which the EKG suggests infarction despite the presence of left bundle branch block.

2. ST-segment elevation in the inferior leads or left lateral leads is compatible with infarction in the presence of a left bundle branch block.

3. In the presence of a left bundle branch block, a Q wave in leads I, aVL, V_5 or V_6 suggests infarction of the septum.

4. In the presence of a left bundle branch block, QRS complexes in the left precordial leads with S waves in the presence of slurred R waves and inverted T waves suggest free wall left ventricular infarction.

5. Progressive diffuse T wave inversion can indicate infarction in the presence of left bundle branch block.

REFERENCES

1. Sodi-Pollares D, Rodriquez MI: Morphology of the unipolar leads recorded at the septal surfaces: Its application to the diagnosis of left bundle branch block complicated by myocardial infarction. Am Heart J 1952;43:27–41.
2. Sodi-Pollares D, Calder RM: New Bases of Electrocardiography. St. Louis, C.V. Mosby, 1956.
3. Hands ME, Cook EF, Stone PH, et al: Electrocardiographic diagnosis of myocardial infarction in the presence of complete left bundle branch block. Am Heart J 1988;116:2330.
4. Sgarbossa EB, Pinski SL, Barbagelata A: Electrocardiographic diagnosis of evolving acute myocardial infarction in the presence of left bundle branch block. N Engl J Med 1996;334:481.

PATIENT 57

A 36-year-old male drug abuser with chest pain

A 36-year-old man presents with substernal chest pain radiating to his left arm. Previously in good health, the patient denies a history of cardiovascular disease. He smokes two packs of cigarettes a day and occasionally snorts cocaine, which he used 24 hours before admission. He denies diabetes, hypertension, or a family history of coronary disease.

Physical Examination: Vital signs: temperature 99.2°; pulse 100 (regular); blood pressure 150/90. General: moderate distress from chest pain. Nose: inflamed nasal membranes. Chest: clear. Cardiac: no murmurs.

Laboratory Findings: EKG: see below.

Question: How did cocaine contribute to this patient's cardiac event?

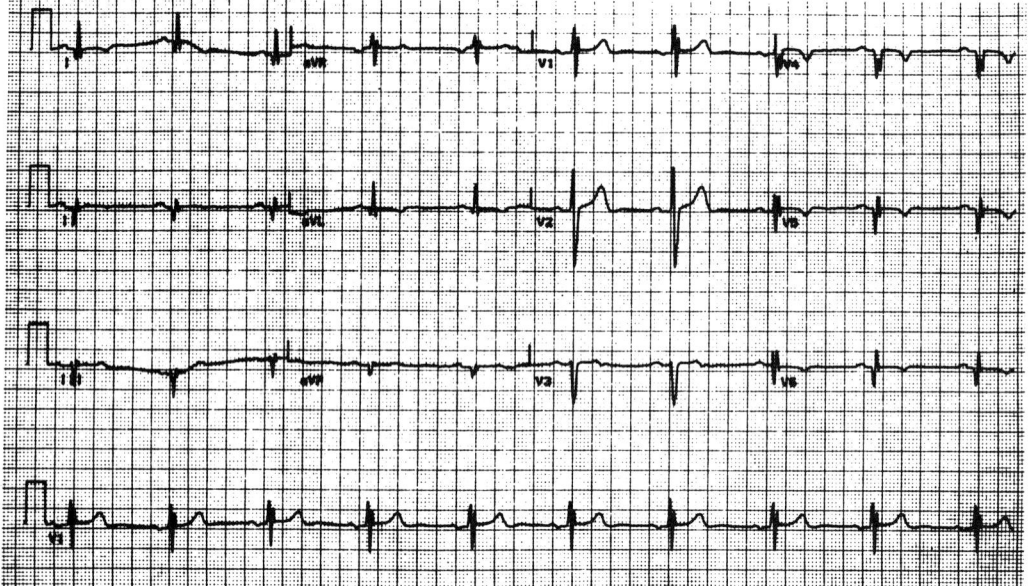

Answer: By potentiating the effects of norepinephrine on the cardiovascular system.

Discussion: Cocaine inhibits re-uptake of norepinephrine by the sympathetic nerve endings. The results are **vasoconstriction, hypertension, increased heart rate and cardiac output, and increased myocardial oxygen consumption.** Increased myocardial oxygen demand together with decreased coronary blood flow due to vasoconstriction can lead to angina pectoris and cardiac arrhythmias in patients with preexisting coronary disease. However, patients with "normal" coronary arteries also may suffer from acute myocardial infarctions after cocaine abuse. Typically such complications occur when doses of cocaine in excess of 1 gm are used, but the sensitivity to the drug is quite variable. Presumably, high doses of cocaine and its nonionic complex form called "crack" induce prolonged coronary spasm, which in turn causes myocardial infarction.

The susceptibility of patients to cocaine-induced cardiac disease seems capricious. Some patients experience serious myocardial sequelae after only brief cocaine use, even in small doses. At least one report indicates that myocardial infarction can occur after the application of topical cocaine as an anesthetic. Other patients may have a myocardial infarction after long-term illicit use of the drug.

Prolonged cocaine abuse can injure the myocardium in a more gradual fashion, presumably through a catecholamine toxicity, as occurs in patients with **pheochromocytoma.** In this condition, as in cocaine abuse, **patchy areas of fibrinoid necrosis** lead to myocardial dysfunction. Myocardial dysfunction in combination with cocaine-induced increases in afterload and coronary vasoconstriction causes congestive heart failure and a dilated cardiomyopathy. The patchy areas of myocardial damage also may produce lethal cardiac arrhythmias and sudden death.

The best therapy for acute cocaine-induced cardiac toxicity is uncertain. Previous reviews recommended beta-blocker therapy to reduce the beta-adrenergic effects of the drug. More recent studies, however, demonstrate that this therapy potentiates vasoconstriction by leaving the alpha-adrenergic effects of cocaine unopposed. This may worsen coronary spasm and even precipitate acute myocardial infarction. In the absence of myocardial failure, calcium channel–blocking agents seem appropriate, considering their ability to cause general vasodilatation and their usefulness in coronary artery spasm. Patients who have suffered myocardial infarction following cocaine abuse are subject to recurrent infarction probably due to recurrent coronary spasm. One case reported thrombus formation, and the coronary vessel was opened with the administration of heparin and GPIIb/IIIa inhibitor (tirofiban).

The present patient's EKG demonstrated acute inferolateral myocardial infarction. He recovered and was lost to followup.

Clinical Pearls

1. Cocaine may induce coronary spasm, leading to acute myocardial infarction even in patients without underlying coronary artery disease.

2. Beta-adrenergic blocking agents may potentiate the risk of coronary spasm in cocaine abuse.

3. The risk of cardiovascular complications is not easily predicted by the length of drug abuse or the dose taken.

REFERENCES

1. Majid PA, Patel B, Kim HS, et al: An angiographic and histologic study of cocaine-induced chest pain. Am J Cardiol 1990;65:812–814.
2. Isner JM, Chokshi SK: Cardiovascular complications of cocaine. Curr Probl Cardiol 1991;16:89.
3. Kloner RA, Hale S, Alker K, et al: The effects of acute and chronic cocaine use on the heart. Circulation 1992;85:407–419.
4. Frangogiannis NG, Farmer JA, Lakkis NM: Tirofiban for cocaine-induced coronary artery thrombosis. A novel therapeutic approach. Circulation 1999;100:1939.

PATIENT 58

A 59-year-old man with recent onset of atrial fibrillation

A 59-year-old man presents with an abrupt onset of palpitations accompanied by a vague complaint of "feeling ill." Mild hypertension is noted, and he is placed on verapamil. A subsequent Holter monitor reveals atrial fibrillation with a ventricular response up to 157 beats/min. The patient denies exertional dyspnea, orthopnea, paroxysmal nocturnal dyspnea, chest pain, heat intolerance, and tremor. He generally abstains from caffeine, smokes a pipe, and drinks alcohol in moderation. He is admitted for further evaluation.

Physical Examination: Vital signs: pulse 108 (irregular); blood pressure 150/94. Neck: thyroid normal; carotid pulsations equal. Cardiac: no jugular venous distention; no extra sounds or murmurs. Chest: clear. Abdomen: liver not enlarged. Extremities: normal peripheral pulses.

Laboratory Findings: CBC, partial thromboplastin time, prothrombin time, urinalysis, blood chemistry, and thyroid function studies: normal. Chest radiograph: normal cardiac size; unfolded aorta. EKG: atrial fibrillation with a ventricular response of 110; nonspecific ST-T changes. Echocardiographic and Doppler studies: normal.

Question: How should this patient be managed?

Answer: Exclude an organic cause for the arrhythmia and begin digoxin and a calcium blocker (verapamil or diltiazem) or a beta-blocker.

Discussion: Atrial fibrillation not associated with rheumatic heart disease or valvular abnormalities affects about 2–4% of persons over the age of 60. The risk for stroke in this group is five to six times that of patients of similar age in normal sinus rhythm. About 30% of patients with atrial fibrillation experience an embolism during their lifetime. However, the stroke risk is not increased for those with atrial fibrillation who are less than 60 years of age and have no evidence of thyrotoxicosis, valvular disease, coronary artery disease, hypertension, or cardiac enlargement. The term **lone atrial fibrillation** was coined for this group.

Consider cardioversion in patients with atrial fibrillation, especially if it has been present for less than 1 year. Exclude definite causes of atrial fibrillation, such as thyrotoxicosis. Echocardiography can be useful to uncover conditions not suspected clinically, such as mitral stenosis. In addition, echocardiography provides a measure of left atrial size, which usually is less than 4.5 cm for successful cardioversion. However, consider cardioversion even if left atrial size is up to 6 cm in diameter, because some of the atrial enlargement may be due to the fibrillation and not structural abnormalities. Transeophageal echo is better for detecting thrombi and for determining left atrial appendage function.

The initial aim in managing patients with atrial fibrillation is to **slow the ventricular rate.** In some patients, atrial fibrillation and rapid heart rate may be the primary cause rather than the consequence of left ventricular dysfunction. The left ventricular dysfunction may be completely reversible with control of the ventricular rate.

Patients with atrial fibrillation who have chest pain, pulmonary edema, or cardiogenic shock should have DC conversion. If those with nonvalvular atrial fibrillation are stable, give digoxin and a calcium blocker (verapamil or diltiazem) or a beta-blocker. These drugs slow the ventricular rate, but do not convert the patient. Digitalis has been considered the standard initial agent for many years. However, because its major effect is via the vagus nerve to block the AV node, the drug's efficacy frequently is low due to the overriding, heightened sympathetic tone with recent-onset atrial fibrillation. In addition, digitalis, through its vague effect, shortens the refractory phase of atrial muscle and may *perpetuate* atrial fibrillation. Calcium blockers (verapamil and diltiazem) and beta-blockers are more effective in reducing the ventricular rate than digoxin. Despite these data, most clinicians still administer digoxin with verapamil, diltiazem, or a beta-blocker because these combinations work well together.

Patients that are admitted to the hospital usually receive IV diltiazem along with digoxin. However, if patients are stable they can be treated as outpatients, since 60–70% will convert spontaneously in the first 24–48 hours. Studies have shown that some of the patients that converted spontaneously did not receive digoxin, verapamil, diltiazem, or a beta-blocker. Therefore, these drugs can be given to control the ventricular rate, and then patients can be sent home. If they do not convert spontaneously by the next day, then they can be admitted for cardioversion. Such treatment within 48 hours of the onset of atrial fibrillation makes anticoagulation unnecessary. Embolization during the first 48 hours is rare.

Many drugs have been used for cardioversion, but today **ibutilide** (a type III drug) is the therapy of choice. One milligram is given intravenously over 10 minutes, followed by a second milligram; if cardioversion does not occur, DC shock can be administered. The major side reaction with ibutilide is torsade de pointes. Check that the magnesium and potassium serum levels are normal and that the QTc is 440 msec or less before administration. Avoid ibutilide if the ejection fraction is very low.

Atrial fibrillation is more common the first 5 days after conversion because atrial fibrillation shortens the refractory period of the atrial muscle. This is due to calcium loading; thus it is preferable with digoxin to initially give verapamil or diltiazem, which may block this effect. Administer anticoagulation if the atrial fibrillation is beyond 48 hours of duration, prior thromboembolism has occurred, valvular disease is present, or a prosthetic heart valve is in place. In such cases, anticoagulation usually is required 3–4 weeks before and after cardioversion, maintaining the INR between 2 and 3. However, if transesophageal echo is available and no thrombus is noted, then only a few days of anticoagulation is needed prior to cardioversion, instead of 3–4 weeks. Transesophageal echo is cost effective, but it may not be logistically possible in many hospitals. After cardioversion, anticoagulation should be continued for 4 weeks.

Give antiarrhythmic drugs to prevent reoccurrence of atrial fibrillation. Quinidine, procainamide, disopyramide, propafenone, flecainide, sotalol, amiodarone, dofetidide, and azimidide (not yet released) are used to prevent recurrences. It generally is best to continue verapamil or diltiazem since they prevent calcium overloading of the atria and shortening of the atrial refractory phase. Along with these, an antiarrhythmic drug is added, depending on the underlying disorder. If there is no structural heart disease, propafenone and flecainide are preferable. Sotalol and amiodarone can be given if there is structural heart disease. In the presence of coronary artery disease, sotalol is the best choice; if congestive heart failure, use amiodarone. If there is no cause for a long QT interval, then quinidine, procainamide, or disopyramide can be given in the event other drugs are not successful in prevention.

The present patient converted spontaneously on digoxin and diltiazem.

Clinical Pearls

1. Recent-onset atrial fibrillation may not respond well to digitalis alone unless congestive heart failure is present. Add a beta-blocker, verapamil, or diltiazem to control the ventricular response.

2. Consider electric cardioversion if sinus rhythm is not pharmacologically restored in all patients with recent-onset nonvalvular atrial fibrillation—regardless of left atrial size.

3. Give oral anticoagulation to patients with nonvalvular atrial fibrillation prior to cardioversion if the arrhythmia occurred beyond 48 hours. Anticoagulation may be given only for a few days prior to conversion if transesophageal echo shows no thrombi.

4. Continue oral anticoagulation for 3–4 weeks after successful cardioversion, because effective atrial contraction may lag weeks behind restoration of normal sinus rhythm of EKG.

5. Atrial fibrillation can shorten the refractory phase for several days post conversion and cause recurrences of the arrhythmia. Calcium loading can be a factor, and this can be blocked by the use of verapamil or diltiazem.

REFERENCES

1. Bjerkelund CJ, Orning OM: The efficacy of anticoagulant therapy in preventing embolism related to DC electrical conversion of atrial fibrillation. Am J Cardiol 1969;23:208–216.
2. Grogan M, Smith HC, Gersh BJ, et al: Left ventricular dysfunction due to atrial fibrillation in patients initially believed to have idiopathic dilated cardiomyopathy. Am J Cardiol 1992;69:1570–1573.
3. Weigner MJ, Caulfield TA, Danias PG, et al: Risk for clinical thromboembolism associated with conversion to sinus rhythm in patients with atrial fibrillation lasting less than 48 hours. Ann Intern Med 1997;126:615–620.
4. Danias PG, Caulfield TA, Weigner MJ, et al: Likelihood of spontaneous conversion of atrial fibrillation to sinus rhythm. J Am Coll Cardiol 1998;31:588–592.
5. De Simone A, Stabile G, Vitale DF, et al: Pretreatment with verapamil in patients with persistent or chronic atrial fibrillation who underwent electrical cardioversion. J Am Coll Cardiol 1999;34:810–814.
6. Oral H, Souza JJ, Michaud GF, et al: Facilitating transthoracic cardioversion of atrial fibrillation with ibutilide pretreatment. N Engl J Med 1999;340:1849–1854.

PATIENT 59

A 67-year-old woman with an acute anterior myocardial infarction treated with thrombolytic therapy

A 67-year-old woman experienced a 2-hour episode of chest fullness, severe diaphoresis, shortness of breath, and nausea. A diagnosis of acute anterior myocardial infarction is made in the emergency department. The patient is given 325 mg of aspirin, and thrombolytic therapy is started. A lidocaine bolus and infusion are administered for complex ventricular ectopy.

Physical Examination: Vital signs: pulse 65; blood pressure 170/110. General: obese; no distress. Cardiac: no jugular venous distention; PMI not palpable; no murmurs; S_4 audible at the apex. Abdomen: obese; no masses or bruits. Extremities: no peripheral edema.

Laboratory Findings: Initial CPK 979 IU/L; serial CPKs increased to 2250 IU/L with 17% MB fraction.

Question: What is the thrombolytic agent of choice for this patient?

Answer: Recombinant tissue plasminogen activator (rt-PA) may be the thrombolytic agent of choice; however, therapeutic advances are changing our approach to the treatment of acute myocardial infarction.

Discussion: Many studies have compared three commonly used thrombolytic agents: **streptokinase** (SK), **recombinant tissue-type plasminogen activator** (rt-PA), and **anistreplase** (APSAC). Although all agents decrease mortality and increase left ventricular ejection fraction, differences between the drugs could lead to differences in effectiveness. For instance, the half-life of the agents is 20 minutes for SK, 5 minutes for rt-PA, and 90–120 minutes for APSAC. The International GISSI II study compared rt-PA and SK, and the ISIS-3 study compared duteplase (a variant of the human rt-PA), SK, and APSAC. No significant difference in hospital or 35-day mortality was found between treatment groups.

These trials have been criticized because heparin was administered subcutaneously and not as a continuous intravenous infusion, as is commonly done in the United States. Most physicians in the United States give 5000 units of heparin as bolus IV initially and then a titrated dose to maintain the partial thromboplastin time 1.5–2 times the control. Of interest, the European trials had a higher mortality than the American Thrombolysis and Thrombin Inhibition in Myocardial Infarction (TIMI) studies.

The Global Utilization of Streptokinase and Tissue Plasminogen Activator for Occluded Arteries (GUSTO) study was designed to compare streptokinase and rt-PA. Patients were randomized to one of four treatment regimens: frontloaded, weight-adjusted rt-PA with IV heparin; streptokinase with IV heparin; streptokinase with subcutaneous heparin; and a combination of rt-PA and streptokinase. There were approximately 10,000 patients of similar demography in each group. Accelerated rt-PA infusion with IV heparin yielded a higher patency rate and saved an additional 9–11 lives per 1000 patients compared with the streptokinase regimen. However, rt-PA resulted in one extra stroke per 1000 patients treated compared with streptokinase. Note that both rt-PA and APSAC are significantly more expensive than SK.

Reteplase (recombinant plasminogen activator) results in a higher incidence of normal flow rates and is easier to administer than rt-PA, but yields no clinical advantage in mortality. Many other thrombolytic agents are being evaluated. The ASSENT II trial is comparing TNK-TPA with rt-PA.

Besides thrombolytic therapy, consider aspirin, beta-blocker, nitroglycerin, heparin, and angiotensin-converting enzyme inhibitors. Ongoing trials are studying the rationale for **combination strategies** (drugs, angioplasties, and stents). Low-molecular-weight heparin (LMWH) and glycoprotein IIb/IIIa antagonists look very promising. Future studies will clarify whether LMWH and GP IIb/IIIa antagonists should be given routinely along with a thrombolytic agent or prior to angioplasty and/or stents. Perhaps a combination of low-dose thrombolysis and GP IIb/IIIa inhibitors can improve results (TIMI 14 trial and GUSTO 4). The Plasminogen-Activator Angioplasty Compatability Trial (PACT) is looking at the combination of low dose rt-PA and angioplasty if after rt-PA the first angiogram does not show TIMI grade 3 flow. Targeting each component of the occlusive coronary thrombus—fibrin (thrombolytic agent), thrombin (heparin), and platelets (aspirin and GP IIb/IIa)—may turn out to be the best combination.

The present patient was given rt-PA and IV heparin, and her chest pain subsided. The ST segments returned to the baseline and her subsequent course was uneventful.

Clinical Pearls

1. Although earlier trials found no difference in the effectiveness of thrombolytic agents, the GUSTO trial suggests that rt-PA is the most effective thrombolytic agent.

2. Reteplase has no advantage over rt-PA, but is easier to administer. Another new thrombolytic agent being studied is TNK-TPA.

3. Consider adjunctive therapy such as aspirin, beta-blockers, nitroglycerin, heparin, and angiotensin-converting enzymes inhibitors.

4. Many trials are targeting each component of the occlusive coronary thrombus: fibrin (thrombolytic agent), thrombus (heparin and LMWH), and platelets (GP IIb/IIIa inhibitors). These and other combinations are being evaluated.

REFERENCES

1. Preliminary Results of the Global Utilization of Streptokinase and t-PA for Occluded Coronary Arteries (GUSTO) Study. Presented at the Annual Meeting of the American Federation for Clinical Research in Washington, D.C., April 30, 1993.
2. The Global Use of Strategies to Open Occluded Coronary Arteries (GUSTO III) Investigators: A comparison of reteplase with alteplase for acute myocardial infarction. N Engl J Med 1997;337:1118–1123.
3. Cannon CP: Overcoming thrombolytic resistance. Rationale and initial clinical experience combining thrombolytic therapy and glycoprotein IIb/IIIa receptor inhibition for acute myocardial infarction. J Am Coll Cardiol 1999;34:1395–1402.
4. van den Merkhof LFM, Zijlstra F, Olsson H, et al: Abciximab in the treatment of acute myocardial infarction eligible for primary percutaneous transluminal coronary angioplasty. J Am Coll Cardiol 1999;33:1528–1532.

PATIENT 60

A 72-year-old man with episodes of lightheadedness

A 72-year-old man has experienced episodes of lightheadedness and near-syncope, which improve with sitting or lying down, for the previous several months. He denies chest pain or dyspnea. Holter monitoring, performed during numerous hospital admissions to evaluate these symptoms, reported sinus arrhythmia but no cardiac causes for his problems. He has been known to have hypertension for several years; it recently was controlled with nifedipine.

Physical Examination: Vital signs: pulse 70 (irregular); blood pressure 160/90; no orthostasis. Neck: carotid sinuses not sensitive to pressure; no carotid bruits. Chest: occasional rhonchi. Cardiac: no murmurs or extra sounds.

Laboratory Findings: CBC, urinalysis, blood chemistries: normal. EKG rhythm strip: see below.

Question: What is the diagnosis?

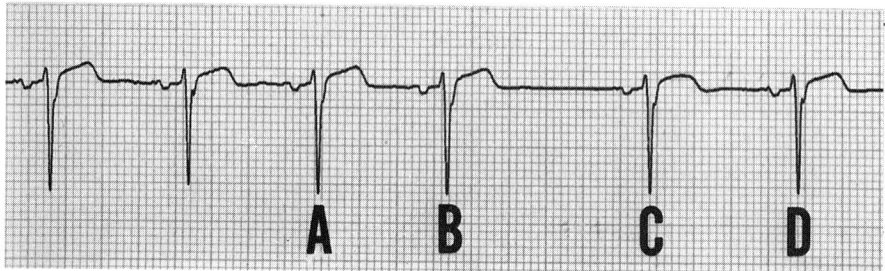

Figure reproduced from Gazes PC: Clinical Cardiology—A Cost-Effective Approach, 4th ed. New York, Chapman and Hall, 1997; with permission.

Diagnosis: Sick sinus syndrome (SSS).

Discussion: During previous evaluations, the present patient's EKG rhythm strips were interpreted as sinus arrhythmia. On closer observation of the EKG shown, however, the QRSs were noted to have typical Wenckebach groupings. The QRS complexes approach each other; the B–C interval is less than twice the preceding RR interval designated A–B; and the A–B interval is less than the RR interval designated C–D. Although this is the typical Wenckebach grouping noted in type I AV block, in this case the PR interval does not change as it does in AV block. Instead, these findings are diagnostic of **sinoatrial (SA) Wenckebach exit block.**

QRS complexes that occur in pairs may often be due to 3:2 Wenckebach block. Because the P-R interval is constant in SA nodal Wenckebach block, this rhythm often is mistaken for atrial bigeminy. In general, when grouped beating is recognized, suspect Wenckebach block as the cause.

To assist in diagnosis of SA node Wenckebach, measure the total Wenckebach period from the first P wave of the group to the first P wave of the next group. Divide this total value by the number of cycles, including the dropped beat that occurs during the total period. This value will give the SA node cycle length, which starts before the first P wave. It will occur with each beat further from the next P wave, giving the SA node progressive conduction time noted with a Wenckebach exit block of the SA node.

Frequently, sinus node dysfunction is suspected but difficult to prove, because the EKG is normal during the period of observation. In assessing the sinus node function, the sinus node recovery time and the SA conduction time can be measured during invasive electrophysiologic studies. While abnormal responses indicate sinus node disease, unfortunately the test is not sensitive. Omit drugs such as beta blockers, verapamil, diltiazem, and clonidine prior to testing, because they may cause SA node dysfunction.

The present patient had a pacemaker inserted and became asymptomatic. His lightheadedness was probably caused by a high-grade SA node exit block that was never recorded.

Clinical Pearls

1. Grouped beating always should raise the suspicion of Wenckebach block.
2. SA node Wenckebach exit block has the same grouping as AV node Wenckebach block, but the PR interval does not change.
3. SA node Wenckebach exit block often is misdiagnosed as sinus arrhythmia.

REFERENCES

1. Breithardt G, Seipel L, Loogen F: Sinus node recovery time and calculated sinoatrial conduction time in normal subjects and patients with sinus node dysfunction. Circulation 1977;56:43–50.
2. Chung EK: Sick sinus syndrome: Current views. Mod Concepts Cardiovasc Dis 1980;49:61–66.
3. Dreifus LS, Hessen SE: Sinoatrial block: Bradycardia-tachycardia syndrome. The Heart House Learning Center 1990;6:1–15.
4. Gergoratos G, Cheitlin MD, Conill AC, et al: ACC/AHA Guidelines for implantation of cardiac pacemakers and antiarrhythmia devices. JACC 1998;31:1175–1209.

PATIENT 61

A 54-year-old man with a basal systolic murmur and right bundle branch block

A 54-year-old man is noted on routine examination to have a basal systolic murmur and right bundle branch block, and he is referred to a cardiologist for further evaluation. He denies chest pain, dyspnea, and peripheral edema. He has been told for many years that he has a functional murmur.

Physical Examination: Vital signs: pulse 80; blood pressure 130/80. General: obese. Cardiac: no palpable lifts; wide fixed splitting of S_2; a systolic ejection murmur in the pulmonic area; a midsystolic click followed by a high-pitched murmur of mitral insufficiency at the apex.

Laboratory Findings: CBC and urinalysis: normal. Chest radiography: a small aortic knob; large pulmonary arteries with prominent tertiary branches. EKG: right bundle branch block. Cardiac catheterization data: see below. The catheter entered a pulmonary vein directly from the right atrium.

Hemodynamic measurements	Pressure (mmHg)	Oxygen saturation (%)
Superior vena cava		65
Inferior vena cava		73
Mid right atrium	11	85
Right ventricle	30/12	85
Pulmonary artery	26/16	84
Pulmonary vein		94
Aorta	110/70	91

Question: What is the diagnosis?

Diagnosis: Atrial septal defect (sinus venous type), partial anomalous pulmonary venous drainage, and mitral valve prolapse.

Discussion: There are three types of atrial septal defects: sinus venous, ostium secundum, and ostium primum. The most common is the **ostium secundum defect,** which occurs in the mid-atrium and often is associated with mitral valve prolapse. The **sinus venous type** occurs higher in the septum near the entrance of the superior vena cava into the right atrium and often is associated with anomalous pulmonary venous drainage. The **ostium primum defect** is located low in the atrial septum; it results from an endocardial cushion defect and may involve the membranous ventricular septum and atrioventricular valves.

An atrial septal defect should be suspected if there are bony abnormalities of the extremities, such as a thumb resembling a finger (Holt-Oram syndrome). Otherwise, findings on physical examination are similar for the three types. Often a hyperdynamic, brief, right ventricular lift is present. The characteristic finding is wide, fixed splitting of the second heart sound. The splitting, which does not vary with respiration, occurs despite the normal increase in systemic venous return with inspiration and decrease during expiration, because there is less flow through the atrial septal defect during inspiration and more flow occurring during expiration. Thus, there is a constant, large, right ventricular stroke volume during inspiration and expiration, which causes a constant delay in pulmonic valve closure.

The systolic ejection murmur of an atrial septal defect is due to the increased flow across the pulmonary outflow tract. There is no murmur generated by the atrial septal defect itself. At times with large shunts, the increased flow across the tricuspid valve can produce a mid-diastolic rumbling murmur at the fourth intercostal space along the left sternal border. This murmur has been confused with mitral stenosis but can be differentiated on the basis that the murmur increases during inspiration in an atrial septal defect. The combination of an atrial septal defect and mitral stenosis is known as **Lutembacher's syndrome.** Perhaps some of these reported in the past did not have mitral stenosis; rather, the diastolic rumbling murmur was that of the tricuspid flow type associated with a large left-to-right atrial shunt.

Partial anamolous pulmonary venous drainage results in the same clinical picture as an uncomplicated atrial septal defect. A mid-systolic click with late apical systolic murmur indicates mitral valve prolapse, which most often is noted with a secundum defect. This type of prolapse associated with a small left ventricle may disappear after surgical closure of the atrial septal defect.

The EKG usually shows outflow tract right ventricular hypertrophy, but right bundle branch block often is noted in adults. An ostium primum defect is suggested if there is first-degree or higher AV block or left axis deviation, since the conduction system is involved by the endocardial cushion defect. The venous type defect may be associated with an ectopic pacemaker focus. Many children can escape to adulthood before the defect is detected because it is well tolerated. In adults, an atrial septal defect typically is noted because of chest radiographic findings of a small aortic knob, large pulmonary arteries with prominent tertiary branches, and right ventricular enlargement. Echocardiographic and Doppler studies demonstrate the enlarged right ventricle, the shunt, and paradoxical systolic motion of the septum. Heart catheterization studies demonstrate a step-up in oxygen saturation in the right atrium. When a high saturation is found in the superior vena cava *or the catheter enters a pulmonary vein directly from the right atrium,* a sinus venosus type defect with partial anomalous pulmonary venous return is most likely. The present patient showed these findings.

Atrial septal defects with significant shunts should be closed even if the patient is over 60 years of age. The left ventricle can have decreased distensibility due to age, associated hypertension, or coronary artery disease. This decreased distensibility impairs left ventricular filling that can increase the shunt, leading to right ventricular volume overload, right ventricular failure, pulmonary and paradoxical systemic embolization, supraventricular arrhythmias, and, rarely, pulmonary hypertension.

Following surgery, patients may have persistent atrial arrhythmias, or arrhythmias may develop for the first time. In selected patients, centrally located defects can be closed by transcatheter devices of the clamshell type.

In the present patient, a sinus venosus defect and anomalous pulmonary venous return were noted at surgery. The sinus venosus defect was repaired with a patch that included the right superior pulmonary vein into the left atrium. A small patent foramen ovale was closed by direct suturing. The patient remains asymptomatic.

Clinical Pearls

1. If a patient has a thumb that resembles a finger or other upper-extremity abnormality, suspect a secundum type atrial defect.
2. Wide, fixed splitting of the second sound almost always indicates atrial septal defect and/or partial anomalous pulmonary venous drainage.
3. A chest radiograph often provides the first clue to the diagnosis of an atrial septal defect in adults and shows a small aortic knob, large pulmonary arteries with prominent tertiary branches, and right ventricular enlargement.
4. A normal width QRS resembling a right bundle branch block often is associated with an atrial septal defect in young patients, and a right bundle block is noted in adults.
5. Atrial arrhythmias are common in atrial septal defect and may persist or appear for the first time after surgical repair.
6. The defect can be closed with transcather devices in selected patients.

REFERENCES

1. Smith AT, Sack GH Jr, Taylor GJ: Holt-Oram syndrome. J Pediatr 1979;95:538–543.
2. Nagata S, Nimura Y, Sakakibara H, et al: Mitral valve lesion associated with secumdum atrial septal defect. Br Heart J 1983;49;51–58.
3. Konstantinides S, Geibel A, Olschewski M, et al: A comparison of surgical and medical therapy for atrial septal defect in adults. New Engl J Med 1995;333:469.

PATIENT 62

A 62-year-old man with syncope after voiding

A 62-year-old man experienced a syncopal episode when voiding after awakening from sleep. He recovered promptly. He denies premonitory symptoms, but states that he consumed 4 ounces of ethanol prior to going to bed. Additionally, he experienced a similar episode 30 years earlier. Otherwise, the patient is in good health and very active, without cardiovascular symptoms.

Physical Examination: Vital signs: pulse 80; blood pressure 130/80. Neck: no bruits. Cardiac: normal. Neurologic examination: normal.

Laboratory Findings: EKG: right bundle branch block with a left axis of −45°. Electrophysiologic studies: normal HV interval of 52 msec; normal SA and AV node function; no inducible arrhythmias. When his groin is infiltrated with local anesthesia in preparation for the procedure, he experiences a vagal episode, with his heart rate dropping to 17 beats/min.

Question: What is the likely cause of the patient's syncope?

Diagnosis: Postmicturition syncope.

Discussion: Postmicturition syndrome is triggered by vagal sensory input from the rapid emptying of the bladder during voiding, which causes **reflex vasodilatation** and **decreased cerebral blood flow.** The syndrome usually occurs in the early morning hours when vascular resistance is low. Alcohol consumption may further reduce peripheral resistance, contributing to the syndrome. Other cardiovascular causes of syncope are the vasovagal faint, autonomic dysfunction (neurally mediated hypotensive bradycardia syndrome), obstruction to cardiac inflow or outflow, and both tachyarrhythmias and bradyarrhythmias.

The pathophysiologic mechanism for syncope in patients with autonomic dysfunction is complex. On assuming an upright position, central volume decreases, which stimulates the baroreceptors and causes central adrenergic stimulation, which in turn increases inotropic state and heart rate. Hypercontraction of the left ventricle activates cardiac mechanical receptors, producing the **Bezold-Jarisch reflex.** In this reflex, signals are carried to the central nervous system by C-fibers, producing an increase in sympathetic outflow and causing vasodilatation, a decrease in blood pressure, and an increase in vagal tone, which decreases the heart rate. This combination of active vasodilatation and bradycardia causes the syncope.

When a cardiac cause for syncope is present, it can be suspected on the basis of history and physical examination alone in 50% of cases. If cardiac abnormalities are detected, Holter monitoring, event loop recording, implantable loop recorder, tilt testing, and electrophysiologic testing may help you arrive at a specific diagnosis. The yield of Holter monitoring is low—it is definitive in only 1% of cases and rules out a cardiac cause in about 15% of cases. The arrhythmic yield is about 40% in preliminary studies with an implantable loop recorder over a period up to 14 months. Results of electrophysiologic testing are of very low yield if the history, physical examination, and resting EKG are normal. The yield of electrophysiologic testing increases significantly, however, in patients with cardiac disease detected by routine examination.

The present patient's syncope was typical for that associated with micturition. It occurred after he had several alcoholic drinks and got out of a warm bed. However, in view of the right bundle branch block and left anterior fasicular block, trifascicular block with transient third-degree AV block and syncope had to be excluded. Therefore, electrophysiologic studies were performed. During the needle puncture of his groin, he experienced a vasovagal reaction that was similar to his postmicturition syncope, but no higher degrees of conduction disturbance were detected.

Clinical Pearls

1. Cardiovascular syncope can be diagnosed in 50% of cases by obtaining a thorough history and conducting a detailed physical examination.

2. Postmicturition syncope often occurs after ingestion of alcohol when the patient arises from a warm bed to void.

3. The yield of Holter monitoring in diagnosing the cause of syncope is quite low.

4. Autonomic dysfunction (neurocardiogenic syncope) is a relatively new diagnosis, accounting for many cases of syncope. It often occurs in individuals without structural heart disease and can be detected by the tilt-table test.

REFERENCES

1. Shaal SF, Nelson SD, Boudoulas H, Lewis RP: Syncope. Curr Probl Cardiol 1992;27:211–264.
2. Kosinski DJ, Wolfe PA, Grubb BP: Neurocardiogenic syncope: A review of pathophysiology, diagnosis, and treatment. Cardiovasc Rev Rep 1993;14:22–29.
3. ACC/AHA Guidelines for Ambulatory Electrocardiography: Executive Summary and Recommendations. A report of the American College of Cardiology/American Heart Association Task Force on Practice Guidelines (Committee to Revised the Guidelines for Ambulatory Electrophysiology). Circulation 1999;100:886–893.
4. Krahn AD, Klein GJ, Yee R, et al: Use of extended monitoring strategy in patients with problematic syncope. Circulation 1999;99:406–410.

PATIENT 63

A 65-year-old woman with an acute inferior infarction and premature ventricular beats

A 65-year-old woman presents to the Chest Pain Clinic with a 1-hour history of substernal chest pain that is radiating to her neck and down both arms. She has known hypertension and diabetes.

Physical Examination: Vital signs: pulse 70 and irregular; blood pressure 140/90. Cardiac: no jugular venous distention; no murmurs or gallops noted. Chest: clear. Abdomen: normal. Extremities: normal.

Laboratory Findings: EKG: acute inferior myocardial infarction; premature ventricular beats (PVBs). Rhythm strip: see below.

Question: Should this patient receive prophylactic lidocaine?

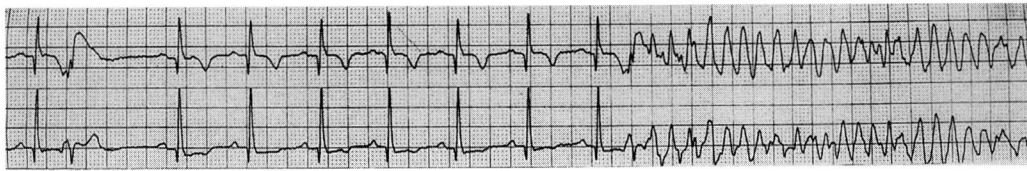

Answer: The decision rests on the type and severity of the ventricular ectopy.

Discussion: If, during the acute stage of a myocardial infarction, the patient has complex ventricular arrhythmias, including runs of ventricular tachycardia, multifocal PVBs, more than six PVBs per minute, or the "R-on-T" phenomenon, most agree that lidocaine should be given, because these arrhythmias may presage ventricular fibrillation. However, administering prophylactic lidocaine in the absence of such arrhythmias is no longer advised, because although primary ventricular fibrillation can be prevented by lidocaine, the drug also increases the risk of aystole. Lidocaine-induced aystole is perhaps more common in inferior infarctions, although this point is unproved.

The impetus to prevent ventricular fibrillation during acute myocardial infarction derives from studies that show that patients who are resuscitated following primary ventricular fibrillation have an increased incidence of in-hospital mortality. However, meta-analysis of randomized trials of lidocaine therapy do not show a decrease in mortality.

The proper dosing schedule is uncertain because different studies used different schedules. We recommend an initial dose of 1.5 mg/kg given as an intravenous bolus injection, followed 15 minutes later by a second bolus injection of 0.5 mg/kg, followed by a constant infusion of 2–4 mg/min. This dose must be decreased in patients over the age of 70, in patients with congestive heart failure, in patients with hepatic dysfunction, and in patients receiving cimetidine, all of whom are more likely to develop lidocaine intoxication because of reduced drug metabolism. Intoxication often produces the neurologic symptoms of slurred speech, obtundation, and seizures.

Since newer forms of therapy for acute myocardial infarction (thrombolytics, adjunctive agents, and invasive procedures) were introduced, the 10% incidence of ventricular fibrillation reported formerly has now been reduced dramatically. Most patients now receive **beta-blockers**, which may not prevent ventricular ectopy, but do reduce ventricular fibrillation and mortality from acute myocardial infarction.

On admission to the coronary care unit, the present patient's EKG showed occasional R-on-T PVBs. She subsequently developed ventricular fibrillation, which responded to DC shock. Her remaining course was uneventful.

Clinical Pearls

1. Give lidocaine for complex ventricular arrhythmias in the setting of an acute myocardial infarction, especially if R-on-T PVBs are present.
2. Routine use of prophylactic lidocaine is no longer indicated.
3. Toxic manifestations of lidocaine are more apt to occur in the elderly or patients with heart failure, hypotension, or liver disease.

REFERENCES

1. Volpi A, Maggioni A, Franzosi MG, et al: In-hospital prognosis of patients with acute myocardial infarction complicated by primary ventricular fibrillation. N Engl J Med 1987;317:257–261.
2. Teo KK, Yusef S, Furberg CD: Effects of prophylactic antiarrhythmic drug therapy in acute myocardial infarction: an overview of results from randomized controlled trials. JAMA 1993;270:1589–1595.
3. Ryan TJ, Anderson JL, Antman EM, et al: ACC/AHA guidelines for the management of patients with acute myocardial infarction. J Am Coll Cardiol 1996;28:1328–1428.

PATIENT 64

A 70-year-old woman with transient ischemic attacks and a cold right hand

A 70-year-old woman with known hypertension experiences two transient cerebral ischemic attacks, followed by the sudden onset of coldness of her right hand. She has no history of acute myocardial infarctions or palpitations.

Physical Examination: Vital signs: pulse 90; blood pressure 155/80. Cardiac: grade II/VI aortic systolic ejection murmur audible in the primary aortic area; no extra sounds. Chest: clear. Extremities: absent right radial pulse; cold right hand with cyanotic finger tips.

Laboratory Findings: CBC and urinalysis: normal. EKG: normal. M-mode and two-D echocardiogram: normal. Transeophageal echocardiogram: see below.

Question: What is your diagnosis?

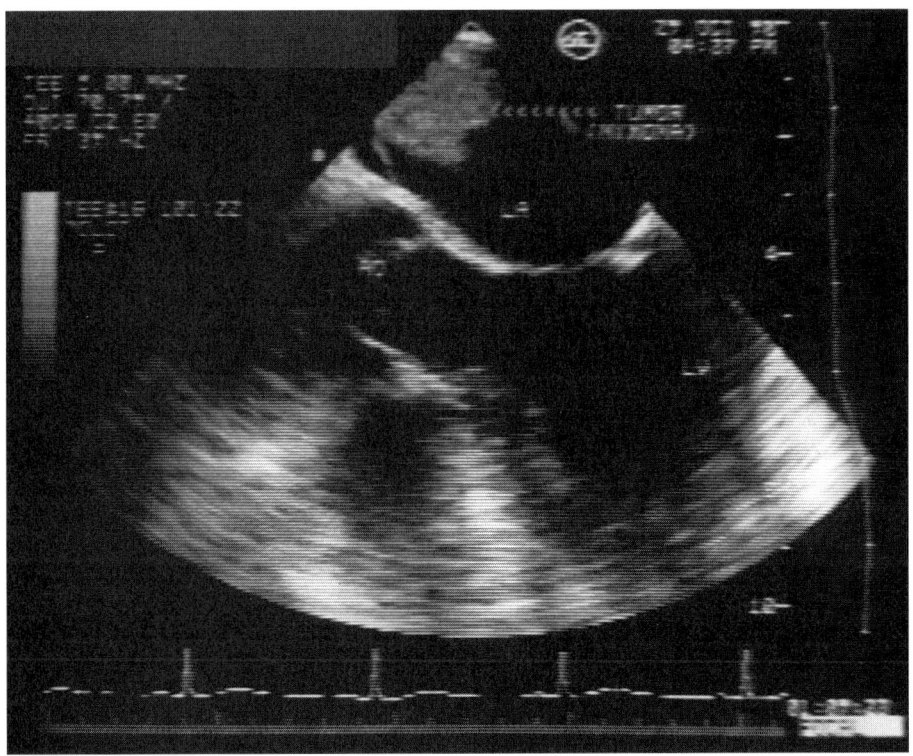

Diagnosis: Left atrial myxoma with emboli to brain and right radial artery.

Discussion: Compared to other conditions affecting the heart, primary cardiac tumors are rare disorders; metastatic tumors are more common. Primary tumors are benign in 75% of patients. Up to 50% of these benign primary cardiac tumors are myxomas. Most myxomas arise from the left atrium where they usually are attached to the fossa ovalis. The cell origin is controversial. Some authorities believe that myxomas have a mesenchymal origin, whereas others think they derive from endocardial cells.

Symptoms of left atrial myxoma fall into three categories: (1) **local mechanical effects,** (2) **embolic consequences,** and (3) **systemic symptoms.** The local effects of the tumor may closely resemble those of mitral stenosis, as the tumor obstructs the mitral orifice and prevents left atria outflow. In distinction to mitral stenosis, however, the tumor effects may be gravity dependent and typically are more severe when the patient is standing upright, allowing gravity to pull the tumor into the mitral orifice. The embolic phenomena often are the first manifestations of the disease. The diagnosis sometimes is made from the material extracted by embolectomy. An embolic stroke or other vascular embolic occlusion in a young person without an obvious source of embolism should arouse suspicion that a myxoma may be present. Approximately one-third of patients also experience fatigue, fever, and weight loss—which, in connection with the embolic phenomena, could easily be mistaken for infective endocarditis. Raynaud's phenomenon, elevated sedimentation rate, and hyperglobulinemia also may be present.

On physical examination, an early diastolic sound (tumor plop) often is followed by a diastolic murmur, further confusing this disease with mitral stenosis. The tumor may damage the mitral valve, leading to the murmur of mitral regurgitation. Atrial fibrillation rarely occurs.

Although myxomas typically arise from the left atrium, they also have been noted to arise (in order of decreasing incidence) from the right atrium, right ventricle, and left ventricle. Suspect right-sided myxomas if syncope, variable tricuspid murmurs, or pulmonary emboli occur. Occasionally, these right-sided myxomas may have pericarditis. Right bundle branch block and atrial flutter or fibrillation occur frequently.

Echocardiography is by far the most direct and accurate way to make the diagnosis. Myxomas also may be revealed by cine CT scanning, MRI, and angiography. Angiographically, the tumor is discerned during the levo phase of pulmonary arteriography when dye fills the left atrium. Occasionally, as in this case, transesophageal echocardiography (TEE) is necessary to make the diagnosis. TEE is a rapidly developing technique that allows superb visualization of the heart and great vessels. TEE is not limited by interference from the chest wall or lungs, which occasionally reduces the image quality of transthoracic echocardiography.

The only effective therapy for atrial myxoma is surgical removal. In 95% of cases, surgery effects a permanent cure. Approximately 5% of patients have recurrences. During surgery, it is important that the stalk and surrounding area is entirely excised. In some cases, this produces a small atrial septal defect that usually can be easily repaired.

In the present patient, embolectomy from the right radial artery showed the obstruction to be due to myxomatous tissue. Although M-mode and two-dimensional echocardiogram did not demonstrate the left atrial myxoma, it was clearly seen on the TEE. Its location on the posterior aspect of the left atrium made surface visualization more difficult. The mass was 4.8 cm^2 in diameter. It did not involve the mitral valve, and its characteristics were consistent with a myxoma, which was subsequently confirmed by microscopy following surgical resection.

Clinical Pearls

1. Atrial myxomas may entirely mimic mitral stenosis or infective endocarditis.
2. Suspect the diagnosis when a stroke or systemic embolization occurs in a healthy, young patient—in whom other causes of embolization are rare.
3. Atrial myxomas must be surgically removed; however, 5% recur following surgery, and postoperative surveillance is required.

REFERENCES

1. Obeid AI, Marvasti M, Parker F, et al: Comparison of transthoracic and transesophageal echocardiography in diagnosis of left atrial myxoma. Am J Cardiol 1989;63:1006–1008.
2. Salcedo EE, Cohen GI, White RD, et al: Cardiac tumors. Diagnosis and management. Curr Probl Cardio 1992;17:79.
3. McAllister HA, Hall RJ, Cooley DA: Tumors of the heart and pericardium. Curr Probl Cardiol 1999;24:63–116.

PATIENT 65

A 70-year-old alcoholic man with sinus bradycardia and confusion

A 70-year-old man with known alcoholism was found outside, semicomatose and confused, on a cold winter day. He had not been known to have cardiac disease. His family states that he drinks almost on a daily basis, but always appears mentally alert.

Physical Examination: Vital signs: rectal temperature 86°F; pulse 34; blood pressure 80/50. General: confused; could not respond to commands. Chest: clear. Cardiac: decreased heart sounds. Abdomen: soft.

Laboratory Findings: Hct 53%; WBC and electrolytes: normal. EKG: see below.

Question: What is the etiology of the patient's EKG abnormalities?

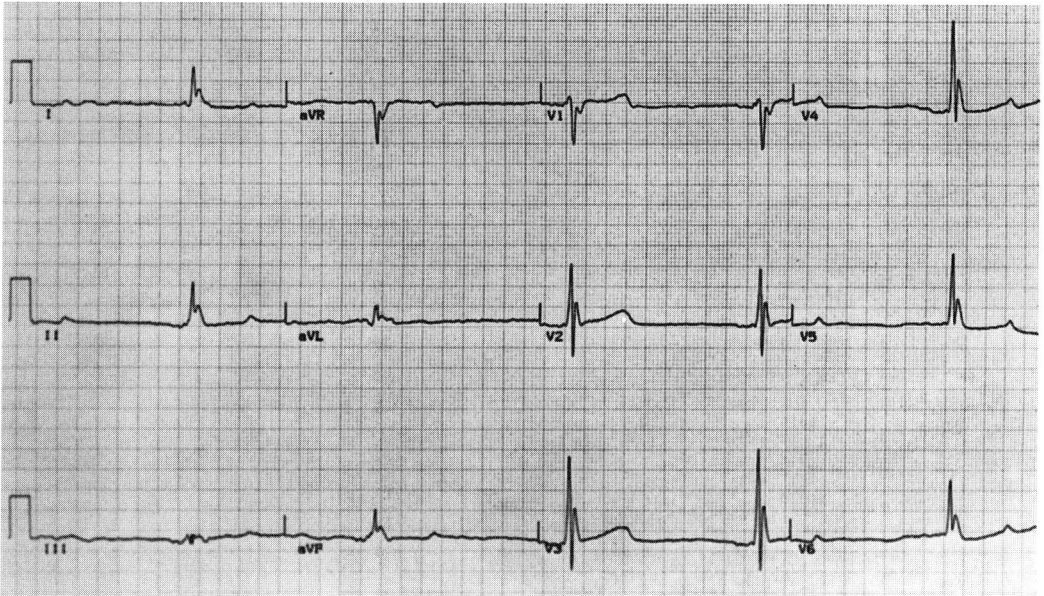

Diagnosis: Hypothermia.

Discussion: Hypothermia is a clinical problem defined as a body temperature <95°F. Common associated conditions include alcoholism, hypothyroidism, and central nervous system disease. The use of phenothiazines and barbiturates contribute to the disorder. The elderly are more prone to hypothermia because of a decreased ability to increase metabolic rate and heat production, decreased muscle mass, and decreased vasoconstrictive response to cold.

The physiologic response to mild hypothermia is an increase in blood pressure, pulse rate, cardiac output, central venous pressure, and peripheral vascular resistance. Few serious complications arise until body temperature falls below 92°. As body temperature drops below 89°F, heart rate, blood pressure, and cardiac output begin to decline. Atrial fibrillation is a common arrhythmia below 90°, and the risk of ventricular fibrillation increases dramatically when body temperature falls below 86°. Circulatory collapse produced by hypothermia causes abnormalities of the myocardium by producing abnormalities of the microcirculation (microinfarcts, subendocardial hemorrhages, and petechiae).

The kidney may be affected by hypothermia and secondarily alters cardiovascular function. Decreased core body temperature reduces renal concentrating ability, leading to a "cold diuresis." This diuresis can lead to intravascular volume depletion, further compounding the hypotension associated with depressed cardiac function. Other consequences of hypothermia include central nervous system (CNS) depression, respiratory alkalosis, hyperglycemia (because insulin secretion is reduced), intestinal ileus, and pancreatitis.

A thermometer must be used that can record in the hypothermic ranges. Evaluation of arterial blood gases is necessary, but the clinician should know whether the reporting laboratory has temperature-corrected blood gas results. The hematocrit is a useful guide in assessing volume depletion by estimating the amount of hemoconcentration.

Treatment of mild hypothermia (temperature >86°F) in a conscious patient is best accomplished by passive rewarming with blankets. Active rewarming by applying warm packs may be dangerous because they cause peripheral vasodilation, which paradoxically can cause worsening of the core hypothermia. Treatment of severe hypothermia requires intensive care. The patient should be intubated and placed on a respirator. Because the patient is likely to be alkalemic, care must be taken not to exacerbate the alkalosis by overventilation. Volume repletion is almost always necessary, and fluids should be warmed to 98.6°F prior to infusion.

If rapid rewarming is necessary because of cardiac instability or severe hypothermia, warm fluids by nasogastric tube or rectal tube may contribute to raising body temperature, but the effect is minor. In severe instances with unstable hemodynamics, rewarming with cardiopulmonary bypass may improve patient outcome. Active external warming should be limited to the trunk, allowing the limbs to remain temporarily vasoconstricted to reduce the chance of paradoxic worsening of central hypothermia. Most arrhythmias resolve upon rewarming, and antiarrhythmic drugs rarely are necessary. Ventricular fibrillation often is refractory until there has been significant rewarming. Patients may appear dead, but should not be pronounced so until rewarming has been accomplished and resuscitation fails.

The present patient demonstrated a typical EKG feature of hypothermia—**sinus bradycardia and J wave**—which is called an **Osborn's wave.** The J wave is noted as a deflection inscribed between the QRS complex and the beginning of the ST segment. The electrophysiologic mechanism of the Osborn wave is not known. The patient underwent passive rewarming and recovered.

Clinical Pearls

1. The elderly, alcoholics, and persons with CNS disease are most prone to hypothermia.
2. Active peripheral rewarming may cause a paradoxic central worsening of the hypothermia.
3. Osborn's wave is the characteristic EKG finding of hypothermia.
4. Clinicians must know whether blood gas results have been temperature-corrected, to accurately assess oxygenation and acid-base disturbances.

REFERENCES

1. Osborn JJ: Experimental hypothermia: Respiratory and blood pH changes in relation to cardiac function. Am J Physiol 1953;175:389–398.
2. Reuler JB: Hypothermia: Pathophysiology, clinical settings, and management. Ann Intern Med 1978;89:519–527.
3. Povoa R, Arroyo JB, Ferreira C, et al: Electrocardiographic changes in accidental hypothermia. Arq Bras Cardiol 1992;58:11–14.

PATIENT 66

A 57-year-old woman with episodes of palpitations not controlled with carotid sinus massage

A 57-year-old woman noted episodes of "rapid heart beat" over the previous 3 months. The episodes stopped abruptly but often recurred several times a day. They appeared to be less frequent upon walking. At times she had sharp left chest pain and dyspnea with exertion. Carotid sinus massage did not abort the arrhythmia.

Physical Examination: Vital signs: pulse irregular, rate 150; blood pressure 120/70. Cardiac: no clicks or murmurs noted with various maneuvers.

Laboratory Findings: CBC, urinalysis, electrolytes, creatinine: normal. EKG: normal with premature atrial beats. Thallium stress test with peak heart rate of 160 beats/min: normal. Echo Doppler studies: normal. Holter monitoring strip: see below.

Question: What arrhythmia is occurring?

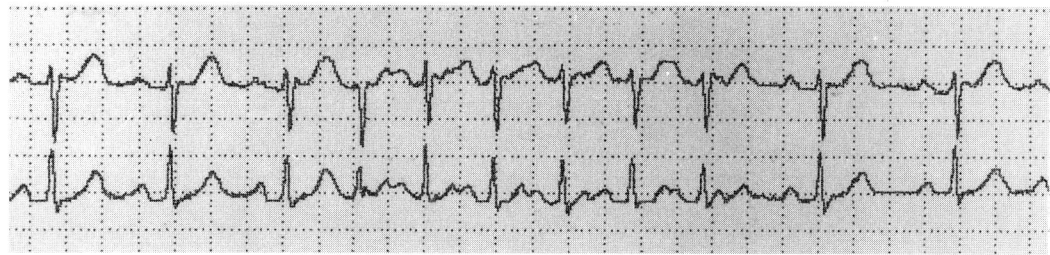

Diagnosis: Recurrent atrial tachycardia.

Discussion: Atrial tachycardia (long RP type) accounts for less than 10% of the supraventricular tachycardias. Atrial tachycardia results from enhanced automaticity, triggered activity, and atrial reentry. The rhythm may be idiopathic or caused by myocardial infarction, ethanol ingestion, chronic lung disease, digitalis intoxication, or metabolic abnormalities.

The rate ranges from 100–200 beats/min; it may be sustained or nonsustained. The arrhythmia is somewhat irregular, with a warm-up period during which the rate increases after the first few beats, and a period of slowing before termination of the arrhythmia. The abnormal P waves, seen before the QRS complexes, are the same throughout the arrhythmia, differing from atrioventricular (AV) nodal reentry tachycardia, in which the initial ectopic P wave differs from the subsequent retrograde P waves. In addition, a premature atrial beat resets but does not convert atrial tachycardia, whereas a premature beat usually terminates the reentry type.

If bundle branch block or aberration is present, the QRS complexes are wide and the tachycardia can resemble ventricular tachycardia, especially if the P waves are buried in the T waves and thus not seen. Atrial tachycardia can have varying degrees of AV block. Although vagal maneuvers may stop reentry in AV nodal tachycardia, it only increases AV block in atrial tachycardia and does not abort the arrhythmia.

Atrial tachycardia with AV block (PAT with block) can be due to **heart disease** alone, but in about 50% of cases it is due to **digitalis toxicity.** This is usually manifested by a 2:1 block, but at times may appear as Wenckebach block. If the atrial rate is closer to 250, it may be difficult to distinguish from atrial flutter. Although the atrial waves in flutter appear as sawtooth waves, this morphology also may be seen with atrial tachycardia. Further confusion arises because the atrial rate in atrial flutter may be slower, and thus in the range of atrial tachycardia, if the patient has been taking an antiarrhythmic agent such as the Class 1A drugs.

Therapy may be difficult. Class 1A drugs (quinidine, disopyramide, procainamide) usually suppress the atrial tachycardia. The automatic types respond to beta blockers. Verapamil or diltiazem increases the AV block but has no effect on the atrial rate. Discontinue digitalis if atrial tachycardia with block occurs. Correct hypokalemia if it is present. The incessant atrial tachycardia (lasting more than half of the day) can result in dilated cardiomyopathy. In such cases, perform radiofrequency ablation.

The present patient was treated successfully with quinidine sulfate.

Clinical Pearls

1. Unlike AV nodal reentrant tachycardia, atrial tachycardia usually has P waves before each QRS and is not aborted by an ectopic beat.

2. Vagal maneuvers and drugs that increase vagal tone increase the AV block in atrial tachycardia, but do not terminate the arrhythmia.

3. Atrial tachycardia with block often is due to digitalis toxicity.

4. The incessant types respond to radiofrequency ablation.

REFERENCES
1. Goldreyer BN, Gallagher JJ, Damato AN: The electrophysiologic demonstration of atrial ectopic tachycardia in man. Am Heart J 1973;85:205–215.
2. Peters RW, Scheinman MM: Emergency treatment of supraventricular tachycardia. Med Clin North Am 1979;63:7392.
3. Chen SA, Chiang CE, Yang CJ, et al: Sustained atrial tachycardia in adult patients. Electrophysiological characteristics, pharmacological response, possible mechanisms, and effects of radiofrequency ablation. Circulation 1994;90:1262.

PATIENT 67

A 60-year-old woman with sluggishness, fatigue, and chest pain

A 60-year-old woman has experienced sluggishness, fatigue, exertional dyspnea, substernal chest pain, and hoarseness for several months. She describes the chest pain as a tightness that occurs with exertion. In addition, the patient cannot tolerate cold weather. She denies hypertension and diabetes.

Physical Examination: Vital signs: pulse 45; blood pressure 100/70. General: moderately obese. Head: coarse hair. Skin: dry and puffy. Neurologic: delayed deep tendon reflexes.

Laboratory Findings: CBC and urinalysis: normal. Cholesterol: 350 mg. Chest radiograph: increased cardiac silhouette. EKG: see below.

Question: What is the probable diagnosis?

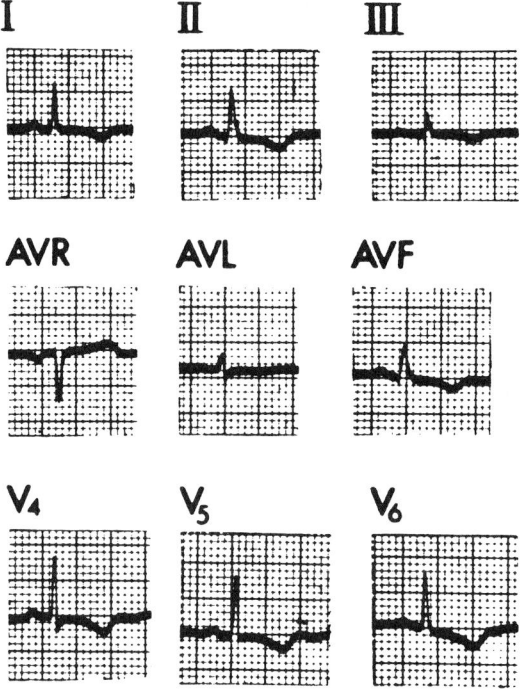

Figure reproduced from Gazes PC: Clinical Cardiology—A Cost-Effective Approach, 4th ed. New York, Chapman and Hall, 1997; with permission.

Diagnosis: Myxedema with coronary artery disease (stable angina).

Discussion: Patients with **hypothroidism** may present with varied manifestations of cardiac disease due to abnormalities of the myocardium, pericardium, and coronary vascular bed. **Pericardial effusions** develop in approximately 50% of patients with longstanding hypothyroidism. The effusions typically progress slowly, allowing the pericardium to stretch and accommodate the fluid collection. Consequently, pericardial tamponade is a rare clinical finding in patients with pericardial effusions due to hypothyroidism.

Additionally, hypothyroidism may depress myocardial contractility and decrease cardiac output partially because of the mucoid infiltration, muscle cell necrosis, and interstitial fibrosis found within the myocardium in patients with **myxedema.** Although contractility is decreased, normal left ventricular filling pressures usually are maintained, so that patients do not often present with clinical manifestations of increased pulmonary or right-sided systemic venous pressures.

Although patients with hypothyroidism appear to be at risk for significant serum lipid abnormalities, it remains unclear whether patients with hypothyroidism have an increased risk for atherosclerotic coronary artery disease. It is probable that coronary disease is more prevalent in myxedema, yet myocardial infarction and angina are less common because of decreased metabolic demands on the myocardium. Bradyarrhythmias are another typical cardiac manifestation of hypothyroidism.

The diagnosis of myxedema is suspected in the presence of the classic signs and symptoms, which include fatigue, dyspnea, hoarseness, coarse hair, slow return of the reflex response, dry puffy skin, and findings of depressed myocardial function. The arterial pulse pressure usually is narrow, and the cardiac sounds are decreased. Paradoxically, hypertension has been noted, especially in the elderly. Some patients demonstrate a cervical scar, indicating a previous thyroidectomy. Interestingly, a new cause of hypothyroidism is amiodarone therapy, which alters thyroid function by inhibiting the peripheral conversion of T4 and T3 and by inhibiting iodine organification.

Suggestive laboratory findings include EKG abnormalities of low voltage and inverted T waves (shown on previous page). The chest radiograph may demonstrate an enlarged cardiac silhouette, which typically is demonstrated by echocardiography to be due to the presence of pericardial effusion.

The present patient had thyroid studies diagnostic of hypothyroidism. Thyroid hormone was replaced slowly because angina, heart failure, and major arrhythmia would likely be precipitated in this patient who had underlying coronary artery disease indicated by a history of angina. With therapy, the patient's heart size returned to normal.

Clinical Pearls

1. The EKG findings of sinus bradycardia, low voltage, and inverted T waves suggest myxedema.

2. Thyroid hormone should be replaced in gradually increasing doses, especially if the patient has underlying coronary artery disease.

3. An enlarged cardiac silhouette is common in myxedema and usually is due to the presence of a pericardial effusion.

4. Amiodarone is a new, relatively common cause of decreased thyroid function.

REFERENCES

1. Shenoy MM, Goldman JM: Hypothyroid cardiomyopathy: Echocardiographic documentation of reversibility. Am J Med Sci 1987;294:1–9.
2. Lee RT, Plappert M, St. John Sutton MG: Depressed left ventricular systolic ejection force in hypothyroidism. Am J Cardiol 1990;65:5236–527.
3. Aronow WS: The heart and thyroid disease. Clin Geriatr Med 1995;11:219–229.
4. Perk M, O'Neill BJ: The effect of thyroid hormone therapy on angiographic coronary artery disease progression. Can J Cardiol 1997;13:273–286.
5. Becerra A, Belliod D, Luengo A, et al: Lipoprotein(a) and other lipoproteins in hypothyroid patients before and after thyroid replacement therapy. Clin Nutr 1999;18:319–322.

PATIENT 68

A 24-year-old man with substernal chest pain that worsened with inspiration

A 24-year-old medical student had sudden onset of substernal pain with radiation to his shoulders and neck. He describes the pain as heavy and squeezing, but at times it has a sharp component, especially if he takes a deep breath or coughs. The patient also noted fever occurring soon after the pain began.

Physical Examination: Vital signs: pulse 100; blood pressure 110/70. Cardiac: three-component pericardial friction rub over the precordium best heard along the left sternal border with the patient sitting up and leaning forward.

Laboratory Findings: CBC, urinalysis, and blood chemistry: normal. Electrocardiogram: see below. Cardiac enzymes: normal.

Question: What is the likely cause of the patient's condition?

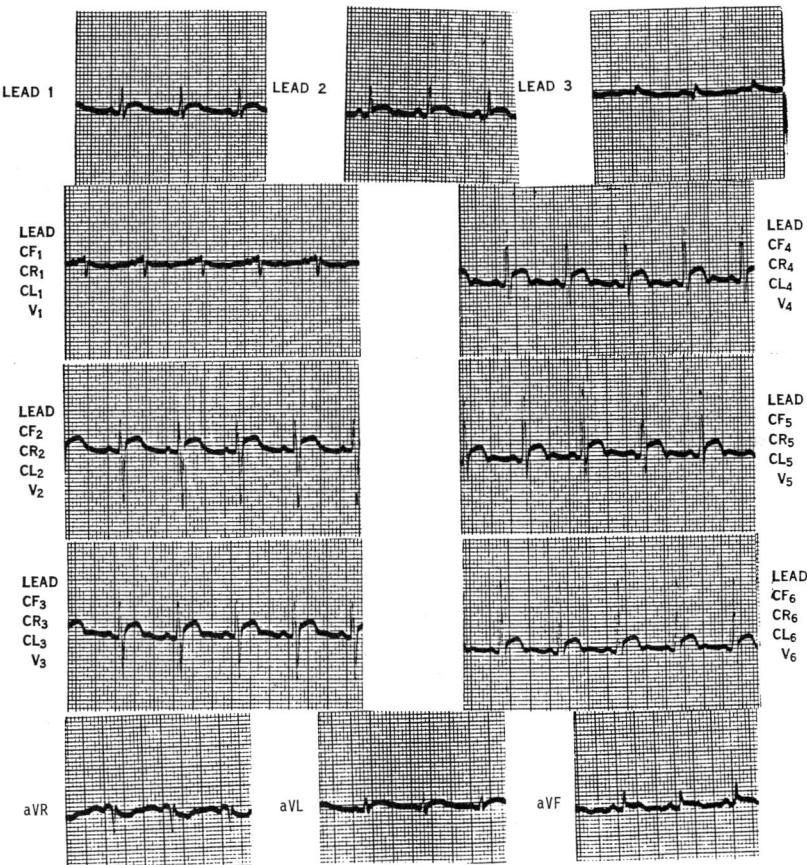

Diagnosis: Acute pericarditis.

Discussion: Acute pericarditis may have the same character and distribution of chest pain as coronary artery disease. However, it often is aggravated by coughing or deep breathing and has a sharp component. The pain typically radiates to the back of the shoulders and neck. The visceral pericardial membrane has no pain fibers. It is the parietal membrane that senses pain through afferent pain fibers carried in the phrenic nerve.

A pericardial friction rub may or may not be present and often is noted intermittently. Generally there are two components (during atrial and ventricular systole), but a third component may be added by ventricular diastole. Occasionally, a one-component rub may be present and is indistinguishable from a systolic murmur. A rub can produce a palpable thrill, especially in patients with uremic pericarditis.

Chest pain, a pericardial rub, and fever occurring early in the course of symptoms are more diagnostic of acute pericarditis than acute myocardial infarction. However, pericardial rubs and fever develop in 20% of patients with an acute transmural myocardial infarction, but they usually occur 24 hours or more after the onset of pain.

The EKG in pericarditis shows diffuse ST elevation except for ST depression in aVR or in the right precordial leads. Spodick described **four EKG stages of pericarditis:** stage 1 shows ST elevation; stage 2 shows ST segments returning to baseline with flattening of the T waves; stage 3 shows inversion of the T waves; and stage 4 shows a return of the tracing to normal. However, some patients retain inverted T waves indefinitely. During the first two stages the PR segment may be depressed. Early repolarization, a normal variant, may mimic the ST-segment changes of acute pericarditis, but usually in such cases the ST segment is concave upwardly, whereas the ST-segment elevation of periocarditis comes straight off of the QRS complex or is concave downwardly.

Unless there is a pericardial effusion, the chest radiograph demonstrates a normal-sized heart. Echocardiography often shows a pericardial effusion, which helps make the diagnosis. Although a viral etiology typically is suspected in the young otherwise healthy patient, no specific etiology usually is established, and further studies may be unnecessary if the pericarditis resolves and does not recur. In ill patients or patients with expanding pericardial effusions, an etiology should be sought. Infection with coxsackievirus or echovirus, influenza, mumps, malignancy, uremia, bacterial infection, myocardial infarction, and collagen vascular disease are common etiologies. Perform blood cultures, fungal serologic tests, cold agglutinin tests, thyroid studies, heterophile antibody titer, serum BUN and creatinine determination, and antinuclear antibody titers (ANA) to establish a cause for the pericarditis. Perform diagnostic pericardiocentesis when: (1) the diagnosis of recurrent or persistent pericarditis has eluded other diagnostic modalities, or (2) infection or malignancy are suspected as the cause.

Patients with viral or idiopathic types usually respond to nonsteroidal antiinflammatory drugs (NSAIDs). IF NSAIDs fail, corticosteroids are indicated. Corticosteroids, immunosuppressive agents, and pericardiectomy have been used for those with recurrent attacks. Colchicine appears to be a promising adjunct to conventional treatment.

The present patient's pericarditis resolved with administration of ibuprofen.

Clinical Pearls

1. The pain of pericarditis may be indistinguishable from that of acute myocardial infarction. Sudden onset of chest pain, a pericardial rub, and fever are distinguishing clues.

2. The two components of the friction rub that usually are heard are atrial systole and ventricular systole.

3. The EKG shows diffuse ST-segment elevation, which usually comes straight off of the QRS or is downward concave, and PR segment depression.

4. Most often no cause can be found, and the pericarditis responds to NSAIDS.

5. Corticosteroids, immunosuppressive agents, colchicine, and pericardiectomy are accepted modalities for those who have recurrent episodes.

REFERENCES

1. Spodick DH: Electrocardiogram in acute pericarditis. Distribution of morphologic and axial changes by stages. Am J Cardiol 1974;33:470–474.
2. Gazes PC: Pericarditis. Cardiovasc Dis Chest Pain 1985;1:2–8.
3. Adler Y, Finkelsein Y, Guindo J, et al: Colchicine treatment for recurrent pericarditis. Circulation 1998;97:2183–2185.

PATIENT 69

A 52-year-old man with early morning chest pain

A 52-year-old man presents with a 6-week history of substernal pain with radiation to his jaw and left arm occurring at rest and lasting for 15–30 minutes. These episodes frequently awaken him from sleep in the early morning. He is admitted to the coronary care unit for further studies and observation. Cigarette smoking is his only risk factor for coronary artery disease.

Physical Examination: Vital signs: pulse 80; blood pressure 124/80. Cardiac: normal.
Laboratory Findings: CBC, urinalysis, electrolytes, and cardiac enzymes: normal. EKG without pain: normal.
Hospital Course: The following day at 3:00 AM he has chest pain. The EKG taken during this episode is shown below. After taking nitroglycerin sublingually, his pain subsides and the EKG returns to normal.

Question: What is the cause of the patient's chest pain?

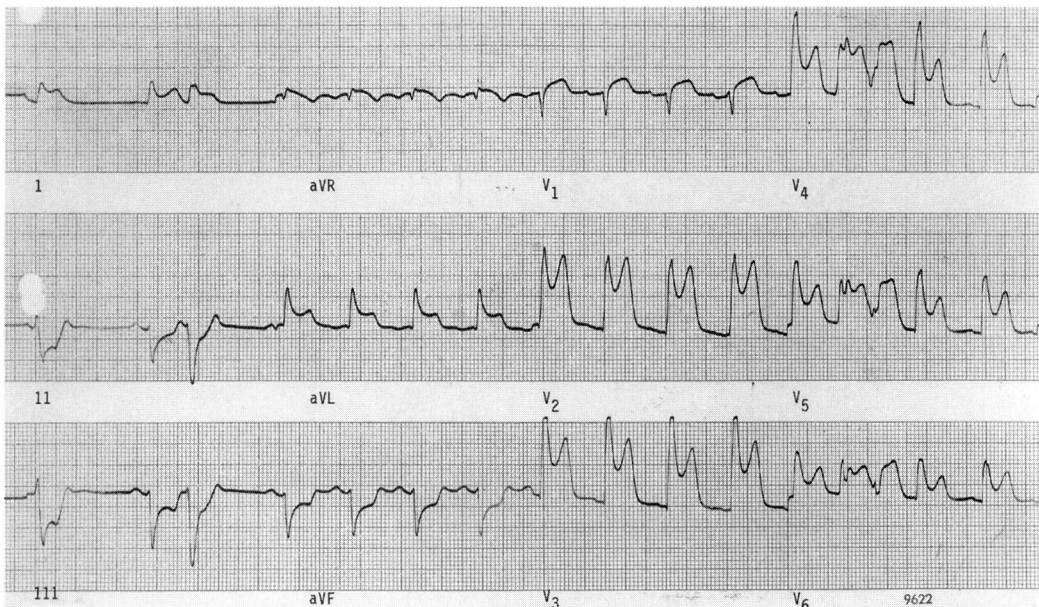

Diagnosis: Variant (Prinzmetal's) angina.

Discussion: Prinzmetal's angina refers to coronary artery lesions with superimposed coronary spasm. Because spasm occasionally occurs in relatively normal coronary arteries, the term variant angina probably is more generally correct. Coronary arteriography in patients with variant angina reveals that 5% have normal vessels, 11% have mild lesions with less than 50% obstruction, 43% have significant single-vessel disease, 21% have double-vessel disease, and 20% have triple-vessel disease.

Classically, angina occurs with exertion when oxygen demand is increased. Conversely, variant angina often occurs at rest, due to reduction in myocardial oxygen supply when coronary spasm occurs. Transmural ischemia results from total occlusion, producing EKG changes of ST-segment elevation, as noted in the present patient's tracing.

The EKG gives a clue as to which artery is involved; spasm alone most often is noted in the right coronary artery. At times, such patients are diagnosed only by ST-segment elevation during Holter monitoring, but because the timing of the attacks is variable, the EKG findings often are difficult to capture. Ventricular arrhythmias frequently occur with episodes, as does heart block, particularly when the right coronary artery is involved.

The cause of coronary artery spasm is unknown. It may be related to **calcium fluxes** that influence coronary artery smooth muscle tone. As calcium availability increases, vasoconstriction increases. Hydrogen ions compete with calcium ions and vasoconstriction also occurs if the hydrogen ion concentration decreases, as might occur with hyperventilation. Conversely, magnesium may suppress variant angina attacks induced by hyperventilation by reducing calcium ion concentration.

Most attacks of variant angina occur in the early morning hours when the patient is recumbent. The pain from hiatal hernia often occurs under similar circumstances, and the two diseases often are confused. An EKG or Holter monitor recorded during the episode usually is required to make the distinction. Early morning exercise may precipitate an attack in a given patient, but afternoon exercise the same day may not. In the early morning, body metabolism is decreased, hydrogen ion concentration is decreased, and calcium ion concentration is increased, producing spasm. Other vasoconstrictors have been implicated in causing spasm, such as leukotrienes, serotonin, and mitogens. Endothelial injury may affect the vasodilator response of the vessel to endothelial-derived relaxant factor and to other agents such as acetylcholine. Cocaine also may produce coronary spasm.

Acute episodes of variant angina respond to nitroglycerin, and long-acting nitrates may prevent attacks. However, **calcium channel blockers** have been the most effective therapy. If the spasm is superimposed on a significant coronary lesion, the fixed lesion should be managed by angioplasty or coronary bypass surgery, as in the other forms of coronary artery disease. Conversely, bypass surgery or angioplasty should not be performed for spasm in a relatively normal coronary vessel. Beta blockers may aggravate the condition, because beta-receptor stimulation causes coronary vasodilatation. Aspirin in high doses also may increase anginal attacks because it blocks production of the vasodilator prostacyclin. Patients with variant angina often have migraine headaches and Raynaud's phenomenon, suggesting a pattern of diffuse arterial spasm.

In the present patient, the ST-segment elevation in the precordial leads suggested that the vessel involved was the left anterior descending (LAD) artery. Coronary arteriography revealed normal coronary arteries, but after ergonovine infusion there was localized spasm in the proximal LAD.

Clinical Pearls

1. Some patients with variant angina suffer from migraine headaches and Raynaud's phenomenon, suggesting a diffuse vasospastic process.

2. Transient ST elevation during chest pain is the characteristic feature of variant angina.

3. The pain syndromes of hiatal hernia and variant angina often are confused, because both occur in the early morning hours when the patient is recumbent.

4. Patients with coronary artery spasm respond to calcium blockers; their attacks may increase with beta blockers or high doses of aspirin therapy.

REFERENCES

1. Prinzmetal M, Kennamer R, Merliss R: Angina pectoris. I. A variant form of angina pectoris. Am J Med 1959;27:375–388.
2. Yasue H, Omote S, Takizawa A, et al: Circadian variation of exercise capacity in patients with Prinzmetal's variant angina: Role of exercise-induced coronary arterial spasm. Circulation 1979;59:938–948.
3. Corcos T, David PR, Bourassa MG, et al: Percutaneous transluminal coronary angioplasty for the treatment of variant angina. J Am Coll Cardiol 1985;5:1046–1054.
4. Shimokawa H, Nagasawa K, Irie I, et al: Clinical characteristics and long-term prognosis of patients with variant angina: A comparative study between western and Japanese populations. Int J Cardiol 1988;18:331–349.
5. Mayer S, Hillis LD: Prinzmetal's variant angina. Clin Cardiol 1998;21:243–246.
6. Vandergoten P, Benit E, Dendale P: Prinzmetal's variant angina: Three case reports and a review of the literature. Acta Cardiol 1999;54:71–76.

PATIENT 70

A 44-year-old man with severe chest pain and an abnormal electrocardiogram

A 44-year-old man has had episodes of mild chest pain for 10 years. The pain is described as occurring in the mid and lower substernal areas, mostly at rest but occasionally with exertion, and lasting variable lengths of time. The EKG is considered to be consistent with an old inferior myocardial infarction. He has no risk factors for coronary disease. The present admission to the coronary care unit was precipitated by a severe, prolonged chest pain.

Physical Examination: Vital signs: pulse 80; blood pressure 130/70. Chest: clear. Cardiac: normal.
Laboratory Findings: CBC, urinalysis, SMA-12 and SMA-7: normal. Chest radiograph: normal. EKG: see below.

Question: What is your diagnosis?

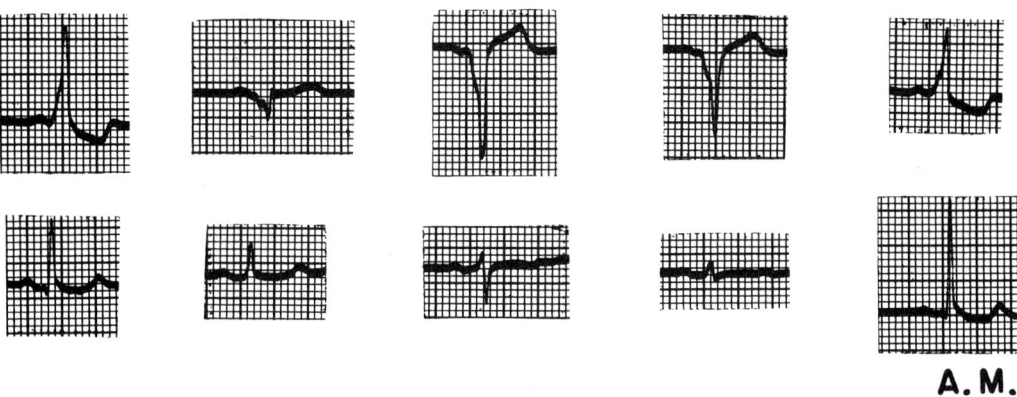

Figure reproduced from Gazes PC: Clinical Cardiology—A Cost-Effective Approach, 4th ed. New York, Chapman and Hall, 1997; with permission.

Diagnosis: Wolff-Parkinson-White (WPW) syndrome with inferior Q waves simulating an inferior infarction.

Discussion: At least 100 clinical conditions have been reported to show EKG changes suggestive of myocardial infarction in the absence of coronary artery disease. Most of these conditions cause ST-T changes, but many produce Q waves. Among those **syndromes producing Q waves in the absence of coronary disease** are myocarditis, emboli to coronary arteries, periarteritis nodosa, brain lesions, cardiac tumors, idiopathic hypertrophic subaortic stenosis, pulmonary embolism, reversal of limb leads, cardiac amyloidosis, neuromuscular disorders, cardiomyopathies, anomalous coronary arteries, and WPW syndrome.

The distribution of Q wave abnormalities in WPW syndrome depends on the location of the aberrant pathway. **Type A** WPW syndrome has upright QRS complexes in all the precordial leads. **Type B** has a negative QRS complex in V1 and a positive QRS complex in V6. **Type C** has a positive QRS complex in V1 and a negative QRS complex in V6. Milstein et al. developed an EKG algorithm for localizing accessory pathways. A combination of this system and types A and B could be as follows: Type A (left ventricular pathways) has a positive delta and QRS complex in V1 for lateral and posteroseptal pathways; the lateral pathway also has isoelectric or negative delta waves in leads 1, aVL, V5, and V6, and the posteroseptal pathway also has negative delta and QRS complex in leads II, III, and aVF. Type B (right ventricular pathways) has negative delta and QRS complexes in V1 and, if located posteroseptal, there also are negative delta and QRS complexes in leads II, III, and aVF. If located anteroseptal, there also is an axis of +30% or more, and if located in the right ventricular free wall, there also is left axis. Type A can be mistaken for right bundle branch block, a true posterior infarction, or an inferior infarction; type B for an anteroseptal infarction, inferior infarction, left ventricular hypertrophy, or left bundle branch block; and type C for right ventricular hypertrophy.

The presence and location of Q waves depend on the direction of the initial conduction through the accessory pathway and how it fuses with the conduction coming through the normal AV pathway. At times a vectorcardiogram is needed to clearly show the WPW changes. Patients with WPW syndrome also often have a false-positive stress test.

In the present patient, EKG findings of WPW syndrome were not noted initially, and he was labeled as having an inferior infarction, much to the patient's anxiety. The top tracing on the previous page shows inferior Q waves and the typical WPW configuration. The lower tracing taken on another occasion shows normal conduction and no inferior Q waves. Coronary arteriograms revealed normal coronary arteries. Additional studies showed that **esophageal spasm** was producing the chest pain.

Clinical Pearls

1. The Q waves normally found in WPW syndrome often lead to the misdiagnosis of myocardial infarction.
2. Noninfarction Q waves also are seen in idiopathic hypertrophic subaortic stenosis and pulmonary embolism.
3. The location of the Q waves in WPW syndrome depends on the location and direction of the aberrant pathway fibers.

REFERENCES

1. Wolff L, Parkinson J, White PD: Bundle branch block with short P-R interval in healthy young people prone to paroxysmal tachycardia. Am Heart J 1930;5:685–704.
2. Gazes PC: False-positive exercise test in the presence of the Wolff-Parkinson-White syndrome. Am Heart J 1969;78:13–15.
3. Giorgi C, Ackaoiu A, Nadesu R, et al: Wolff-Parkinson-White VCG patterns that mimic other cardiac pathologies: A correlative study with the preexcitation pathway localization. Am Heart J 1986;111:891–902.
4. Milstein S, Sharma AD, Guiraudon GM, et al: An algorithm for the electrocardiographic localization of accessory pathways in the Wolff-Parkinson-White syndrome. PACE 1987;10:555.
5. Al-Khatib SM, Pritchett EL: Clinical features of Wolff-Parkinson-White syndrome. Am Heart J 1999;138:403–413.
6. Basiouny T, de Chillou C, Fareh S, et al: Accuracy and limitations of published algorithms using the twelve-lead electrocardiogram to localize overt atrioventricular accessory pathways. J Cardiovasc Electrophysiol 1999;10:1340–1349.

PATIENT 71

A 32-year-old woman with episodes of rapid heart beat

A 32-year-old woman has experienced several episodes of rapid heart beat over the previous 5 years. Recently, the frequency of the episodes has increased. The only symptom associated with these episodes is "feeling weak." At times, she is able to stop an attack by straining, and physicians have aborted attacks by right carotid pressure. Several EKGs reveal a regular, narrow, QRS complex supraventricular tachycardia. She is admitted to the hospital for further studies because of an episode of sustained tachycardia.

Physical Examination: Vital signs: heart rate 187 beats/min; blood pressure 100/60. Cardiac: no jugular venous distention; no unusual sounds or murmurs.

Laboratory Findings: CBC, urinalysis, and routine chemistry: normal. EKG: see below.

Question: What is the diagnosis?

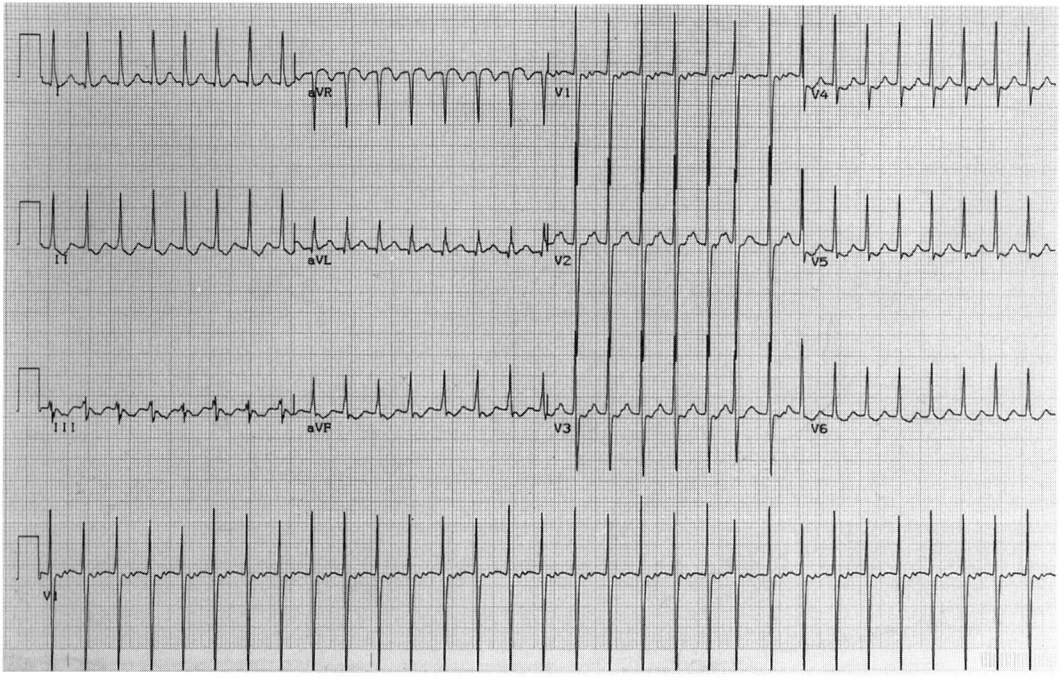

Diagnosis: Atrioventricular reentrant tachycardia (WPW type).

Discussion: Atrioventricular reentrant tachycardia (AVRT) occurs in the Wolff-Parkinson-White (WPW) syndrome with the AV bypass tract either concealed or manifested. The arrhythmia often is referred to as a **reciprocating or circus-movement tachycardia,** and accounts for about 20–30% of supraventricular tachycardias. Conduction is down the AV node and returns retrograde through the accessory pathway to the atrium (orthodromic) in at least 90% of patients. In such cases, the QRS has a normal configuration because the normal antegrade pathway is used.

These regular tachycardias usually have a rate of 180–250 beats/min. The P wave follows the QRS, with an RP interval of greater than 70 msec, or the P wave is located about 140 msec after the beginning of the QRS complex.

Occasionally, it is difficult to differentiate this arrhythmia from the more common AV nodal reentrant tachycardia (AVNRT), which accounts for over 50% of regular supraventricular tachycardias. With the latter arrhythmia, the retrograde P waves may be hidden in or are seen just after the QRS, but are usually less than 70 msec from the R wave.

If bundle branch block is present and is on the same side as the accessory pathway, the AVRT is slower than when the block is absent because the impulse takes longer to reach the accessory pathway. The bundle branch block does not affect the length of the tachycardia cycle in AVNRT. In addition, if there is evidence of AV dissociation or block, AVRT is ruled out, for it should have a 1:1 relationship.

The accessory pathway has a long refractory period and faster conduction than the AV node. Therefore, a critically timed premature beat can block the accessory pathway and conduct down the AV node, then return to the atria by the accessory pathway and initiate the tachycardia.

This type of AV reentrant tachycardia responds to therapies that increase AV nodal block, e.g., vagal maneuvers, intravenous verapamil, digoxin, or adenosine, or to therapies that slow conduction in the WPW pathway, such as procainamide. Frequent attacks that respond poorly to medical therapy should be evaluated with electrophysiologic studies, and the accessory pathway should be ablated by radiofrequency current. This procedure has low morbidity and mortality compared with surgery.

The present patient had P waves located greater than 70 msec (short RP type) after the R wave. The diagnosis of WPW syndrome was suspected and then confirmed by electrophysiologic studies. Subsequently, the bypass tract was ablated successfully by radiofrequency current.

Clinical Pearls

1. The WPW syndrome accounts for 20–30% of supraventricular tachycardias. However, in 90% of these instances, conduction is orthodromic; thus the QRS pattern is normal instead of characteristic of WPW.

2. If the P waves are visible after the QRS complex and the RP interval is greater than 70 msec, the supraventricular tachycardia most likely is due to a concealed WPW pathway.

3. In arrhythmias manifesting WPW configuration, digoxin should not be used. However, orthodromic arrhythmias respond well to any therapy that blocks conduction through the AV node, including digoxin and verapamil. Adenosine is the agent of choice.

4. The bypass tract can be ablated by radiofrequency current.

REFERENCES

1. Manolis AS, Estes NA III: Supraventricular tachycardia: Mechanisms and therapy. Arch Intern Med 1987;147:1706–1716.
2. Prystowsky EN: Diagnosis and management of the preexcitation syndrome. Curr Probl Cardiol 1988;13:231–310.
3. Jackman WM, Wang XZ, Friday KJ, et al: Catheter ablation of accessory atrioventricular pathways (Wolff-Parkinson-White syndrome) by radiofrequency current. N Engl J Med 1991;324:1605–1611.
4. Pieper SJ, Stanton MS: Narrow QRS complex tachycardia. Mayo Clin Proc 1995;70:371.

PATIENT 72

A 67-year-old man with chest pain following a motor vehicle accident

A 67-year-old man was involved in a head-on collision with a tractor-trailer. The patient did not lose consciousness, but did suffer blunt chest trauma from the steering wheel. His past medical history is significant only for hypertension.

Physical Examination: Vital signs: pulse 115 (regular); respirations 18; blood pressure left arm 161/89, right arm 155/90. General: alert; oriented; complaining of chest pain. Head: minor contusions of the face; otherwise normal. Chest: marked contusion and swelling of the mid-sternum with no bony disruption; equal bilateral breath sounds. Cardiac: no jugular venous distention; regular rate and rhythm; no rub, murmur, or gallop.

Laboratory Findings: EKG: sinus tachycardia; left anterior hemiblock. Aortogram: see below.

Question: What is the treatment for this man's condition?

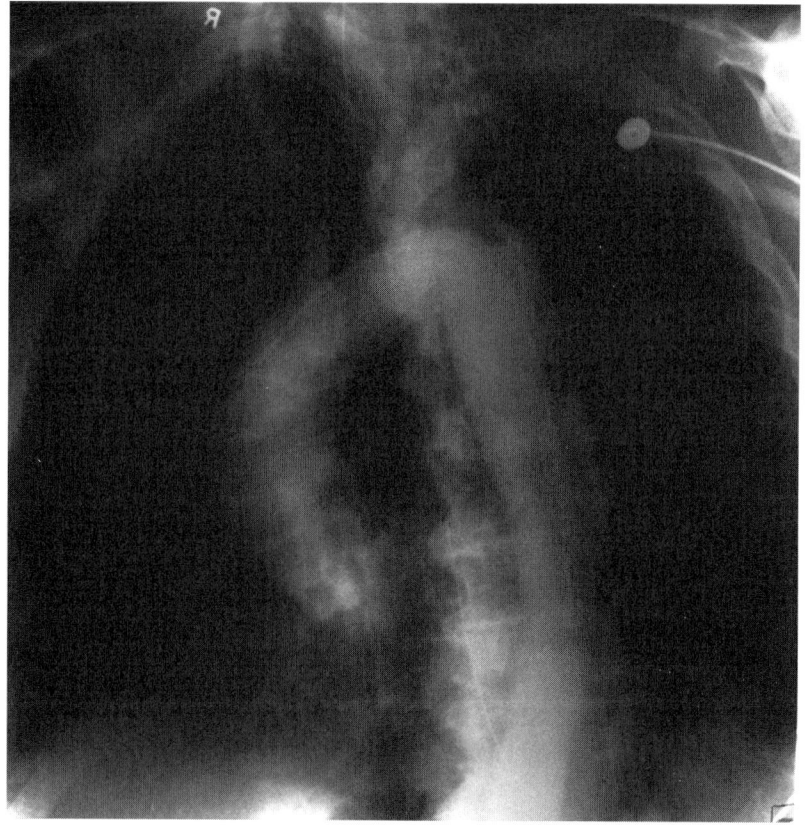

Answer: Aortic repair.

Discussion: Motor vehicle accidents are the most common causes of **nonpenetrating cardiovascular trauma.** Rupture of the thoracic aorta due to blunt chest trauma leads to immediate death in 70–90% of cases. It accounts for up to 18% of deaths in motor vehicle accidents. Blunt chest trauma generally results from a combination of forces, including a direct blow to the chest wall, sudden deceleration at the moment of impact, and an increase in intracardiac and intravascular pressure due to chest compression. The right ventricle and the aorta are the most frequently ruptured structures. As typified by this patient, aortic rupture usually occurs just distal to the left subclavian artery at the site of the ligamentum arteriosum. Other important nonpenetrating injuries include left ventricular rupture and myocardial contusion.

Myocardial contusion occurs in up to 15% of victims of motor vehicle accidents when sudden deceleration produces cardiac injury as the heart contacts the sternum. Chest pain, the most common symptom, usually is due to chest wall trauma. However, the chest pain may be similar in nature to that of myocardial ischemia or pericarditis. While the epicardium is the most likely myocardial layer to be damaged, contusion can affect all layers. Healing usually occurs without permanent sequelae, but large contusions can damage enough myocardium to produce congestive heart failure. Contusion also can lead to hemopericardium and subsequent cardiac tamponade. Serious cardiac arrhythmias also can develop as a consequence of contusion. They typically arise several days after the injury.

In addition to a careful physical examination, a **chest radiograph** and **electrocardiogram** should be standard diagnostic studies for any patient who has suffered significant nonpenetrating chest trauma. The EKG is particularly helpful in making the diagnosis of myocardial contusion when ST-segment elevation indicates a periepicarditis. Initially, the EKG may be normal, but changes may evolve over several days. The chest radiograph may demonstrate a widened mediastinum, which should raise suspicion of aortic trauma.

If nonpenetrating cardiac trauma is suspected, perform an echocardiogram to examine for pericardial effusion, left ventricular dysfunction, intracardiac structural abnormalities, and aortic abnormalities. CT scanning with contrast material and MRI are particularly helpful in making the diagnosis of aortic rupture or dissection. Once traumatic aortic rupture is diagnosed, **surgical repair** is the most effective therapy. Note, however, that **stent grafting** is emerging as a viable therapeutic option for traumatic aortic rupture. The right femoral and left external iliac arteries have been used for introducing the stent graft. Such endovascular grafting needs controlled prospective studies before its widespread use can be recommended.

The present patient had a widened mediastinum on chest radiograph, and the aortogram demonstrated the aortic rupture. He underwent successful aortic repair and was discharged after a long period of recuperation.

Clinical Pearls

1. Blunt cardiac trauma is common but often unsuspected following motor vehicle accidents. Myocardial contusion is the most common lesion, followed in order of frequency by ventricular rupture and aortic rupture.
2. Myocardial contusion usually causes only modest epicardial damage; in some cases, however, severe transmural damage may lead to congestive heart failure.
3. Serious ventricular arrhythmias are common after myocardial contusion and may occur relatively late after the injury.
4. Surgery usually is indicated; however, stent grafting is emerging as a viable option for traumatic aortic rupture.

REFERENCES
1. Mattox KL, Limacher MC, Feliciano DV, et al: Cardiac evaluation following heart injury. J Trauma 1985;25:758–765.
2. Symbas PN: Traumatic heart disease. Curr Probl Cardiol 1991;16:539–582.
3. Rousseau H, Soula P, Perreault P, et al: Delayed treatment of traumatic rupture of the thoracic aorta with endoluminal covered stent. Circulation 1999;99:498–504.

PATIENT 73

A 62-year-old man with hypertension, atypical chest pain, and an abnormal electrocardiogram

A 62-year-old man with partially controlled hypertension is admitted because of an episode of sharp precordial pain with radiation to his left shoulder. The patient has a heavy smoking history and a strongly positive family history for coronary artery disease.

Physical Examination: Vital signs: pulse 80; blood pressure 160/100. General: uncomfortable with chest pain. Cardiac: no extra sounds or murmurs.

Laboratory Findings: CBC, urinalysis, blood chemistries: normal. EKG: see below.

Question: What is the etiology of the abnormal EKG?

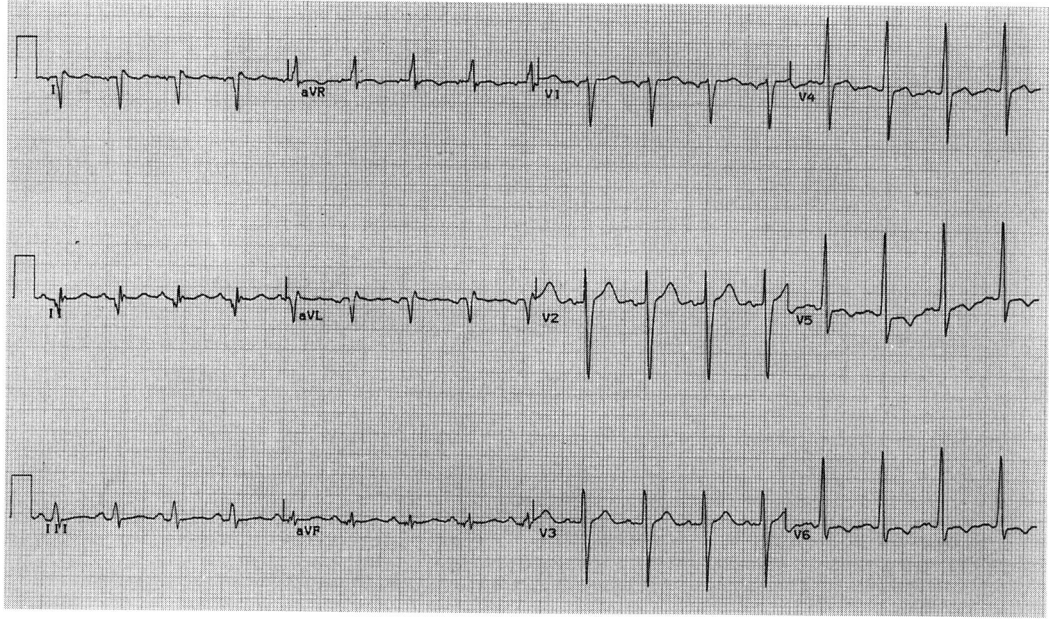

Diagnosis: Reversal of the right and left EKG arm leads.

Discussion: Despite the technical advances in the portable equipment used to generate EKGs, operator and system errors still can complicate EKG interpretation. On a busy clinical service, even experienced operators may reverse the arm leads and inadvertently challenge EKG readers. Recognition of **EKG signs of limb lead reversal** allows the reader to detect the error quickly, to prevent cardiac misdiagnoses, and to determine which leads have been reversed.

If an aVL pattern is noted in the aVR lead or an aVR pattern is noted in the aVL lead, the right and left arm leads have been reversed. If an aVF pattern is noted in the aVR lead and an aVR pattern is present in the aVF lead, the right arm and left leg leads have been reversed. If an aVL pattern is noted in the aVF lead and an aVF pattern appears in the aVL lead, the left arm and left leg leads have been reversed. Even the right leg ground lead can be improperly placed.

In this era of "managed care," with hospital workers being cross-trained in a broader array of responsibilities, less experienced personnel may be performing EKGs, and a greater incidence of lead placement errors may complicate diagnosis. In addition, improper precordial lead placement and improper standardization may cause wrong clinical impressions and ultimately lead to healthy patients being diagnosed as having heart disease. Other misleading artifacts can be produced by loose cables, body tremors (as with parkinsonism), surrounding instrumentation, and hiccoughs, to name a few. Telemetrically transmitted tracings often have artifacts that may simulate a serious arrhythmia. Computer-generated reports, which are inaccurate approximately 20% of the time, are another source of EKG misinterpretation. Such reports should always be reviewed by a physician for accuracy.

In the present patient, the inverted P waves and QRS complexes in lead I suggested lead reversal. Although these EKG findings could have indicated dextrocardia, patients with dextrocardia have reversal of the precordial patterns, which was not present. If the lead reversal had not been suspected, the presence of Q waves in leads I, II, and aVL could have led to a diagnosis of myocardial infarction. The inverted T waves in the precordial leads did not evolve with serial EKGs and were due to repolarization changes related to the patient's longstanding hypertension.

Clinical Pearls

1. The right and left arm leads may be reversed if the P waves and QRS complexes are inverted in lead I.
2. The right arm and left leg leads may be reversed if aVR pattern is noted in aVF.
3. The left arm and left leg lead may be reversed if the aVL pattern is noted in aVF.
4. Inexperienced readers and computer-generated reports can lead to wrong clinical impressions.

REFERENCES
1. Simonson E: Differentiation Between Normal and Abnormal Electrocardiography. St. Louis, Mosby, 1961, p 262.
2. Castellanos A, Saoudi NC, Schwartz A, et al: Electrocardiographic patterns resulting from improper connections of the right leg (ground) cable. PACE 1985;8:364–368.
3. Hurst JS: Crotchets. Clin Cardiol 1999;22:611–613.

PATIENT 74

A 52-year-old man with an anterior myocardial infarction managed with thrombolytic therapy

A 52-year-old man was pulling up a crab trap into his boat when he experienced sudden onset of severe retrosternal pain that radiated down both arms. He is a heavy smoker and has a past history of occasional effort-related angina.

Physical Examination: Vital signs: pulse 80; blood pressure 130/80. Chest: clear. Cardiac: apical S_4 sound; normal S_1 and S_2; no S_3 or murmur.

Laboratory Findings: Peak CPK 2250 IU/L with 17% MB fraction. EKG: anterior ST segment elevation.

Hospital Course: The patient was treated for an anterior myocardial infarction with tPA within 1–1.5 hours after the onset of symptoms. His chest pain resolved immediately, after which he had an episode of accelerated idioventricular rhythm. Several days later coronary arteriography was performed.

Question: Can you predict from the above findings this patient's coronary anatomy and ventricular function?

Answer: No, but results of coronary arteriography will allow prediction.

Discussion: In patients with acute myocardial infarction (MI) treated with thrombolytic therapy, it is almost impossible to predict if the occluded vessel has opened, how much residual stenosis remains, and the status of coronary vessels unrelated to the infarct. The relief of pain, the return of ST segments to baseline, and the onset of arrhythmias (often accelerated idioventricular rhythm) are suggestive but not conclusive signs of reperfusion.

The inability to use bedside clinical data to determine reperfusion suggests the potential importance of **routine coronary arteriography** after thrombolytic therapy. Several multi-center trials recommend a conservative approach in patients who have a satisfactory response to therapy, using coronary arteriography only if signs of spontaneous or exercise-induced ischemia occur. Routine coronary arteriography after thrombolytic therapy, however, has shown that 30% of patients have a patent infarct vessel and two- or three-vessel disease, whereas 5% of patients have a patent infarct vessel and left main disease. These findings and the possibility of rescue angioplasty if the vessel is not open support the value of routine coronary arteriography.

Many ongoing studies will answer the question of whether all patients should have coronary arteriography. Different combination trials of low-molecular-weight heparin, GP IIb/IIIa inhibitors, low-dose thrombolytic agents, angioplasty and/or stents, and direct angioplasty are in progress. It now appears that coronary arteriography will be done early after an MI in most patients. This is necessary since preliminary studies show better results with combinations that include angioplasty and stents. Such combinations require coronary arteriography.

An interesting finding in patients undergoing post-thrombolytic therapy is that the culprit coronary lesion responsible for the infarction may not be severe. In fact, coronary arteriograms obtained in patients several months before their infarctions show severe culprit preinfarction coronary artery lesions in only a third of patients. After successful thrombolytic therapy, 11% of patients have minimal residual coronary obstruction. The ability of thrombolytic therapy to return a coronary artery occlusion to its noncritical baseline severity underlies the improvement that occurs in posttreatment ventricular functions: one third of all patients show improvement in ventricular function from the 3rd to 10th days, with some further improvement up to 45 days. Improvement may be delayed until resolution of myocardial stunning. Echocardiography is valuable in monitoring the course of changes in ventricular function in such patients.

The present patient's coronary arteriograph revealed a 20% proximal lesion in the left anterior descending artery, with an intraluminal defect consistent with thrombus. The remaining coronary arteries unrelated to the infarct were normal. The ventriculogram showed anterolateral akinesis and apical dyskinesis, with an ejection fraction of 25%.

Clinical Pearls

1. After thrombolytic therapy, the relief of pain, resolution of ST segment elevation, and reperfusion arrhythmias are suggestive yet inconclusive signs that the infarct-related vessel has opened.

2. A coronary plaque of 50% or less can rupture, develop a thrombus, and completely occlude the vessel.

3. Combinations of low-molecular-weight heparin, GP IIb/IIIa inhibitors, low-dose thrombolytic agents, angioplasty, stents, and direct angioplasty are being evaluated.

4. It appears that most patients with an acute MI will receive early coronary arteriography, in view of the ongoing trials of combination therapy.

5. Akinetic or dyskinetic myocardium after thrombolytic therapy may represent stunned myocardium. Improvement in ventricular function may not be noted until days 3 to 10, with some further improvement occurring between days 10 and 45.

REFERENCES

1. Nierste D, Little WC: Morphology of the culprit coronary artery lesion preceding myocardial infarction. Circulation 1989;80(Suppl II):II–349.
2. Kereiakes DJ, Topol EJ, George BS, et al: Myocardial infarction with minimal coronary atherosclerosis in the era of thrombolytic reperfusion: The Thrombolysis and Angioplasty in Myocardial Infarction (TAMI) Study Group. J Am Coll Cardiol 1991;17:304–312.
3. Ohman EM, Kleiman NS, Gacioch G, et al.: Combined accelerated tissue-plasminogen activator and platelet glycoprotein IIb/IIIa integrin receptor blockade with integrilin in acute myocardial infarction. Results of a randomized, placebo-controlled, dose-ranging trial. Circulation 1997;95:846–854.
4. Antoniucci D, Santoro GM, Bolognese L, et al.: A clinical trial comparing primary stenting of the infarct-related artery with optimal primary angioplasty for acute myocardial infarction. Results from the Florence Randomized Elective Stenting in Acute Coronary Occlusions (FRESCO) Trial. J Am Coll Cardiol 1998;31:1234–1239.

PATIENT 75

A 28-year-old man with hypotension and a continuous murmur

A previously healthy, 28-year-old construction worker collapses suddenly while on the job. He has no previous cardiac symptoms, and a physical examination performed a year earlier was normal. There is no family history of heart disease.

Physical Examination: Vital signs: pulse 120 and regular; blood pressure 80/40. General: no acute distress or diaphoresis. Chest: basilar crackles. Cardiac: III/VI continuous murmur with a loud diastolic component heard in the aortic area radiating across the sternum.

Laboratory Findings: WBC 9900/μl. Chest radiograph: normal cardiac size; normal aorta; increased vascular markings. EKG: normal. Echocardiogram: technically difficult study. Cardiac catheterization: see data below.

	O_2 saturation	Pressure (mmHg)
Right atrium	55%	8
Right ventricle	85%	40/8
Pulmonary artery	84%	40/12/15
Pulmonary capillary wedge	95%	11
Left ventricle	95%	80/12

Question: What congenital abnormality best explains these data, the clinical history, and the physical examination?

Diagnosis: Ruptured sinus of Valsalva aneurysm.

Discussion: Aneurysms of the sinus of Valsalva occur as a result of congenital weaknesses of the sinuses. Rupture usually occurs before the age of 30, but some aneurysms may exist for a lifetime without rupture. The rupture is usually spontaneous but may be precipitated by increased aortic pressure, as occurs in isometric exercise, or may occur secondary to infective endocarditis. The present patient's occupation of construction worker may have produced frequent episodes of isometric exercise leading to the tear. An aneurysm of the noncoronary sinus ruptures into the right atrium, whereas the right coronary sinus ruptures into the right ventricle. Occasionally, the rupture is directly into the pericardium, where it leads to pericardial tamponade and death.

The continuous murmur found in this disease indicates continuous flow from the aorta to the right ventricle or right atrium because the pressure in the aorta is always higher than the pressure in those chambers. Continuous murmurs also occur in patent ductus arteriosus and coarctation of the aorta, but these entities do not produce precipitous deterioration or an oxygen step-up in the right ventricle. The common association of ventricular septal defect with aortic insufficiency may cause confusion at physical examination, but catastrophic deterioration would be distinctly unusual with that combination of lesions.

The present patient had an oxygen step-up at the level of the right ventricle, indicating rupture of the right coronary sinus of Valsalva. Oximetry data indicated a 4:1 left-to-right shunt. This large transfer of blood from the aorta to the right ventricle reduced forward cardiac output and led to hypotension. Immediate surgical correction was successful in the present patient. However, small perforations may be observed for years without additional therapy besides prophylaxis for endocarditis. Moderate-sized tears may lead to gradual right and left ventricular volume over-loads, resulting in the more gradual onset of congestive heart failure. These should be repaired when symptoms develop or when left ventricular dilatation becomes prominent. Operative mortality is approximately 4%. Patients with active endocarditis account for most of these deaths.

Clinical Pearls

1. The acute onset of a continuous murmur that produces hemodynamic compromise usually indicates a ruptured sinus of Valsalva aneurysm.

2. An oxygen step-up that occurs at the right atrial or right ventricular level together with a continuous murmur makes the diagnosis likely.

3. Prophylaxis against endocarditis is required in patients with sinus of Valsalva aneurysms.

REFERENCES

1. Mayer ED, Ruffman K, Saggau W, et al: Ruptured aneurysms of the sinus of Valsalva. Ann Thorac Surg 1986;42:81–85.
2. Perloff JK: Potential longevity in unoperated adults. In Roberts WC (ed): Adult Congenital Heart Disease. Philadelphia, F.A. Davis, 1987, pp 29–48.
3. Takach TJ, Reul GJ, Duncan JM, et al: Sinus of Valsalva aneurysm or fistula: Management and outcome. Ann Thorac Surg 1999;68:1573–1577.

PATIENT 76

A 7-year-old boy with an acute myocardial infarction

A 7-year-old boy presents with the sudden onset of anterior chest pain, vomiting, and general malaise. One year earlier, the patient experienced a febrile illness that had been associated with conjuctivitis and peeling of the skin on the hands and feet.

Physical Examination: Vital signs: temperature 99°; pulse 110; respirations 22; blood pressure 110/60. General: mild distress. Fundi: no hemorrhages. Skin: normal. Chest: clear. Cardiac: normal S_1 and S_2. Extremities: no petechiae or splinter hemorrhages.

Laboratory Findings: WBC 8900/µl; Hct 35%. EKG: ST segment elevation in the right precordial leads consistent with an anterior myocardial infarction. Echocardiogram: see below.

Question: What is the patient's underlying disease?

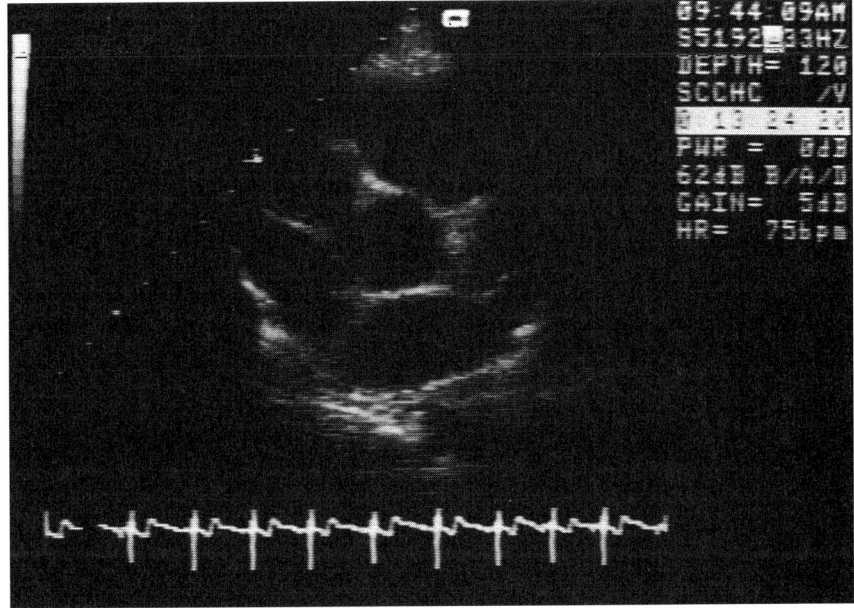

Diagnosis: Mucocutaneous lymph node syndrome (Kawasaki's disease).

Discussion: Kawasaki's disease is a febrile illness of early childhood of unknown etiology. Typically, patients present with a febrile illness that does not respond to antibiotic therapy. The skin on the palms and feet becomes erythematous and desquamates. Additional findings include bilateral congestion of the ocular conjuctiva, dry fissured lips and strawberry tongue, cervical lymphadenopathy, and a diffuse erythematous rash unassociated with vesicles.

The most important morbidity attached to Kawasaki's disease results from a perivasculitis that occurs in small arteries, particularly the coronary vascular bed. The vasculitis eventually leads to coronary aneurysmal dilatation, as demonstrated on the echocardiogram of the present patient. These aneurysms may subsequently thrombose, producing acute coronary insufficiency and myocardial infarction. It is unknown whether aneurysms may spontaneously resolve in some patients.

Patients who develop a myocardial infarction usually experience their cardiac event within 6 months of the initial febrile symptoms. As in the present patient's case, however, a myocardial infarction may occur several months or years following the onset of the disease. Some patients develop aneurysms in all three major coronary arteries and experience recurrent myocardial infarctions in different vascular distributions. Unlike coronary atherosclerotic aneurysms in the adult, Kawasaki aneurysms may rupture, causing acute hemopericardium and death. Other cardiac manifestations of the disease include pericarditis and myocarditis, which may precipitate arrhythmias and, occasionally, congestive heart failure.

All patients diagnosed with Kawasaki's disease within 10 days of the onset of fever should receive intravenous gamma globulin and high-dose salicylates, which will reduce the arteritis and aneurysm formation. Corticosteroids appear to be detrimental and should not be used. Although some patients have undergone bypass surgery, the rate of saphenous bypass closure is high at approximately 30%. Currently it is unclear whether bypass surgery prolongs life.

The present patient recovered from his anterior myocardial infarction and left the hospital on long-term salicylate therapy. The diagnosis of Kawasaki's disease was confirmed by echocardiogram, which demonstrated coronary artery aneurysmal dilatation.

Clinical Pearls

1. The initial manifestations of Kawasaki's disease are a febrile illness with an erythematous rash on hands and feet that progresses to desquamation. Additional findings include conjunctival congestion, fissured lips, strawberry tongue, cervical lymphadenopathy, and a diffuse nonvesicular erythematous rash.

2. Coronary aneurysm formation is the most serious consequence of Kawasaki's disease.

3. Therapy includes salicylates and gamma globulin. Steroids should be avoided.

4. Myocardial infarction usually occurs within 6 months after the onset of the illness. In some patients, however, cardiac events may occur several years later.

REFERENCES

1. Hiraishi S, Yashiro K, Oguchi K, et al: Clinical course of cardiovascular involvement in the mucocutaneous lymph node syndrome. Am J Cardiol 1981;47:323–330.
2. Kato H, Ichinose E, Kawasaki T: Myocardial infarction in Kawasaki disease: Clinical analyses in 195 cases. J Pediatr 1986;108:923–927.
3. Nakano H, Saito A, Ueda K, et al: Clinical characteristics of myocardial infarction following Kawasaki disease. Report of 11 cases. J Pediatr 1986;108:198–203.
4. Klassen TP, Rowe PC, Gafni A: Economic evaluation of intravenous immune globulin therapy for Kawasaki syndrome. J Pediatr 1993;122:538–542.

PATIENT 77

A 68-year-old man with recurrent heart failure and a systolic murmur

A 68-year-old man is evaluated for recurrent episodes of congestive heart failure over the previous 6 months that were refractory to furosemide and digoxin. A trial of captopril (12.5 mg p.o. t.i.d.) produced near-syncope.

Physical Examination: Vital signs: pulse 115; respirations 26; blood pressure 100/50. Neck: jugular venous distention; minimal delay of carotid upstrokes. Chest: bibasilar rales. Cardiac: S_3; I/VI late-peaking systolic murmur.

Laboratory Findings: EKG: sinus tachycardia; left atrial enlargement; left ventricular hypertrophy with strain pattern. Pressure tracings from cardiac catherization: see below.

Questions: What is the cause of the patient's soft heart murmur? Why did captopril produce near-syncope?

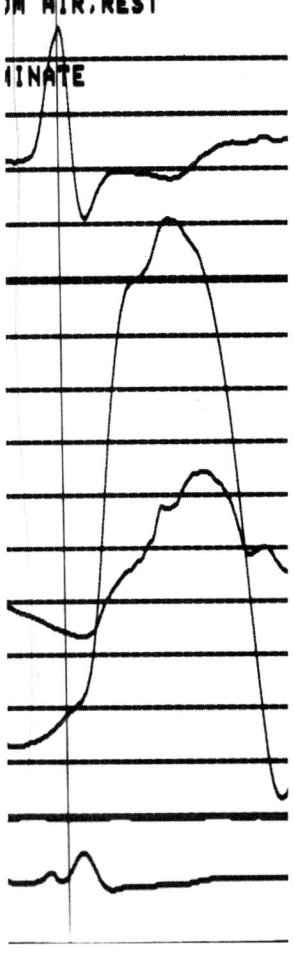

Diagnosis: Aortic stenosis.

Discussion: Asymptomatic patients with aortic stenosis have an excellent prognosis. Once the symptoms of angina, syncope, or congestive heart failure develop, however, the prognosis worsens dramatically unless surgical correction is performed. On average, 50% of patients who develop angina will be dead within 5 years, 50% of patients who develop syncope will be dead in 3 years, and 50% of patients who develop congestive heart failure will die within 2 years unless the aortic valve is replaced.

Failure to recognize that aortic stenosis is the cause of the patient's heart failure can produce tragic results. Although vasodilators have become the mainstay of therapy in the treatment of congestive heart failure, they are contraindicated in severe aortic stenosis. Vasodilators used in aortic stenosis produce a fall in total peripheral resistance without leading to the expected increase in cardiac output because output is fixed by the severe obstruction to left ventricular outflow. These hemodynamic circumstances can lead to severe hypotension, syncope, and even death. Thus, it is crucial to diagnose aortic stenosis before therapy for congestive heart failure is begun. The most important clues are the delayed carotid upstrokes, the late-peaking quality of the systolic ejection murmur, and the second heart sound, which is often single because aortic valve leaflet mobility is restricted. In elderly patients, inelasticity of the carotid arteries may cause the upstroke to feel relatively normal. The murmur in aortic stenosis may not be impressive in intensity, especially after congestive heart failure has ensued and total forward output has been reduced.

When aortic stenosis is suspected, the first diagnostic study should be an echocardiogram with Doppler interrogation of the aortic valve. The echocardiogram will provide clues about overall left ventricular function, the degree of hypertrophy, and aortic valve motion. The Doppler study can accurately measure the transvalvular gradient and, thus, helps to better quantify the severity of the disease. A peak flow velocity of ≥ 4.0 m/sec across the aortic valve in asymptomatic patients indicates that symptoms are likely to develop within 2 years. When history, physical examination, and the echocardiogram indicate that severe aortic stenosis is the cause of the patient's heart failure, cardiac catheterization, in consideration of surgery, should be performed in a timely fashion to perform coronary arteriography and confirm the hemodynamic status. Aortic valve area and aortic valve resistance can be calculated to further guide the clinician in estimating the severity of the disease.

No effective medical therapy exists for aortic stenosis. Aortic valve replacement is the only satisfactory definitive therapy. Balloon aortic valvotomy may be employed as a palliative measure in extreme cases, when the patient is deemed not to be a surgical candidate.

In the present patient, the pressure tracing demonstrated a large pressure gradient across the aortic valve. Aortic valve replacement was performed, and the ejection fraction, which was 0.22 preoperatively, increased to 0.45 postoperatively. The patient's heart failure improved dramatically.

Clinical Pearls

1. The murmur of severe aortic stenosis may be soft in intensity but is long in duration and peaks late in systole.
2. The elderly may not have the classic peripheral finding of a delayed carotid upstroke.
3. The development of congestive heart failure in aortic stenosis is an ominous sign, with a 50% mortality within 2 years without valve replacement.
4. In any patient with congestive heart failure in whom vasodilator therapy is about to be initiated, the diagnosis of aortic stenosis (in which vasodilators are contraindicated) must be excluded.
5. No medical therapy exists for aortic stenosis. Attempts to temporize or delay surgery after the development of symptoms of angina, syncope, or heart failure may lead to sudden death.

REFERENCES

1. Ross J Jr, Braunwald E: Aortic stenosis. Circulation 1968;38(Suppl V):V68–V67
2. Carabello BA: Timing of surgery for acquired aortic stenosis. Cardiovasc Rev Rep 1987;8:15–20.
3. Karavan MP, Carabello BA: Clinical controversies in aortic stenosis. Mod Concepts Cardiovasc Dis 1991;60:61–66.
4. Otto CM, Burwash IG, Legget ME, et al: Prospective study of asymptomatic valvular aortic stenosis. Clinical, echocardiographic, and exercise predictors of outcome. Circulation 1997;95:2262–2270.

PATIENT 78

A 45-year-old woman with exertional angina

A 45-year-old woman with a history of hypertension notes a 3-month history of angina occurring usually after extreme exertion. She has no prior cardiac history. Her risk factors for atherosclerosis include obesity, a positive family history, and hypertension.

Physical Examination: Vital signs: pulse 80; respirations 16; blood pressure 150/80. General: obese female in no distress. Chest: clear. Cardiac: S_4. Extremities: 2+ symmetric distal pulses.

Laboratory Findings: Cardiac catheterization: see below.

Questions: What is the coronary anatomy? How might it explain the patient's ischema?

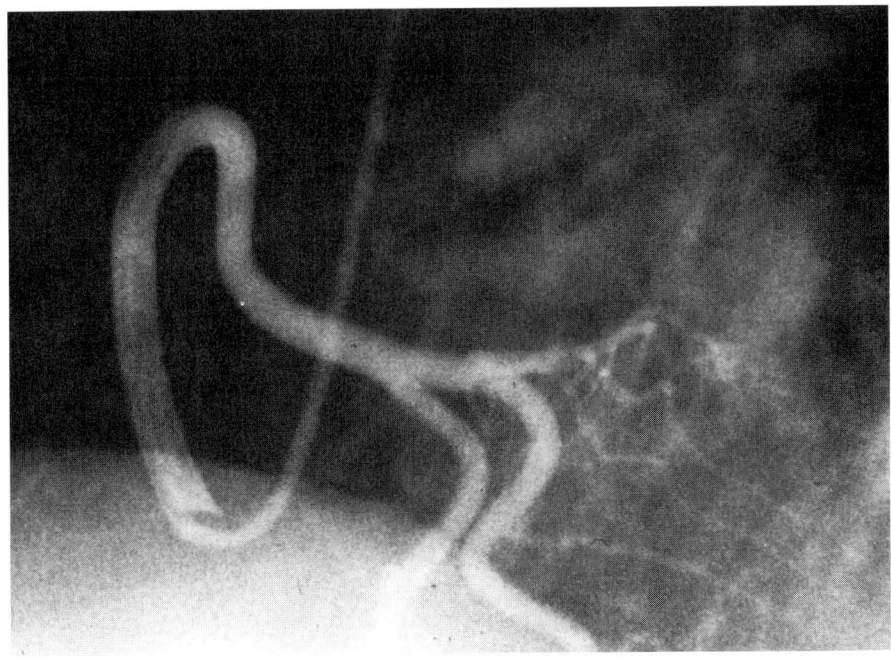

Diagnosis: Anomalous origin of the left coronary artery.

Discussion: Coronary arteriograms in the present patient demonstrated that the left coronary artery originated from the right coronary cusp and passed between the right ventricular outflow tract and aorta en route to the left ventricle. In this anomaly, although the coronary vessels are anatomically free of disease, myocardial ischemia may develop perhaps because the coronary vessels are pinched between the right ventricular outflow tract and the aorta as pressure rises in these structures during exercise. Angina, thallium perfusion defects, and sudden death have been reported, supporting the existence of true ischemia. Coronary bypass surgery with ligation of the proximal portion of the vessels has been advocated to alter the pathway for coronary blood flow away from this anomalous pattern. Anomalous origin of the right coronary artery from the left sinus of Valsalva also may cause ischemia.

Three other anomalous coronary lesions may cause ischemia: (1) congenital coronary stenosis; (2) origin of the left coronary artery from the pulmonary artery; and (3) coronary artery to coronary vein fistulas. In congenital coronary stenosis the lesions are not atherosclerotic, but congenitally stenotic. The coronary narrowing limits flow, producing ischemia. Origin of the left coronary from the pulmonary artery causes low perfusion pressure and reduced oxygen content, and leads to myocardial ischemia and/or infarction. Only 25% of patients survive into adulthood without surgery. Coronary artery to coronary vein fistulas (a left-to-right shunt) may produce ischemia distal to the fistula as flow is diverted into the fistula rather than into the myocardium. Most fistulas drain into the right ventricle. A large fistula may create a substantial left-to-right shunt that leads to volume overload and left ventricular failure. Other complications of fistulas are bacterial endocarditis and rupture.

Several other coronary anomalies occur but do not produce hemodynamic or ischemic sequelae. The most common of these is origin of the circumflex artery from the right coronary cusp. Because the circumflex artery does not course between the aorta and right ventricular outflow tract, reduced coronary blood flow does not occur. Other common anomalies include separate origin of the first septal perforator, origin of the left anterior descending artery from the right coronary cusp where the course is around rather than between the right ventricular outflow tract and aorta, and single coronary arteries. Although these lesions do not by themselves create coronary ischemia, like any vessel, they are subject to coronary atherosclerosis. During cardiac catheterization, the failure to recognize and engage an aberrant artery arising from an unsuspected ostia will result in failure to diagnose symptomatic coronary disease in that vessel.

The present patient was treated with a beta blocker and became asymptomatic on therapy.

Clinical Pearls

1. At the time of cardiac catheterization all vessels must be accounted for after the standard coronary arteriograms have been performed. If the three major arteries cannot be defined, a search for an anomalous takeoff must be undertaken.

2. Several coronary anomalies have hemodynamic consequences. Although most are detected during childhood, passage of the left coronary between the right ventricular outflow tract and aorta is a potential cause of sudden death in the adult.

3. Patients with left coronary arteries that pass between the right ventricular outflow tract and aorta may improve with beta blockers.

REFERENCES

1. Engel HJ, Torres C, Page HL: Major variations in anatomical origin of the coronary arteries: Angiographic observations in 4,250 patients without associated congenital heart disease. Cathet Cardiovasc Diagn 1975;1:157.
2. Roberts WC. Major anomalies of coronary arterial origin seen in adulthood. Am Heart J 1986;111:941–963.
3. Click RL, Holmes Jr DR, Vlietstra RE, et al: Anomalous coronary arteries: Location, degree of atherosclerosis and effect on survival—a report from the Coronary Artery Surgery Study. J Am Coll Cardiol 1989;13:531–537.
4. Grollman Jr JH, Mao SS, Weinstein SR: Arteriographic demonstration of both kinking at the origin and compression between the great vessels of an anomalous right coronary artery arising in common with a left coronary artery from above the left sinus of Valsalva. Cathet Cardiovasc Diagn 1992;25:46–51.

PATIENT 79

A 30-year-old man with fever, chills, and a new heart murmur

A 30-year-old man presents with 1 week of fever, chills, general malaise, and arthralgia. He denies intravenous drug abuse, heavy alcohol intake, or other significant past medical history, including a history of rheumatic fever. He does report a recent history of fever and a sore throat that resolved in 4 days.

Physical Examination: Vital signs: temperature 102°; pulse 110 and regular; blood pressure 110/60. General: thin male in moderate distress. Throat: pharyngeal erythema with small pustules. Chest: clear. Cardiac: no gallop; II/VI diastolic murmur at the base radiating down the left sternal border. Extremities: fine erythematous rash over the distal extremities; erythematous swollen carpal, prepatellar, and ankle joints.

Laboratory Findings: ESR: 92 mm/hr. Throat culture: positive for group A hemolytic streptococcus. Blood cultures: negative. Echocardiogram: aortic and mitral insufficiency without vegetations.

Question: What is the cause of this patient's symptom complex?

Diagnosis: Acute rheumatic fever.

Discussion: Clinical diagnosis of acute rheumatic fever is based on the presence of two major Jones criteria or one major and two minor Jones criteria together with evidence of a recent streptococcal infection. The five major Jones criteria are carditis, polyarthritis, chorea, erythema marginatum, and subcutaneous nodules. Minor criteria are fever, arthralgia, history of rheumatic fever, elevated erthrocyte sedimentation rate, and a prolonged PR interval. Evidence of a preceding streptococcal infection includes a positive culture, increased anti-streptolysin O titer, or increased anti-DNase B titer.

In evaluating the major Jones criteria, carditis is thought to be present when a new murmur is found, when there is evidence of a new pericardial effusion or friction rub, or when there is evidence of severe newly developed myocardial dysfunction. Carditis is most commonly diagnosed by finding a new murmur of mitral regurgitation. The new murmur of aortic regurgitation, as noted in the present patient, is also a common occurrence.

Chorea usually occurs only in young children; its incidence decreases rapidly after the age of 10. It may also occur as an isolated entity, with rheumatic heart disease developing years later. Erythema marginatum is a rash confined to the trunk and arms that appears as a pink ring that spreads through the skin. It is not painful or indurated and blanches upon pressure. It may appear transiently, fade, and then reappear after the acute rheumatic episode has subsided. The arthritis typically occurs in older patients and usually involves the large joints, such as the elbows, ankles, knees, and wrists. It often improves with aspirin therapy.

The incidence of rheumatic fever has declined dramatically in the last three decades, although sporadic outbreaks still occur. Antibiotic usage was thought to be important in the decline of rheumatic fever; however, the decline began before antibiotics were readily available. The etiology and pathophysiology of the disease are not entirely clear. The most widely held theory is that antigens which crossreact with the streptococcus are also present in the heart, resulting in autoimmune attack.

In the United States, the major sequela of rheumatic fever is valvular heart disease. Acutely, mitral and aortic regurgitation occur as the leaflets become inflamed and incompetent. However, the hemodynamic disturbance produced by the acute disease is usually mild. Several years after the acute event, possibly due to "smoldering" disease, the valvular disease becomes more severe. The most common manifestation is severe mitral stenosis, which usually occurs in women. Aortic insufficiency, mitral insufficiency, and aortic stenosis follow in an order of decreasing incidence.

Acutely, penicillin therapy to eradicate the streptococcal infection together with aspirin to treat the arthritis or arthralgia form the basis of therapy. If aspirin is not effective in suppressing the inflammatory manifestations of the disease, corticosteroids can be added. Once one episode of acute rheumatic fever has occurred, secondary prophylaxis with 1.2 million units of benzathine penicillin G injected monthly is the treatment of choice. Prophylaxis should probably continue until age 50.

In the present patient, the murmur of aortic regurgitation was new and fulfilled the major Jones criterion, carditis. Three minor criteria—fever, arthralgia, and increased sedimentation rate—were also present. He responded to aspirin therapy and was placed on penicillin prophylaxis. He recovered and is currently receiving prophylactic penicillin and yearly evaluation of his valvular heart disease.

Clinical Pearls

1. The diagnosis of acute rheumatic fever today is usually made by the appearance of a new heart murmur, which represents one major Jones criterion (carditis), together with two minor Jones criteria.

2. Although mitral stenosis is the most common sequela of rheumatic fever, acutely, valvular regurgitation predominates.

3. Antibiotic usage was thought to be important in the decline of rheumatic fever; however, the decline began before antibiotics were readily available.

REFERENCES

1. Kaplan MH: Immunologic relation of streptococcal and tissue antigens. I. Properties of an antigen in certain strains of group A streptococci exhibiting an immunologic crossreaction with human heart tissue. J Immunol 1963;90:595–606.
2. Roberts WC, Virmani R: Aschoff bodies at necropsy in valvular heart disease. Evidence from an analysis of 543 patients over 14 years of age that rheumatic heart disease, at least anatomically, is a disease of the mitral valve. Circulation 1978;57:803–807.
3. Gordis L: The virtual disappearance of rheumatic fever in the United States: Lessons in the rise and fall of disease. Circulation 1985;72:1155–1162.
4. Khanna AK, Buskirk DR, Williams RC Jr, et al: Presence of a non-HLA B cell antigen in rheumatic fever in patients and their families as defined by a monoclonal antibody. J Clin Invest 1989;83:1710–1716.

PATIENT 80

A 45-year-old man with intractable congestive heart failure

A 45-year-old physician was first diagnosed in 1971 as having congestive cardiomyopathy. One year later he sustained an embolism to the left middle cerebral artery, with resulting transient right hemiparesis and persistent aphasia. In 1984 he began having exertional dyspnea and coughing spells, especially upon lying down. His symptoms of congestive failure have become progressively worse and respond poorly to digitalis, diuretics, and preload and afterload reducing agents. Several members of his family have varying types of hypertropic cardiomyopathy.

Physical Examination: Vital signs: pulse 80; blood pressure 100/70. Neck: at 45° position, deep jugular vein pulsations to the angle of the jaw. Cardiac: S_3 and S_4 gallops; no murmurs. Chest: bibasilar rales. Abdomen: hepatomelgaly. Extremities: peripheral edema.

Laboratory Findings: CBC and urinalysis: normal. Cr: 1 mg/dl. Serum electrolytes: normal. Chest radiograph: generalized cardiomegaly with superior pulmonary venous congestion. EKG: first-degree AV block; right bundle branch block; Q wave in leads II, III, AVF, and V_1 and V_4; biatrial enlargement. Echocardiogram: consistent with a congestive cardiomyopathy; generalized hypokinesis; all chambers dilated. MUGA: ejection fraction 19%.

Question: What would you recommend for this patient?

Diagnosis: Heart transplantation is indicated for this patient with familial congestive cardiomyopathy.

Discussion: Long-term survival after cardiac transplantation has steadily improved during the last 20 years. The 1-year survival is now 82%, and the 5-year survival is 65%. Despite this clinical success, the majority of candidates never undergo surgery because of the limited donor supply. About 20,000 patients under 70 years of age are potential heart recipients in the U.S. each year, but only 2,500 donor hearts become available.

In order to rank transplant recipients on the basis of need, waiting lists are computerized nationally and patients must undergo thorough evaluation. The diagnosis of heart disease should be established and the potential for reversibility investigated. Hemodynamic monitoring and laboratory tests determine potential reversibility of any pulmonary, renal, and hepatic dysfunction resulting from congestion and poor perfusion. The majority of patients referred for heart transplantation have ejection fractions less than 20–25%, but this in itself is an insufficient indication. Exercise testing is important for patients without cardiac compromise at rest. **General indications** for transplantation are irreversible cardiac disease that is not responding to medical therapy and has no surgical option, and high risk of death within the next 1 year. There should be no noncardiac conditions that would shorten the patient's life expectancy or increase the risk of rejection.

Contraindications to cardiac transplantation include age over 65 years, active infection, severe diabetes, severe peripheral vascular disease, active ulcer disease, FEV_1 or FVC <60% of predicted, history of chronic bronchitis, serum creatinine >2 mg/dl, creatinine clearance <50 ml/min, bilirubin >2.5 mg/dl, transaminase > twice normal, pulmonary artery systolic pressure >60 mmHg, mean transpulmonary gradient >15 mmHg, and high level of patient noncompliance. Some organ dysfunction may be allowed if it can be reversed with optimal hemodynamic function produced by using nitroprusside and/or dobutamine for 72 hours. In some instances ventricular assist devices may be used for refractory failure as temporary support until a donor is available. The upper limit of cardiac *donor* age is 60 years, and those over 45 years should have coronary arteriography to exclude the presence of coronary artery disease.

Following successful transplantation, detection of rejection is one of the most critical aspects. Endomyocardial biopsy is one of the best ways to diagnose rejection. Most rejections occur within the first 2 months and 90% occur by the first 6 months. Therefore, biopsies are scheduled weekly for the first 4–6 weeks, then biweekly for a month, then monthly for 3 months, then every 2 months for a year. After the first year, biopsies are performed every 3 months, every 6 months in the third year, and then annually at the time of catherization. Continuous immunosuppressive therapy with azathioprine, cyclosporine, corticosteriods, or antilymphocyte antibodies is necessary. Accelerated graft atherosclerosis has become the leading cause of death in long-term survivors. Such patients are denervated and do not experience angina. This atherosclerosis differs from the usual variety in that it is more diffuse, distal, and cellular, with less lipid accumulation. Collateral vessels are rare.

The present patient had progressive congestive failure that did not respond to medical therapy, and his chances of surviving even a few months were unlikely. After routine studies for heart transplantation, he had cardiac catheterization and endomyocardial biopsy. His coronaries were normal. Findings at catheterization were those of a dilated cardiomyopathy and biopsy showed substantial myocardial fibrosis. The patient had cardiac transplantation and has done very well.

Clinical Pearls

1. One-year survival after cardiac transplantation is 82%, and 5-year survival is 65%.
2. The age limit for recipients of transplanted hearts is up to 65 years, and the age limit for donors is up to 60 years of age.
3. Rejection is still the major problem in the care of transplantation patients and is monitored by frequent endomyocardial biopsies.

REFERENCES

1. Gao SZ, Alderman EL, Schroeder JS, et al: Accelerated coronary vascular disease in the heart transplant patient: Coronary arteriographic findings. J Am Coll Cardiol 1988;12:334–340.
2. Grattan MT, Moreno-Cabral CE, Starnes VA, et al: Eight-year results of cyclosporine-treated patients with cardiac transplants. J Thorac Cardiovasc Surg 1990;99:500–509
3. Stevenson LW, Miller LW: Cardiac transplantation as therapy for heart failure. Curr Probl Cardiol 1991;16:223–305.
4. Hosenpud JD, Bennett LE, Keck BM: The Registry of the International Society for Heart and Lung Transplantation: Fifteenth official report—1998. J Heart Lung Transplant 1998;17:656–668.

PATIENT 81

A 23-year-old retarded woman with acute chest pain

A 23-year-old woman presents to the emergency room with substernal chest pain that radiates to her left arm. She has mild diaphoresis, but no nausea or vomiting. There is no previous history of angina or myocardial infarction. She has mild mental retardation, but is progressing well in a school for the mentally handicapped. She also has a history of bilateral optic lens dislocation.

Physical Examination: Vital signs: pulse 70 and regular; blood pressure 100/60. General: tall, slender woman with moderate chest pain. Cardiac: S_4; no murmurs. Extremities: elongated digits that are not hyperextensible.

Laboratory Findings: EKG: see below.

Question: What is the most likely diagnosis?

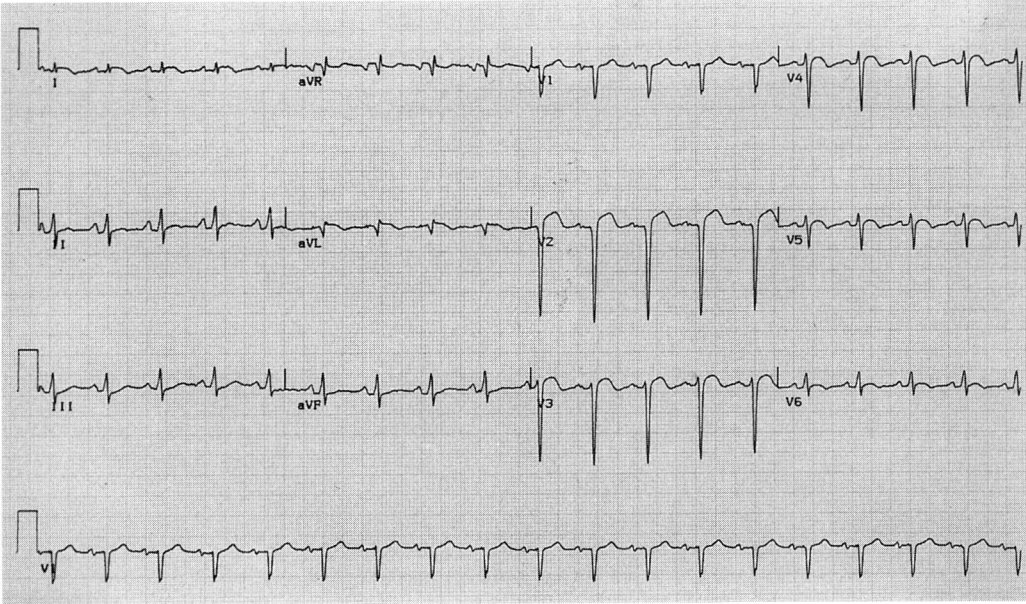

187

Diagnosis: Myocardial infarction associated with homocystinuria.

Discussion: Homocystinuria is usually due to a deficiency of cystathionine beta-synthase. Patients with this deficiency often are misdiagnosed as having Marfan syndrome. A tall body habitus, ectopia lentis, and pectus deformities are, in fact, features common to both Marfan syndrome and homocystinuria. Unlike Marfan syndrome, in homocystinuria the joints are not hyperextensible and the palate is usually not highly arched. Mental retardation is not a feature of Marfan syndrome but is common in homocystinuria. The major differences between the two syndromes, however, lie in their cardiovascular manifestations. Marfan syndrome produces mitral valve prolapse, aortic root dilatation, aortic dissection, and aortic valve insufficiency, whereas the major feature of homocystinuria is a hypercoagulable state. Hypercoagulability in turn leads to premature myocardial infarction, pulmonary embolism, and thrombotic stroke.

Once the syndrome is suspected clinically, the diagnosis is made by biochemical testing. The deficiency in cystathionine beta-synthase prevents homocysteine from reacting with serine to form cystathionine. Instead, two molecules of homocysteine combine to form homocystine; a high urinary homocystine level confirms the diagnosis.

If the disease is suspected in newborns because of a positive family history, methionine restriction reduces the incidence of mental retardation and seizures. Approximately half of the older patients with the disease respond to large doses of vitamin B6 (pyridoxine) and folate, which reduces the homocystinemia and homocystinuria. Antithrombotic therapy with aspirin and/or warfarin also seems advisable, but their value is unproven.

More recently, there has been intense interest in less blatant forms of the disease. Heterozygotes have none of the outward characteristics, but do have elevated homocysteine levels. Such patients are at risk for vascular thrombosis, and the role of homocysteine as a coronary risk factor is now undergoing active scrutiny.

The present patient recovered from her myocardial infarction and began therapy with pyridoxine and warfarin.

Clinical Pearls

1. Homocystinuria is a rare inherited disease that phenotypically resembles Marfan syndrome.

2. The cardiovascular consequences of homocystinuria are different from those of Marfan syndrome and include arterial and venous thrombosis.

3. Treatment with pyridoxine is effective in approximately half of patients with homocystinuria.

REFERENCES

1. Wilcken DEL, Wilcken B, Dudman NPB, et al: Homocystinuria—the effects of betaine in the treatment of patients not responsive to pyridoxine. N Engl J Med 1983;309:448–453.
2. Boers GHJ, Smals AGH, Trijbels FJM, et al: Heterozygosity for homocystinuria in premature peripheral and cerebral occlusive arterial disease. N Engl J Med 1985;313:709–715.
3. Mudd SH, Skovby F, Levy HL, et al: The natural history of homocystinuria due to cystathionine-β-synthase deficiency. Am J Hum Genet 1985;37:1–31.
4. Selhub J, Jacques PF, Bostom AG, et al: Association between plasma homocysteine concentrations and extracranial carotid-artery stenosis. N Engl J Med 1995;332:286–291.

PATIENT 82

A 25-year-old intravenous drug user with fever, chills, anorexia, and weight loss

A 25-year-old woman, who is an intravenous drug abuser, reports a 3-week history of persistent fever with night sweats, a 10-pound weight loss, anorexia, increasing fatigue, and minimal dyspnea.

Physical Examination: Vital signs: pulse 120 (regular); temperature 101.5°; blood pressure 100/60. Fundi: Roth spot in left eye. Chest: clear. Cardiac: no neck vein distention; II/VI holosytolic murmur along left sternal border that increased with inspiration; II/VI systolic ejection murmur at the base; no gallop or rub. Extremities: scattered needle tracks.

Laboratory Findings: Blood cultures: 4 of 4 bottles positive for *Staphylococcus epidermidis,* methicillin resistant. Chest radiograph: multiple 5–8 mm nodular densities in the periphery of both lung fields. Echocardiogram: see below.

Question: What is the diagnosis and the patient's prognosis?

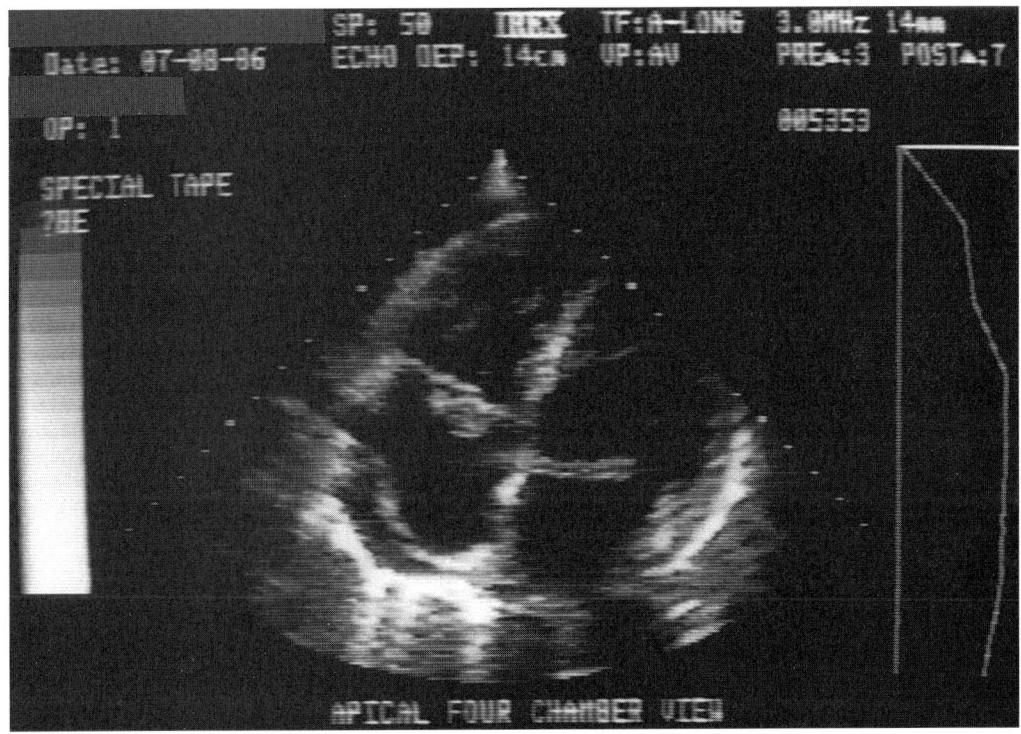

Diagnosis: Tricuspid valve endocarditis with septic pulmonary emboli related to intravenous drug abuse.

Discussion: When drug abuse is the cause of infective endocarditis, it dramatically alters the bacteriology, mortality, and sites of the disease compared with other etiologies. Staphylococcal species, which are introduced into the venous system by contaminated needles through contaminated skin, are the most common causative organisms, accounting for 60% of cases. In nonaddicts, *Streptococcus viridans* is the predominant infectious agent. Tricuspid valve involvement in non-addicts is rare; in drug addicts, tricuspid infection is present in approximately 75%. The left-sided valves are still commonly infected—about one third of all cases.

A common consequence of tricuspid endocarditis is septic pulmonary embolism, as in the present patient. If antimicrobial therapy is delayed, the emboli frequently become lung abscesses. As with systemic emboli in infective endocarditis, septic pulmonary emboli are not treated with anticoagulants because thrombosis is not the cause of the pulmonary embolization.

The prognosis for right-sided endocarditis in addicts is good, with a 90% survival rate. However, the risk of death in left-sided endocarditis in addicts is increased compared with nonaddicts, and the mortality is 40%. The high mortality reflects delay in seeking therapy, the high incidence of *Staphylococcus aureus* as the infective agent, and the tendency toward multiple-valve infections and ring abscess formation. If appropriate antibiotics fail to cure endocarditis in the addict, surgical therapy is complicated by the likelihood of reinfection of a prosthetic valve. In the case of the tricuspid valve, total removal of the valve is well tolerated hemodynamically, at least initially, and obviates the need for a prosthesis. One strategy is to remove the valve entirely, wait for bacteriologic cure, and perform a second operation for tricuspid valve replacement if the symptoms of right-sided congestive heart failure develop. An exception is when multiple emboli have caused pulmonary hypertension, impeding forward flow and worsening the amount of tricuspid regurgitation that will be present when the valve is removed. In these cases, valve replacement is necessary.

Recent emphasis on mitral valve repair in patients with mitral regurgitation has led to renewed interest in tricuspid valve repair. When possible, debridement and repair of the tricuspid valve allow for bacteriologic cure without insertion of a prosthesis and without the severe tricuspid regurgitation of valve excision.

In the present patient, bacteriologic cure was effected with vancomycin. She continued her intravenous drug abuse, however, and died of staphylococcal sepsis 8 months later.

Clinical Pearls

1. Although tricuspid valve endocarditis is rare, in drug addicts it constitutes most of the infected sites.

2. Right-sided endocarditis is associated with a much lower mortality than is left-sided endocarditis.

3. Total tricuspid valve excision to effect bacteriologic cure is remarkably well tolerated, at least initially.

4. Septic pulmonary emboli from infected tricuspid valves are treated with antibiotics and not anticoagulants.

REFERENCES

1. Arbulu A, Thomas NW, Wilson RF: Valvulectomy without prosthetic replacement: A lifesaving operation from tricuspid Pseudomonas endocarditis. J Thorac Cardiovasc Surg 1972;64:103–107.
2. Robbins MJ, Soeiro R, Frishman WH, et al: Right-sided valvular endocarditis: Etiology, diagnosis, and approach to therapy. Am Heart J 1986;111:128–135.
3. Stern HJ, Sisto DA, Strom JA, et al: Immediate tricuspid valve replacement for endocarditis: Indications and results. J Thorac Cardiovasc Surg 1986;91:163–167.
4. Arbulu A, Holmes RJ, Asfaw I: Surgical treatment of intractable right-sided infective endocarditis in drug addicts: 25 years of experience. J Heart Valve Dis 1993;2:129–137.

PATIENT 83

A 51-year-old man with poorly controlled hypertension and pulmonary edema

A 51-year-old man had been in his usual state of health until the day of admission, when he notes the acute onset of dyspnea. There has been no previous orthopnea, and he denies angina, palpitations, or syncope. He has a 3-year history of hypertension poorly controlled by hydrochlorothiazide. The patient reports occasional episodes of diaphoresis and flushing.

Physical Examination: Vital signs: pulse 110 and regular; blood pressure 240/120. General: moderate respiratory distress. Fundi: arterial narrowing; arteriovenous nicking but no papilledema. Chest: diffuse bilateral rales. Cardiac: summation gallop, no murmurs.

Laboratory Findings: CBC: normal. Na^+ 140 mEq/L; K^+ 4.2 mEq/L; Cl^- 102 mEq/L; HCO_3^- 26 mEq/L; BUN 30 mg/dl; Cr 1.2 mg/dl. EKG: normal sinus rhythm; left ventricular hypertrophy.

Hospital Course: After administration of oxygen, furosemide 40 mg intravenously, and nitroglycerin sublingually, the patient improves rapidly.

Question: What test or measure should be included in the evaluation of the patient's severe hypertension?

Diagnosis: Pheochromocytoma. The evaluation should include measurement of urine and plasma catecholamines and their metabolites.

Discussion: Pheochromocytomas are tumors of the chromaffin cells of the adrenergic nervous system. Most are benign tumors arising from the cortex of one of the adrenal glands; however, approximately 10% are malignant and occasionally the tumors are bilateral. Pheochromocytomas may also arise from sympathetic ganglia anywhere in the body or from chemoreceptors. While pheochromocytomas usually present as an isolated disease, they also occur in neurofibromatosis or constitute part of multiple endocrine adenomatosis syndrome II in association with hyperparathyroidism and thyroid C cell hyperplasia or medullary carcinoma.

Adrenal tumors usually produce epinephrine, whereas norepinephrine is usually secreted by most nonadrenal pheochromocytomas. Wide fluctuations in blood pressure due to episodic tumor secretion of catecholamines are considered typical of the disease. However, only about 50% of patients with pheochromocytoma experience widely fluctuating blood pressure; the remainder maintain constant levels of hypertension.

Most patients with pheochromocytoma have other associated symptoms that include flushing, diaphoresis, weight loss, and hyperglycemia. Epinephrine-secreting tumors produce intravascular volume contraction, causing affected patients to suffer from paradoxic orthostatic hypotension, especially if a diuretic is administered. Pulmonary edema, as seen in the present patient, occurs when excess afterload produced by the hypertension impairs cardiac performance. Additionally, chronic high levels of circulating catecholamines may cause direct myocardial damage manifested as fibrinoid necrosis and patchy areas of fibrosis causing myocardial dysfunction. Hypertensive crises can be precipitated by administration of beta blockers (leaving alpha receptor stimulation unopposed), histamine, caffeine, glucocorticoids, and tricyclic antidepressants.

The diagnosis of pheochromocytoma rests on detecting in the urine high levels of plasma catecholamines or high levels of their metabolites, vanillylmandelic acid and metanephrine. Determination of plasma catecholamines has the highest sensitivity but may produce false-negative results if episodic catecholamine release is missed at the time of sampling. On the other hand, the 24-hour urine collection produces summary information about catecholamine release during the day and enhances diagnostic accuracy. Once there is biochemical evidence of a pheochromocytoma, the tumor is usually localized by abdominal CT scanning. In most cases, the typically well-defined adrenal tumors are easily diagnosed. With extraadrenal tumors, scanning with ^{131}I-labeled iodobenzlguanidine, which concentrates in the tumor, is a useful technique to localize the neoplasm. Following identification, the tumors should be removed surgically. Preoperative control of blood pressure with alpha- and beta-adrenergic blocking agents is crucial in ensuring a good surgical outcome.

The present patient had high circulating catecholamines and vanillylmandelic acid, suggesting the diagnosis. His test showed vanillylmandelic acid, 24-hr urine collection, 23 mg (nl <7 mg/d); epinephrine, 24-hr urine collection, 50 μg (nl <15 μg/d); and plasma 433 pg/ml (nl <90 pg/ml). A CT scan demonstrated a 2-cm right adrenal mass that was removed successfully and proved to be a pheochromocytoma. His blood pressure normalized following surgery.

Clinical Pearls

1. Although many patients with pheochromocytoma have episodic elevations in blood pressure thought typical of the disease, in about 50% of cases the blood pressure is constantly elevated without distinct variations.

2. Other symptoms, including palpitations, headache, and diaphoresis, are common in pheochromocytoma. but are usually absent in other forms of hypertension.

3. CT scanning is an excellent diagnostic tool for localizing the tumor once biochemical evidence has established its existence.

REFERENCES

1. Gifford RW, Kvale WF, Maher FT, et al: Clinical features, diagnosis and treatment of pheochromocytoma: A review of 76 cases. Mayo Clin Proc 1964;39:281–302.
2. Bravo EL, Gifford RW: Pheochromocytoma: Diagnosis, localization and management. N Engl J Med 1984;311:1298–1303.
3. Imperato-McGinley J, Gautier T, Ehlers K, et al: Reversibility of catecholamine-induced dilated cardiomyopathy in a child with a pheochromocytoma. N Engl J Med 1987;316:793–797.
4. Graves JW: Management of difficult-to-control hypertension. Mayo Clin Proc 2000;75(3):278–284.

PATIENT 84

A 56-year-old woman with palpitations and chest pain

A 56-year-old woman has had intermittent palpitations and substernal tightness with radiation to her back for 4 years. The chest discomfort usually occurs after walking about one city block and subsides with rest. The longest the discomfort lasts is 10 minutes.

Physical Examination: Vital signs: pulse 80; blood pressure 130/80. Cardiac: multiple midsystolic clicks followed by high-pitched apical systolic murmur; accentuation of murmur, onset of premature beats, and movement of clicks toward first heart sound with standing; murmur inaudible and movement of clicks toward second heart sound with squatting.

Laboratory Findings: EKG: normal. Stress test using the Bruce protocol: 2-mm horizontal ST segment depression in the inferolateral leads and occasional premature ventricular beats. EKG changes resolved immediately upon lying down. Echocardiogram: see below.

Question: What is the patient's diagnosis?

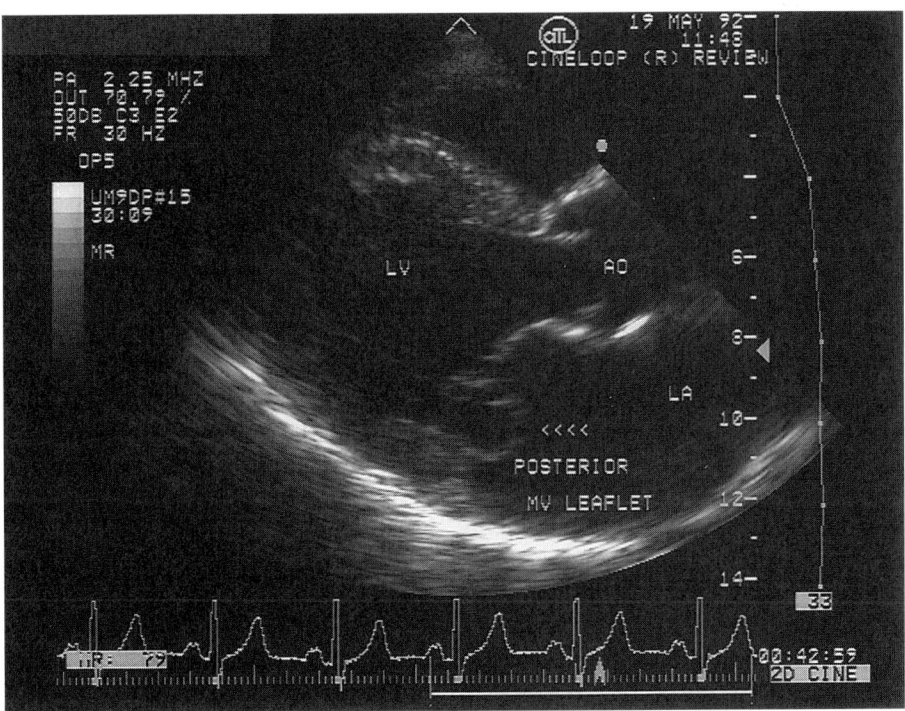

Diagnosis: Mitral valve prolapse (MVP).

Discussion: The true incidence of MVP is difficult to ascertain because the majority of patients are asymptomatic. Previous estimates of a 5% incidence were based upon echocardiographic misinterpretation, and it was not until 1987 that the presence of true mitral valve prolapse was defined echocardiographically. Whether there are any symptoms directly attributable to MVP continues to be widely debated. Although atypical chest pain, anxiety, fatigue, and palpitation have been associated with MVP, cause and effect remain unproven.

Patients with MVP often have a slender body habitus with associated skeletal deformities. The thoracic examination may reveal a pectus excavatum, scoliosis, or a "straight back." The auscultatory findings include one or more high-pitched clicks that occur most typically in midsystole but at various times can move to late or even early systole. In some but not all patients, the midsystolic click is followed by a late systolic murmur. The auscultatory findings can be varied by altering ventricular volume, contractility, and pressure. Left ventricular volume is reduced on standing, which accentuates the prolapse and causes the click and murmur to move closer to the first heart sound. Squatting increases the venous return, systemic vascular resistance, and left ventricular volume. Because of these changes, the prolapse is delayed and the click and murmur move toward the second heart sound and may even disappear. Often these findings are clearer when the patient stands from the squatting position. At times, a systolic honk or whooping sound may also occur.

Focal neurologic findings, such as transient ischemic attacks, amaurosis fugax, retinal artery occlusion, and, rarely, hemiparesis, have been reported in patients with MVP. These neurologic findings probably occur as a result of thromboemboli from the prolapsing valve.

The EKG at rest frequently shows inferolateral T-wave inversion. False-positive EKG stress tests occur in up to 50% of patients with MVP. Premature beats are most common, although practically any arrhythmia can occur, including sinoatrial and atrioventricular node conduction defects. The cause of the arrhythmia is not known but may be related to autonomic dysfunction or mechanical effects of the floppy valve. Syncope correlates poorly with the presence of arrhythmias.

Strict echocardiographic criteria should be used to detect MVP because needless patient anxiety can be created by overdiagnosing the condition. Echocardiographic signs of MVP should be interpreted in light of the patient's physical findings; the echocardiogram is not clinically useful if the patient has no evidence of the disease on careful auscultation. Doppler echocardiography is useful for the detection and quantitation of the severity of mitral regurgitation.

The prognosis is excellent in the majority of patients. Some patients, however, will develop major arrhythmias, sudden death, infective endocarditis, thromboemboli, ruptured chordae, or progressive mitral insufficiency that requires valve replacement. Most complications are noted in patients with significant mitral regurgitation and thickened redundant valves who have left atrial and left ventricular enlargement.

Many patients with MVP do well without therapy. Propranolol can be administered effectively to patients with supraventricular arrhythmias or frequent premature ventricular contractions. If a murmur is present or if the valve leaflets are redundant or thickened, standard antibiotic prophylaxis against infective endocarditis is required.

The present patient's echocardiogram and Doppler study showed MVP and mild mitral insufficiency. Because of persistent chest pain, a thallium stress test was performed, and results were normal. Despite reassurance from her physicians, the patient requested coronary arteriography because of her concern about coronary disease in light of her brother's history of coronary bypass surgery. The coronary arteries were normal and the left ventriculogram showed mild mitral insufficiency.

Clinical Pearls

1. Patients with MVP experience nonspecific types of chest pains that are nonanginal in quality, but cause and effect is unproven.
2. Patients with suggestive echocardiographic studies should not be labeled with the diagnosis of MVP unless auscultatory evidence of the disease is present or unless the valve is clearly structurally abnormal.
3. The majority of the patients with MVP have an excellent prognosis. Complications occur primarily in those who have thickening of their leaflets and redundancy of the valve.

REFERENCES

1. Marks AR, Choong CY, Chir MBB, et al: Identification of high-risk and low-risk subgroups of patients with mitral valve prolapse. N Engl 3 Med 1989;320:1031–1036.
2. Fontana ME, Sparks EA, Boudoulas H, Wooley CF: Mitral valve prolapse and the mitral valve prolapse syndrome. Curr Probl Cardiol 1991;16:309–375.
3. Dollar AL, Roberts WC: Morphologic comparison of patients with mitral valve prolapse who died suddenly with patients who died from severe valvular dysfunction or other conditions. J Am Coll Cardiol 1991; 17:921–931.

PATIENT 85

A 54-year-old man with low voltage on electrocardiogram

A 54-year-old man complains of dyspnea on exertion and ankle edema that has progressively worsened over the previous 6 months. The patient is begun on digoxin and furosemide, with little improvement.

Physical Examination: Vital signs: pulse 80; respirations 24; blood pressure 110/60. Neck: jugular venous distention with estimated central venous pressure of 14 cm of water. Chest: bibasilar rales. Cardiac: quiet precordium; S_3 gallop; II/VI holosystolic murmur at the apex. Abdomen: consistent with ascites. Extremities: 2+ peripheral edema.

Laboratory Findings: EKG: low voltage; right bundle branch block. Echocardiogram: see below.

Question: What is the most likely cause of the patient's heart failure?

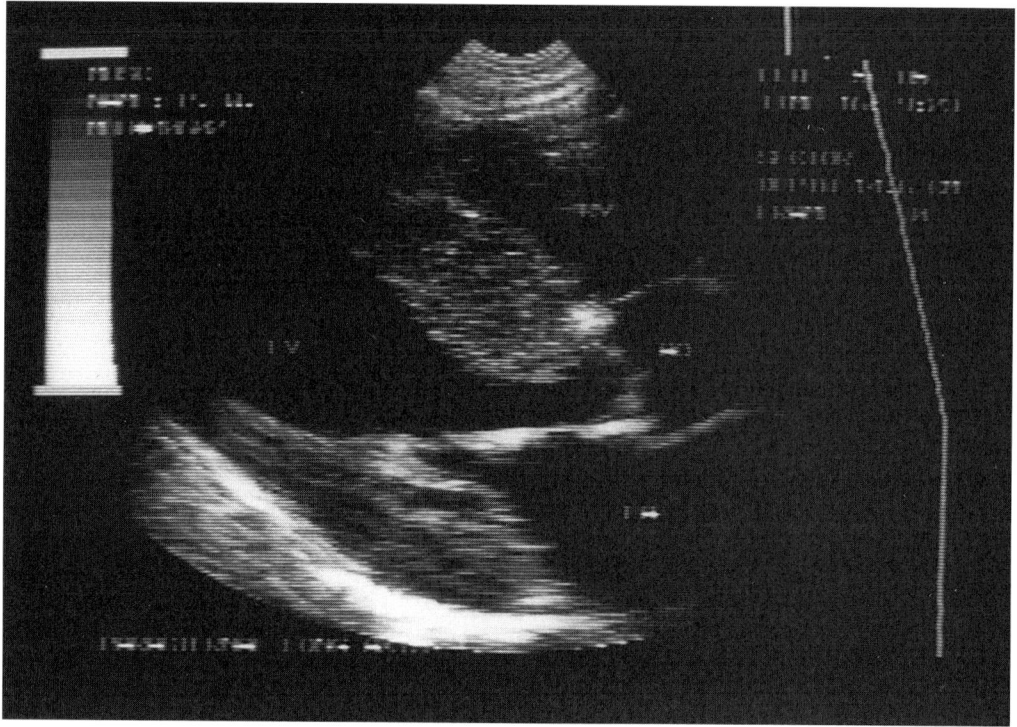

Diagnosis: Amyloid cardiomyopathy.

Discussion: Amyloidosis is an infiltrative disease of the myocardium that initially produces diastolic dysfunction followed by systolic dysfunction later in the course of the disease. Many patients with amyloid cardiac disease, as with other restrictive cardiomyopathies, present with findings of right-sided congestive heart failure out of proportion to left-sided failure. Although amyloid infiltrates both sides of the heart, it is perhaps the ease of detection of right ventricular failure, such as jugular venous distention, edema, and ascites, that makes the right-sided findings seem so prominent.

The echocardiogram in patients with amyloid cardiomyopathy frequently demonstrates a "sparkling" appearance within the myocardium. Additionally, the left ventricular walls and interatrial septum are thickened. The thickening of the cardiac chambers as they become infiltrated with amyloid requires increased filling pressure at a given volume (diastolic dysfunction). In turn, increased filling pressure of the left and right ventricles produces the symptoms of pulmonary and systemic congestion.

Usually, an increase in left ventricular wall thickness, as occurs in hypertrophy, causes increased voltage on the EKG. In amyloidosis, however, increased wall thickness is associated with decreased voltage. This paradox is an important diagnostic clue to the presence of amyloidosis and other cardiac infiltrative disease.

The protein fibrils deposited in amyloidosis are of the AL or AA varieties. AL deposition is the most common and is produced by plasma cell dyscrasias ranging from so-called benign monoclonal gammopathy to multiple myeloma. AL deposition typically involves the heart, tongue, rectum, lymph nodes, spleen, and peripheral nerves. Immunoglobulin electrophoresis is usually abnormal in patients with AL disease. AA deposition occurs in chronic inflammatory diseases such as rheumatoid arthritis and tuberculosis. AA deposition typically involves the liver, spleen, and kidneys. The source of AA protein is not clear. AA and AL deposition may not follow the pattern described above and either type of protein can be deposited in either group of organs.

The clinical diagnosis of amyloid cardiomyopathy rests upon the presentation of a patient with diastolic dysfunction, thickened left ventricular walls, and reduced voltage on EKG. Differentiation from constrictive pericarditis often is difficult, but may be aided by marked respiratory variation in Doppler mitral flow velocity, which is seen in constriction but not in amyloidosis. In advanced disease, systolic dysfunction may coexist with diastolic dysfunction. A tissue diagnosis of amyloidosis can be obtained from biopsy of the rectum, skin, or heart. Therapy is primarily supportive because no specific remedy exists. The restrictive filling pattern in this disease makes patients very susceptible to hypotension induced by vasodilators or diuresis because reduced filling pressure leads to reduced end-diastolic volume and thus reduced cardiac output. Digitalis is usually ineffective and may actually be contraindicated since it is bound by the amyloid, increasing the risk of digitalis intoxication.

The present patient appeared to have diastolic dysfunction as the etiology of the congestive symptoms because of the preservation of an adequate ejection fraction. The low voltage and left bundle branch block with the echocardiographic findings suggested amyloidosis, which was confirmed by rectal biopsy. He died 2 months later from intractable heart failure.

Clinical Pearls

1. The combination of thickened left ventricular walls and low EKG voltage should raise the suspicion of amyloidosis.

2. The most common form of cardiac amyloidosis comes from AL protein produced by plasma cells and is associated with a positive immunoelectrophoresis.

3. Increased filling pressures are required in patients with restrictive cardiomyopathies and diastolic dysfunction to maintain cardiac output. Therapies that reduce filling pressures must be managed with great caution.

4. Digitalis is usually ineffective and may actually be contraindicated because it is bound by the amyloid, increasing the risk of digitalis intoxication.

REFERENCES

1. Carroll JD, Gaasch WH, McAdam KPWJ: Amyloid cardiomyopathy: Characterization by a distinctive voltage/mass relation. Am J Cardiol 1982;49:9–13.
2. Shabetai R: Pathophysiology and differential diagnosis of restrictive cardiomyopathy. Cardiovasc Clin 1988;19:123–132.
3. Gertz MA, Kyle RA: Primary systemic amyloidosis—a diagnostic primer. Mayo Clin Proc 1989;64:1505–1519.
4. Nishimura RA, Tajik AJ: Evaluation of diastolic filling of left ventricle in health and disease: Doppler echocardiography is the clinician's Rosetta stone. J Am Coll Cardiol 1997;30:8–18.

PATIENT 86

A 40-year-old man with decreased exercise tolerance and a diastolic heart murmur

A 40-year-old man with a past medical history of rheumatic fever and a known heart murmur since age 20 complains of dyspnea on exertion.

Physical Examination: Vital signs: pulse 90; respirations 20; blood pressure 150/50. Chest: clear. Cardiac: PMI sixth intercostal space anterior axillary line; S_3; III/VI diastolic murmur radiating down left sternal border; I/VI systolic ejection murmur.

Laboratory Findings: EKG: left ventricular hypertrophy with strain pattern. Cardiac catheterization pressure tracing: see below.

Questions: What is the name of the cardiac catheterization finding? What is the underlying diagnosis?

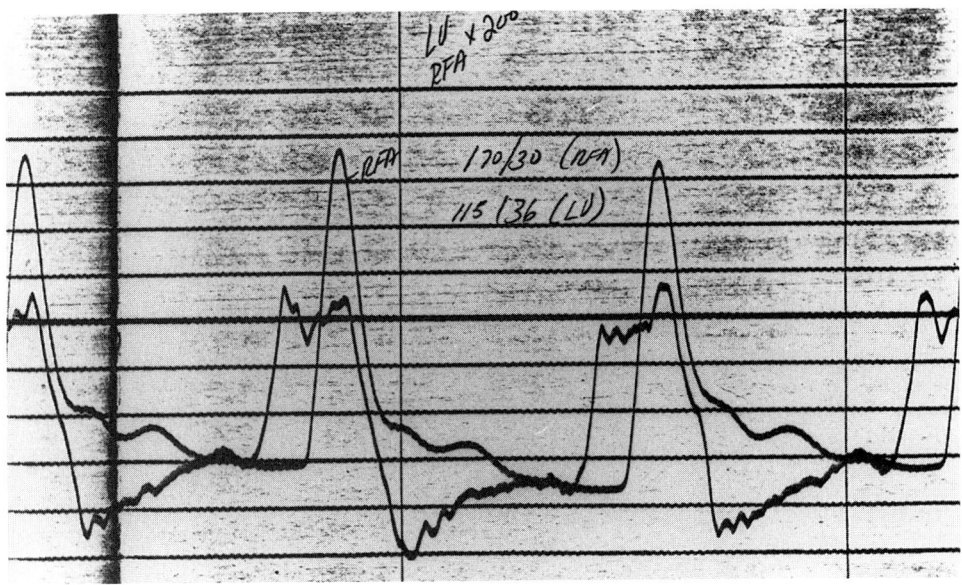

Diagnosis: Hill's sign of chronic aortic insufficiency.

Discussion: Chronic aortic insufficiency places both a volume and pressure overload on the left ventricle. The volume overload occurs because the left ventricle must expel a large enough total stroke volume to compensate for the aortic regurgitant flow during diastole. This increase in total stroke volume is accomplished by the development of eccentric cardiac hypertrophy in which sarcomeres are laid down in series, causing the left ventricle to dilate. Thus over time, if ejection fraction remains constant (for example 50%), an increase in end-diastolic volume from 150 to 300 cc will lead to an increase in total stroke volume from 75 to 150 cc. This large stroke volume accounts for many of the physical signs of aortic insufficiency.

Because pulse pressure (systolic pressure minus diastolic pressure) increases in parallel with stroke volume, patients with chronic aortic insufficiency have wide pulse pressures. Other commonly found signs related to the high total stroke volume and high pulse pressure include de Musset's sign (head bobbing), Duroziez's sign (a to-and-fro bruit heard in a femoral artery that is compressed by the bell of the stethoscope), Corrigan's pulse (rapid carotid upstroke and downstroke), and Quincke's pulse (cyclical blanching and erythema in the capillary bed of the fingertips during nail compression).

Hill's sign, extreme augmentation of systolic blood pressure in the femoral artery compared with the proximal aorta, is the most quantifiable and reliable sign of severe aortic insufficiency. Although the discrepancy of pressures in the present patient was noted during cardiac catheterization, Hill's sign can also be detected by sphygmomanometry during the physical examination by measuring the difference in systolic blood pressure between the arm and leg.

Hill's sign probably results from the summation of the pulse wave with standing waves along the aorta as it travels distally. These standing waves reinforce systolic pressure and cause it to increase. However, in patients with acute aortic insufficiency before the ventricle has had time to dilate, total stroke volume is not increased and Hill's sign, in addition to the other clinical features of chronic aortic insufficiency, may not be present, even though the aortic insufficiency is severe.

The present patient's pressure tracings demonstrated a systolic femoral artery pressure that was 60 mmHg higher than left ventricular pressure. He underwent successful aortic valve replacement with resolution of his dyspnea on exertion.

Clinical Pearls

1. Most of the physical findings of chronic aortic insufficiency result from the compensatory increase in left ventricular stroke volume.

2. Hill's sign, an extreme augmentation of systolic pressure in the leg compared with the proximal aorta or brachial artery, is the most reliable sign that severe aortic regurgitation is present.

3. All of these signs may be absent in acute aortic insufficiency because the left ventricle has not yet had time to dilate, and thus total stroke volume is not augmented.

REFERENCES
1. Sapira JD: Quincke, de Musset, Duroziez, Hill: Some aortic regurgitations. South Med J 1981;74:459–467.
2. Perloff JK: Acute severe aortic regurgitation: Recognition and management. J Cardiovasc Med 1983;8:209–218.
3. Carabello BA: Aortic regurgitation: Hemodynamic determinants of prognosis. In Cohn LH (ed): Aortic Regurgitation. New York, Marcel Dekker, 1986, pp 87–106.

PATIENT 87

A 35-year-old woman with a deep venous thrombosis and a cold right arm

A 35-year-old woman is admitted with a 2-day history of pain and swelling in her right calf. She broke her right tibia in a fall 6 months previously.

Physical Examination: Vital signs: pulse 80; respirations 16; blood pressure 130/80. Chest: clear. Cardiac: normal S_1 and S_2. Extremities: tenderness to deep palpation of the right calf, circumference of the right calf 1 cm larger than the left.

Laboratory Findings: Noninvasive vascular studies: suggest deep venous occlusion at level of right popliteal fossa.

Hospital Course: The diagnosis of thrombophlebitis was made, and the patient was begun on intravenous heparin. The dose was adjusted so that the partial thromboplastin time was approximately 65 seconds. Oral anticoagulation was begun with warfarin, but heparin was continued for 7 days. On the seventh day she complained of pain and pallor in her right arm. Examination demonstrated that the right arm was cool to the touch, and no brachial pulse could be palpated. A hemogram showed the following: Hct 36%; WBC 6600/μl; platelets 32,000/μl.

Question: What caused the vascular compromise in the patient's right arm?

Diagnosis: Heparin-induced thrombocytopenia with arterial thrombosis.

Discusssion: Heparin-induced thrombocytopenia (HIT) occurs in 1–5% of patients treated with intravenous heparin for more than 5 days. Two types of HIT are recognized. HIT1 is a mild thrombocytopenia probably secondary to direct procoagulent effects of heparin. The platelet count usually remains above 100,000/μl; there are no clinical sequelae, and no therapy is required. Heparin usually can be continued or changed to oral anticoagulants. HIT2 is a severe, rarer disease induced by heparin antibodies, which cause platelet aggregation as seen in this patient. The antibodies may injure either the platelets or the endothelium, leading to thrombocytopenia. Higher molecular weight heparin, administration of beef heparin, and previous heparin therapy predispose the patient to heparin-induced thrombocytopenia.

The platelet count should be monitored frequently in all patients receiving heparin. The decision to continue or discontinue heparin depends on the severity of thrombocytopenia, the risks of embolization, and the duration of oral anticoagulant therapy. If only mild thrombocytopenia has occurred and oral anticoagulants have not yet become therapeutic, the risks of embolization are the most important consideration. In deep vein thrombophlebitis that does not extend proximal to the popliteal fossa, the risk of embolism is low, and discontinuing heparin may be advisable if the platelet count is steadily declining. If there is proximal deep vein thrombophlebitis and the thrombocytopenia is only mild, heparin should probably be continued until oral agents have produced effective anticoagulation. On the other hand, heparin must be discontinued if the platelet count drops below 50,000/μl. If heparin must be discontinued in patients at high risk for thromboembolism, and oral anticoagulation has not yet become effective, hirudin should be substituted.

In some patients, severe platelet activation may lead not only to thrombocytopenia but also to platelet aggregation and paradoxical thrombosis of the major arteries, a serious complication of heparin therapy. Depending on the site and extent of thrombosis, the mortality rate is as high as 30%. Thrombosis in the presence of heparin therapy may also eventually lead to limb amputation. Therapy includes the immediate discontinuation of the heparin and mechanical thrombectomy of the vessel. Aspirin and oral anticoagulation should be started immediately, but unfortunately the oral anticoagulant preparations will not become effective for several days. In this case, a nonheparin anticoagulant such as hirudin is substituted.

This patient was begun on aspirin and underwent right brachial thrombectomy. The appearance of the thrombus was consistent with a "white thrombus" composed primarily of platelets with little thrombin deposition.

Clinical Pearls

1. A mild degree of thrombocytopenia is common in patients receiving heparin therapy.
2. Mild thrombocytopenia should be treated by early institution of oral anticoagulants and discontinuance of the heparin as soon as possible.
3. Severe thrombocytopenia or thrombocytopenia with thrombosis requires immediate discontinuation of heparin and the institution of antiplatelet agents. Limb loss and mortality rates are high under these circumstances.

REFERENCES

1. Bell WR, Royall RM: Heparin-associated thrombocytopenia: A comparison of three heparin preparations. N Engl J Med 1980;303:902–907.
2. King DJ, Kelton JG: Heparin-associated thrombocytopenia. Ann Intern Med 1989;100:535–540.
3. Favaloro EJ, Bernal-Hoyos E, Exner T, et al: Heparin-induced thrombocytopenia: Laboratory investigation and confirmation of diagnosis. Pathology 1992;24:177–183.
4. Grau E, Linares M, Olaso MA, et al: Heparin-induced thrombocytopenia: Response to intravenous immunoglobulin in vivo and in vitro. Am J Hematol 1992;39:312–313.
5. Kaplan KL, Francis CW: Heparin-induced thrombocytopenia. Blood Rev 1999;13:1–7.

PATIENT 88

A 40-year-old man with dyspnea and acyanotic congenital heart disease

A 40-year-old man with a known heart murmur since childhood has experienced atrial fibrillation, worsening dyspnea on exertion, and pedal edema over the previous year. He is begun on digoxin, diuretics, and vasodilator therapy, with some improvement, and he is referred for further evaluation.

Physical Examination: Vital signs: pulse 77 (irregular); blood pressure 115/80. Height 73″; weight 116 lbs. General: slim male with pectus carinatum. Cardiac: no jugular venous distention; PMI displaced laterally; thrill palpable at third and fourth intercostal spaces just to left of sternum; V/VI holosystolic murmur at area of thrill. Abdomen: hepatosplenomegaly.

Laboratory Findings: EKG: right bundle branch block; left ventricular hypertrophy; atrial fibrillation. Chest radiograph: prominent main pulmonary arteries. Heart catheterization: see data below.

Hemodynamic measurement	Pressure (mmHg)	Oxygen saturation (%) Room air
Right atrium	12	73
Right ventricle	70/5	
Pulmonary artery	70/30	91
Pulmonary capillary wedge	12	
Aorta	120/60	96
Pulmonary vascular resistance	1040 dynes sec cm^{-5}	
Systemic vascular resistance	1933 dynes sec cm^{-5}	

Question: What is the diagnosis?

Diagnosis: Ventricular septal defect (VSD).

Discussion: Congenital heart lesions usually present in childhood or spontaneously resolve if not severe. Occasionally, however, congenital cardiac conditions may be overlooked until adulthood, when they may be mistaken for acquired cardiac conditions. Atrial septal defects and bicuspid aortic valves are the most common congenital lesions that escape detection during childhood. Less common congenital lesions that present in adults include patent ductus arteriosus, pulmonary stenosis, coarctation of the aorta, tetralogy of Fallot, Eisenmenger's syndrome, and Ebstein's anomaly. Congenital VSDs are seldom observed in adults because the early onset of cardiac symptoms leads to diagnosis and surgical repair in childhood. Occasionally, however, a VSD can remain undetected until it produces cardiac dysfunction later in the patient's life.

Congenital cardiac lesions that present in adulthood commonly simulate other cardiac conditions. Atrial septal defects are often mistaken for mitral stenosis, VSDs may simulate mitral insufficiency or idiopathic hypertrophic subaortic stenosis, and coarctation of the aorta may present with systemic hypertension. Cyanotic lesions may be misdiagnosed as chronic lung disease. The first clues to congenital heart disease in the adult often are the abnormal contour of the heart and the abnormal pulmonary vasculature seen on chest radiograph.

Many congenital cardiac lesions can be repaired in adults. Minor VSDs should not be repaired if the patient is asymptomatic and has a left-to-right shunt ratio of less than 1.5 to 1. Surgery is contraindicated if the pulmonary vascular disease is so severe that the pulmonary to systemic vascular resistance is greater than 0.9. Operation may be advised if the ratio is between 0.75 and 0.9 and bidirectional shunt is present with a small net left-to-right shunt. If the ratio is less than 0.75, pulmonary hypertension is not a contraindication to surgery.

Congenital cardiac lesions may produce symptoms in adults even when successfully repaired in childhood. Patients with atrial septal defects may experience atrial arrhythmias after surgical repair. Patients with repaired VSDs may develop progressive pulmonary hypertension, especially if preoperative pulmonary vascular resistance was moderately elevated. Arrhythmias, conduction defects, heart failure, and endocarditis may occur even after successful repair.

Echocardiographic and Doppler studies in the present patient were consistent with a volume overload of the left ventricle due to a large septal defect in the membranous ventricular septum. Cardiac catheterization showed a 4.6 to 1 left-to-right shunt and a pulmonary to systemic vascular resistance ratio of 0.54. The patient underwent successful closure of his VSD with improvement in his heart failure.

Clinical Pearls

1. In adults, the first clues to a congenital heart lesion are often an abnormal cardiac contour and abnormal pulmonary vasculature on chest radiograph.

2. Adult congenital lesions can be repaired if the pulmonary to systemic vascular resistance ratio is less than 0.75. Patients may still have residual problems, however, including arrhythmias, heart failure, pulmonary hypertension, and endocarditis following surgery.

3. Echocardiographic Doppler studies are the initial diagnostic modality of choice for localizing intracardiac shunts. If tricuspid regurgitation is present, the pulmonary artery pressure can also be estimated.

REFERENCES
1. Hoffman JIE, Rudolph AM: The natural history of ventricular septal defects in infancy. Am J Cardiol 1965;16:634–653.
2. Gazes PC (ed): Clinical Cardiology, 3rd ed. Philadelphia, Lea & Febiger, 1990.
3. Somerville J: The physician's responsibilities: Residua and sequelae. J Am Coll Cardiol 1991;18:325–327.

PATIENT 89

A 55-year-old man with an aortic valve prosthesis, fever, and first-degree atrioventricular block

A 55-year-old man presents with a 6-week history of malaise, weight loss, arthralgias, and a periodic fever beginning 1 week after a dental extraction. Six months earlier, he underwent an aortic valve replacement with a St. Jude's prosthesis for aortic stenosis. Prophylactic antibiotics are prescribed for the dental extraction, but the patient fails to fill his prescription. He denies dyspnea, orthopnea, paroxysmal nocturnal dyspnea, and chest pain.

Physical Examination: Vital signs: temperature 100.8°; pulse 100 (regular); blood pressure 120/60. Eyes: bilateral subconjunctival petechiae. Cardiac: II/VI systolic ejection murmur heard along the left sternal border; normal opening and closing sounds of his prosthetic valve; no diastolic murmur. Extremities: splinter hemorrhage under the nail on the third digit of the right hand.

Laboratory Findings: Previous EKG: normal. Admission EKG: see below.

Hospital Course: Antibiotics are begun. Two days after admission, two of three blood cultures grow *Streptococcus viridans*.

Question: What is the likely cause of the patient's EKG changes?

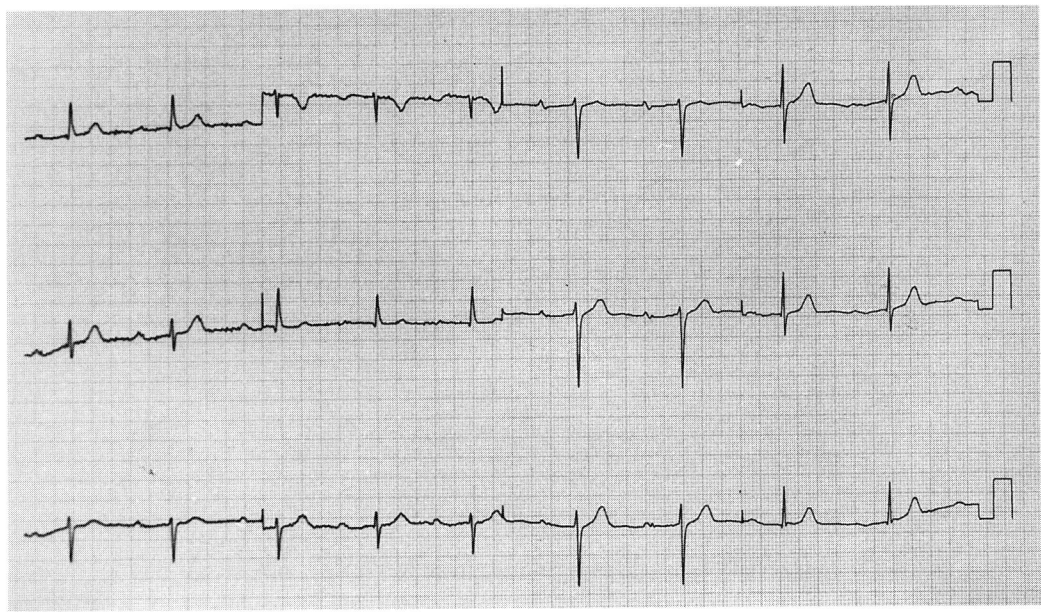

Diagnosis Prosthetic infective endocarditis with probable ring abscess.

Discussion: Endocarditis occurs in approximately 3% of patients with prosthetic valves within 5 years after insertion. Early cases (less than 2 months after operation) are probably due to contamination at the time of surgery or following it. The infecting organism is usually staphylococcus. Remarkably, patients undergoing native valve surgery for endocarditis have only a 10% incidence of reinfection of the prosthesis with the same organism.

Cases of endocarditis late after valve replacement are usually due to infection from dental or genitourinary procedures. As in the present patient, the most common cause of endocarditis is failure of the patient to receive the proper prophylactic antibiotic therapy. Although no controlled study has been performed (or should be performed) to test the efficacy of prophylaxis, infection is rare after adequate prophylaxis but occurs commonly in its absence.

The present patient demonstrated many of the common manifestations of infectious endocarditis. Fever, anorexia, weight loss, and a heart murmur are present in 80% of patients with infective endocarditis. Arthralgias are also a frequent complaint. Petechiae and splinter hemorrhages noted in this case are common, whereas Osler's nodes (tender nodules on the fingers and toes) and Janeway lesions (nontender hemorrhages often occurring on the thenar eminence) are seen in less than 25% of the cases. Debate persists as to the etiology of the cutaneous manifestations of the disease. They may be due to small septic emboli or to deposition of circulating immune complexes. Both mechanisms have been demonstrated.

The diagnosis of infective endocarditis changed dramatically with the implementation of **echocardiography.** The combination of transthoracic and transesophageal echocardiography increases the diagnosis rate from definite endocarditis in 50% of suspected cases using clinical criteria, to 85% when echocardiography is added. In the case of ring abscess, transesophageal echocardiography has a sensitivity of about 90%, compared to about 30% for transthoracic echocardiography.

The usual indications for surgery for infective endocarditis include failure of appropriate antibiotics to effect a bacteriologic cure, congestive heart failure, systemic embolism, and the presence of staphylococcal or fungal infection on a prosthetic valve.

The major EKG finding in the present patient was prolongation of the PR interval. With obvious signs of infective endocarditis and in the absence of therapy with digitalis or beta-blocker agents, the likely diagnosis is a ring abscess affecting the cardiac conducting system. The patient underwent re-replacement of his aortic valve and debridement of a ring abscess. Despite successful surgery, the patient died of adult respiratory distress syndrome 1 month later.

Clinical Pearls

1. The most common late cause of endocarditis in a patient with a prosthetic valve is failure to take appropriate prophylactic antibiotics for dental or genitourinary procedures.
2. An increased PR interval is an ominous sign, suggesting the presence of a ring abscess that may lead to complete heart block.
3. The cutaneous manifestations of infective endocarditis may be due to embolic phenomena, deposition of circulating immune complexes, or both.
4. Reinfection of a prosthetic valve inserted for the bacteriologic cure of endocarditis is rare even in the face of positive blood cultures.

REFERENCES
1. Rutledge R, Kim BJ, Applebaum RE: Actuarial analysis of the risk of prosthetic valve endocarditis in 1,598 patients with mechanical and bioprosthetic valves. Arch Surg 1985;120:469–472.
2. Calderwood SB, Swinski LA, Waternaux CM, et al: Risk factors for the development of prosthetic valve endocarditis.
3. Durack DT, Lukes AS, Bright DK: New criteria for diagnosis of infective endocarditis: utilization of specific echocardiographic findings. Duke Endocarditis Service. Am J Med 1994;96:200–209.
4. Leung DY, Cranney GB, Hopkins AP, et al: Role of transesophageal echocardiography in the diagnosis and management of aortic root abscess. Br Heart J 1994;72:175–181.

PATIENT 90

A 58-year-old man with weight loss and a heart murmur

A 58-year old man presents with a 35-pound weigh loss, intermittent flushing of the face and neck, episodic bronchospasm, diarrhea, and peripheral edema.

Physical Examination: Vital signs: pulse 90; respirations 20; blood pressure 107/60. General: cachectic and ill appearing. Chest: few bibasilar rales; no wheezes. Cardiac: distended neck veins; right ventricular heave; II/VI holosystolic murmur at left sternal border. Abdomen: slightly distended; liver edge pulsatile and palpable 8 cm below the right costal margin. Extremities: 3+ edema to mid-thigh.

Laboratory Findings: Echocardiogram: see below.

Question: What syndrome does this patient manifest?

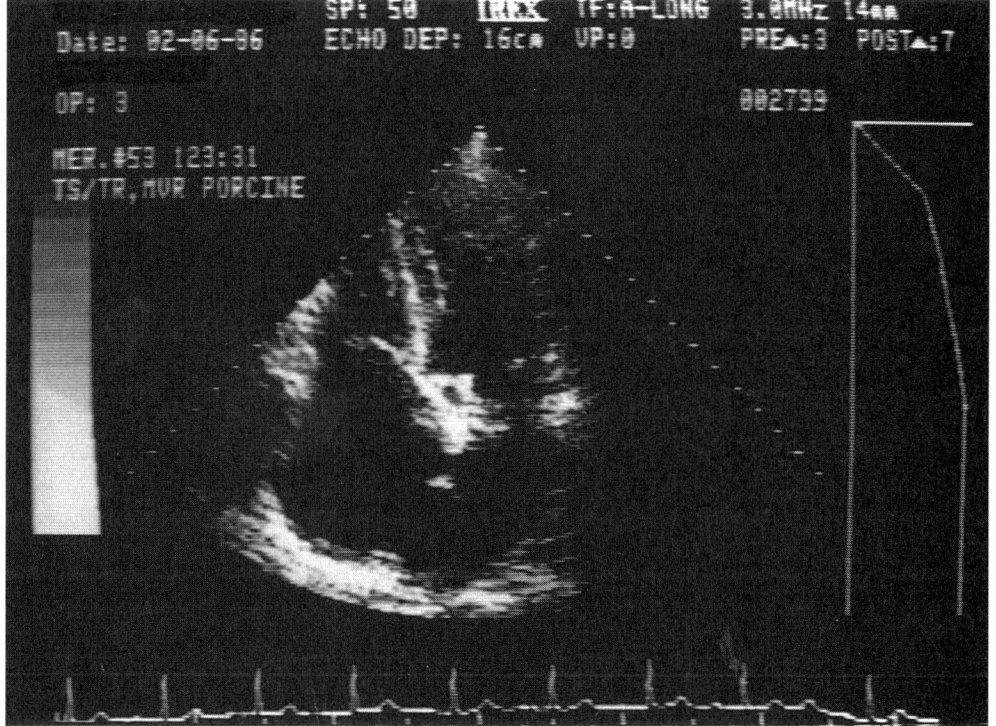

Diagnosis: Tricuspid stenosis and regurgitation due to carcinoid syndrome.

Discussion: Besides rheumatic fever, carcinoid is one of the few diseases that can cause tricuspid stenosis, although the usual cardiac sequela of carcinoid is tricuspid regurgitation. Carcinoid tumors are derived from enterochromaffin cells and usually reside in the ilium or appendix. Although the tumor produces several hormones, including bradykinin, histamine, and prostaglandins, serotonin is thought to be the agent responsible for the valve destruction and most of the other clinical manifestations. If hepatic metastases do not occur, the liver is capable of detoxifying the tumor's humoral products, and cardiac disease does not usually ensue. However, hepatic metastases bypass the liver's detoxifying ability, and the products of the tumor can then produce cardiac pathology.

Occasionally, the high right-sided pressure produced by the tricuspid valve disease may cause a right-to-left shunt across a patient foramen ovale, in turn allowing the left-sided valves to be affected by the serotonin excess. Besides tricuspid valve disease, right ventricular endocardial fibrosis may also occur, leading to right ventricular restrictive physiology. Pulmonic stenosis, usually a congenital defect, may be acquired from this disease. The other major manifestations of carcinoid syndrome, flushing and diarrhea, probably result from serotonin excess. Flushing occurs in 90% of patients. It may occur spontaneously or be brought on by hepatic palpation, ethanol ingestion, stress, or infusion of catecholamines. Other sequelae include bronchospasm and retroperitoneal fibrosis. Occasionally the tumor converts so much of the body's tryptophan stores into serotonin that nicotinic acid normally produced from tryptophan becomes deficient and pellagra may develop.

Once suspected, the diagnosis is confirmed by detecting large quantities of a serotonin metabolite, 5-hydroxyindoleacetic acid (5-HIAA), in the urine. Mild elevation of 5-HIAA not diagnostic of carcinoid syndrome occurs after ingestion of chocolate, walnuts, bananas, and acetaminophen. CT scanning generally reveals metastases to the liver.

The cardiac symptoms of the disease usually respond to diuresis. Valve replacement is rarely indicated. Specific serotonin antagonists such as methysergide may be useful in therapy, although methysergide may lead to retroperitoneal fibrosis just as serotonin excess itself. Phenothiazines, H_2 blockers, cyproheptadine, and alpha-adrenergic antagonists have been used to control diarrhea.

Because carcinoid syndrome typically develops only after hepatic metastases have occurred, resection of the primary tumor in patients with systemic manifestations is usually not indicated unless the tumor has produced intestinal obstruction. The tumors are typically slow-growing and not sensitive to radiation therapy or chemotherapy.

The present patient responded well to administration of furosemide and lost 35 pounds by diuresis. His diarrhea responded partially to cimetidine.

Clinical Pearls

1. Acquired tricuspid and pulmonic stenosis are rare diseases and should raise suspicion of carcinoid syndrome.
2. A history of flushing will almost always be obtained from patients with the disease.
3. Determination of urinary 5-HIAA is the diagnostic test of choice, but many foods and acetaminophen produce mild elevation of this serotonin metabolite.

REFERENCES
1. Ross EM, Roberts WC: The carcinoid syndrome: Comparison of 21 necropsy subjects with carcinoid heart disease to 15 necropsy subjects without carcinoid heart disease. Am J Med 1985;79:339–354.
2. Lundin L, Norheim I, Landelius J, et al: Carcinoid heart disease: Relationship of circulating vasoactive substances to ultrasound-detectable cardiac abnormalities. Circulation 1988;77:264–269.
3. Pellikka PA, Tajik AJ, Khandheria BK, et al: Carcinoid heart disease: Clinical and echocardiographic spectrum in 74 patients. Circulation 1993;87:1188–1196.

PATIENT 91

A 73-year-old man with pulmonary edema and a normal ejection fraction

A 73-year-old man with known hypertension for many years is admitted for evaluation of progressive exertional dyspnea that developed over several days, and for the sudden onset of severe dyspnea. He denies recent chest pain, but does note that 1 year earlier he experienced several episodes of nonspecific chest pain. He underwent coronary arteriography at that time, which demonstrated normal coronary arteries. He has no history of diabetes and has never smoked.

Physical Examination: Vital signs: pulse 100; blood pressure 220/120. General: severe dyspnea. Neck: no venous distention. Chest: crackles throughout all lung fields. Cardiac: no S_3 or murmur.

Laboratory Findings: Cardiac enzymes: normal. Chest radiograph: pulmonary edema with normal heart size. EKG: normal. Echocardiogram and Doppler study: normal chamber sizes with some left ventricular hypertrophy and an ejection fraction of 60%; mitral flow revealed a reduction of the E to A ratio.

Question: What is the cause of this patient's acute pulmonary edema?

Diagnosis: Pulmonary edema secondary to hypertension with diastolic dysfunction.

Discussion: Approximately one-third of patients with signs of congestive heart failure have diastolic dysfunction as the primary cause of the heart failure. Diastolic dysfunction is likely when there is normal systolic function demonstrated by careful clinical and laboratory evaluation. It is important to correctly identify diastolic dysfunction in patients with congestive symptoms because the management differs from that applied when the more commonly recognized systolic dysfunction is the cause of the heart failure. For instance, inotropic agents and afterload-reducing agents commonly used in patients with systolic dysfunction are ineffective in diastolic dysfunction and may actually be harmful.

It can be difficult to distinguish systolic from diastolic dysfunction by history, physical examination, EKG, or routine radiographic data. Therefore, echocardiography, radionucleotide ventriculography, or cardiac catheterization most often must be used to make the diagnosis. Typically, the diagnosis is suggested in patients who present in pulmonary edema with a normal-sized heart and normal ejection fraction. In addition, diastolic dysfunction is suggested by a reduction in the ratio of the velocity of mitral flow during early (E) filling to flow velocity during atrial (A) systole. Normally, the E to A ratio is greater than 1. No noninvasive method (in contrast to cardiac catheterization) measures both intracardiac pressures and volumes needed to calculate compliance, which best evaluates diastolic dysfunction. In the setting of suggestive clinical findings, however, noninvasive demonstration of a normal ejection fraction and an abnormal mitral valve inflow velocity can adequately confirm the diagnosis of diastolic dysfunction.

The purpose of therapy in patients with diastolic dysfunction is to reduce left ventricular diastolic pressure with diuretics and nitrates; maintain regular sinus rhythm; reduce heart rate with beta blockers, verapamil, or diltiazem; manage hypertension; and treat and prevent myocardial ischemia. Antihypertensive therapy should eventually lead to regression of left ventricular hypertrophy with improvement in diastolic dysfunction. Unfortunately, left ventricular mass reduction averages only 11% following institution of antihypertensive therapy. This compares unfavorably to the 50% reduction in mass that occurs following reduction of left ventricular pressure with aortic valve replacement for aortic stenosis. These data suggest that more aggressive therapy or new therapy for hypertension is required.

Traditionally, positive inotropic agents have been viewed as unhelpful in patients with diastolic dysfunction. However, a recent study of digitalis found equal benefit for patients with an ejection fraction greater than 0.45 versus less than 0.45. Perhaps effects of digitalis other than its inotrophy were operative.

In the present patient, intravenous nitroprusside, morphine, and furosemide reduced the patient's blood pressure, and the pulmonary edema cleared. Diastolic dysfunction appeared to be the cause of his congestive symptoms, as demonstrated by his normal heart size, normal ejection fraction, and reduction of the E to A ratio.

Clinical Pearls

1. One-third of patients with signs of congestive heart failure have diastolic dysfunction and normal systolic function.
2. Diastolic dysfunction should be suspected in a patient with signs and symptoms of congestive heart failure who has a normal-sized heart and normal ejection fraction.
3. The goals of therapy are to maintain sinus rhythm, lower filling pressure, and slow the heart rate.

REFERENCES

1. Zile MR: Diastolic dysfunction: Detection, consequences and treatment. I. Definition and determination of diastolic function. Mod Concepts Cardiovasc Dis 1989;58:67–72.
2. Zile MR: Diastolic dysfunction: Detection, consequences and treatment. II. Diagnosis and treatment of diastolic dysfunction. Mod Concepts Cardiovasc Dis 1990;59:1–6.
3. Dahlof B, Pennert K, Hansson L: Reversal of left ventricular hypertrophy in hypertensive patients. A meta-analysis of 109 treatment studies. Am J Hypertens 1992;5:95–110.
4. The Digitalis Investigation Group: The effect of digoxin on mortality and morbidity in patients with heart failure. N Engl J Med 1997;336:525–533.

PATIENT 92

A 28-year-old man with progressive fatigue, dyspnea, and cyanosis

A 28-year-old man was well until 2 years previously, when he noted easy fatigability and dyspnea on exertion. These symptoms gradually progressed until 2 weeks before admission, when he noted abdominal swelling and ankle edema. His family members note that his lips and hands turn blue with minimal exertion. He denies chest pain or hemoptysis. He is receiving no medications.

Physical Examination: Vital signs: pulse 110; respirations 22; blood pressure 90/60. Neck: veins elevated with estimated central venous pressure of 18 cm of water. Chest: clear. Cardiac: a right ventricular heave; increased P2; III/VI holosystolic murmur along the right sternal border that increased with inspiration. Abdomen: distended with a fluid wave. Extremities: 2+ peripheral edema.

Laboratory Findings: EKG: right ventricular hypertrophy. Echocardiogram: technically difficult study that demonstrated normal left ventricular function and no evidence of intracardiac shunting or valvular pathology. Pulmonary function studies: normal. Lung scan: low probability for pulmonary embolism. Right heart catheterization: see data below.

	Pressure (mmHg)	O_2 saturation (%)
Right atrium	20	48
Pulmonary artery	96/48/63	49
Pulmonary capillary wedge	16	92
Cardiac index	1.8 L/min/m^2	

Question: What is the patient's diagnosis and probable prognosis?

Diagnosis: Primary pulmonary hypertension.

Discussion: Primary pulmonary hypertension is a disease of unknown etiology characterized by the presence of increased pulmonary vascular pressures without any demonstrable cause. It is two to three times more common in women than in men and may occur at any age, although it is most common in the third to sixth decades of life. Because no laboratory or imaging features are diagnostic of the disease, the diagnosis is one of exclusion that requires careful patient examination for underlying conditions. Conditions requiring exclusion include left ventricular failure, mitral stenosis, primary lung disease, intracardiac shunts, peripheral pulmonary stenosis, chronic thrombotic pulmonary hypertension, veno-occlusive disease, and vasculitis.

The histopathology of the pulmonary vessels in patients with primary pulmonary hypertension demonstrate microthrombi, initial thickening in an onion-skin-like pattern, medial thickening, and plexiform lesions. These histologic changes act in concert to increase pulmonary vascular resistance and pulmonary arterial pressure. The presence of microthrombi has led some investigators to speculate that thrombosis is a primary event in the disease. This seems unlikely, however, because in many patients thrombosis is limited in extent while the plexiform lesions predominate.

The average survival of patients with primary pulmonary hypertension from the onset of symptoms is approximately 2 years. There is a spectrum of survivorship, however, that can be approximated by examining the patient for prognosticating indices derived by Eysmann and colleagues. A heart rate greater than 87/min, a large pericardial effusion, cardiac index of less than 2.3 L/min/m^2, and a mean pulmonary artery pressure of greater than 61 mmHg are important negative predictors of outcome in the disease. The greater the number of these predictors that are present in a given patient, the sooner death win most probably occur.

Efforts to treat the disease medically have met with limited success. Because thromboembolism is present in almost all patients and predominates in some patients, anticoagulation is recommended unless there is a contraindication. Whether or not anticoagulation extends longevity is unknown. Several vasodilators have been employed with variable success. Some patients have responded to calcium channel blockers, with long-term reduction in pulmonary arterial pressure and pulmonary vascular resistance. These patients, however, appear to be in the minority. Intravenous prostacyclin administered through a constant infusion pump also reduces pulmonary artery pressure, improves quality of life, and also may increase survival. Because abnormalities in nitric oxide (NO) generation have been implicated in this disease, inhaled NO has been employed. It lowers pulmonary pressure only transiently, but may hold promise for development of future therapies. Because a major feature of histopathology of the disease is the presence of lesions that block the pulmonary arteries and arterioles, however, it is understandable why vasodilators often fail to be effective. In the absence of a response to vasodilators, pulmonary transplantation is the only other alternative. Often such patients do not respond well to single lung transplantation, and many such patients have a stormy postoperative course.

This patient had three of the four negative predictors and died while awaiting lung transplantation.

Clinical Pearls

1. Because thromboembolism and local thrombosis play a role in most patients with primary pulmonary hypertension, anticoagulation is usually employed.
2. Infused prostacyclin, although expensive, is the therapy of choice if simpler measures fail.
3. Although some patients respond to vasodilators, many do not, and lung transplantation is the only other effective form of therapy.

REFERENCES

1. Eysmann SB, Palevsky HI, Reichek N, et al: Two-dimensional and Doppler-echocardiographic and cardiac catheterization correlates of survival in primary pulmonary hypertension. Circulation 1989;80:353–360.
2. Pasque MK, Trulock EP, Kaiser LR, et al: Single-lung transplantation for pulmonary hypertension. Circulation 1991;84:2275–2279.
3. Barst RJ, Rubin LJ, Long WA, et al: A comparison of continuous intravenous epoprostenol (prostacyclin) with conventional therapy for primary pulmonary hypertension. The Primary Pulmonary Hypertension Study Group. N Engl J Med 1996;334:296–302.
4. Channick RN, Newhart JW, Johnson FW, et al: Pulsed delivery of inhaled nitric oxide to patients with primary pulmonary hypertension: An ambulatory delivery system and initial clinical tests. Chest 1996;109:1545–1549.

PATIENT 93

A 24-year-old African-American woman with dyspnea on exertion and fatigue following childbirth

A 24-year-old African-American woman is referred for evaluation of congestive heart failure 6 weeks following the delivery of her fourth child. The patient has not been hypertensive and has three previous uncomplicated deliveries. She denies recent symptoms of an upper respiratory tract illness.

Physical Examination: Vital signs: pulse 110 and regular; respirations 24; blood pressure 110/70. General: thin, in moderate respiratory distress. Neck: jugular venous distention. Chest: bibasilar rales. Cardiac: PMI sixth intercostal space anterior axillary line; S_3 gallop; III/VI holosystolic apical murmur. Extremities: 3+ edema to mid-thigh bilaterally; pulses 2+.

Laboratory Findings: EKG: sinus tachycardia; left axis deviation; left ventricular hypertrophy. Echocardiogram: see below.

Question: What is the probable cause of the patient's heart disease?

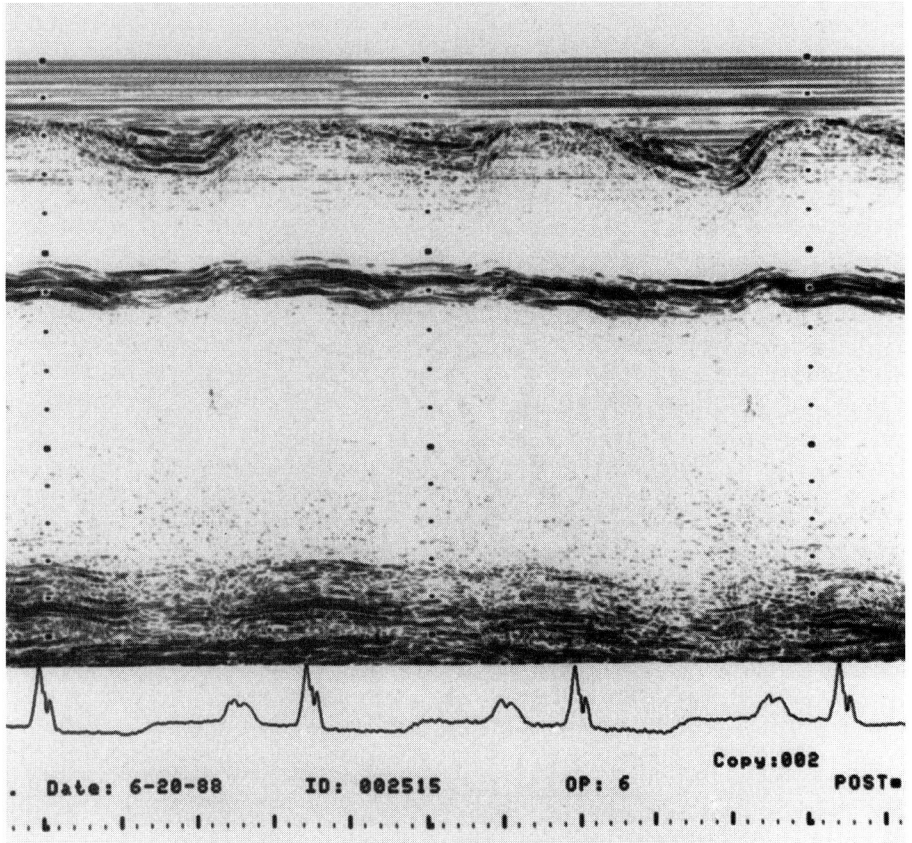

Diagnosis: Peripartum cardiomyopathy.

Discussion: Peripartum cardiomyopathy is an idiopathic dilated cardiomyopathy that may develop during the last 3 months of pregnancy through the first 6 weeks after delivery. As in the present patient, it typically occurs in black multiparous women generally over the age of 30. Although the etiology is unknown, approximately 25% of patients have acute myocarditis on myocardial biopsy specimens. The pathophysiologic connection between pregnancy and the myocarditis is unknown.

There appear to be two different varieties of peripartum cardiomyopathy—reversible and irreversible. In Africa, the disease has been estimated to occur in as many as 1% of all pregnancies. The prognosis is good in Africa, however, with the majority of women showing an improvement in left ventricular function and a decrease in cardiac size in the first year following development of the disease. A large salt intake seems to be related to the disorder.

The prognosis in the United States is less favorable. Some women may have a full recovery, but many have persistent severe left ventricular dysfunction. The prognosis is worse if an increased left ventricular end-diastolic diameter is present in the acute phase of the disease and if symptoms develop in the late postpartum period. If recovery does occur, myopathy may recur with subsequent pregnancies. Thus, women who have developed peripartum cardiomyopathy should be counseled against future pregnancies. In the United States, peripartum cardiomyopathy usually develops 1 month after delivery and has an incidence of approximately 1 in 10,000 deliveries.

Peripartum cardiomyopathy should be suspected when the symptoms and signs of heart failure develop late in pregnancy or after delivery. The EKG shows nonspecific findings. Echocardiography, as seen in the present patient, shows left ventricular dilatation and reduced shortening fraction typical of any dilated cardiomyopathy. With recent pregnancy and an absence of other cardiac pathology or drug abuse, the diagnosis can probably be made echocardiographically without the need for catheterization or biopsy.

Standard therapy for peripartum cardiomyopathy includes digitalis, diuretics, and ACE inhibitors as indicated. Although immunosuppressive therapy may improve the histopathology by light microscopy, these changes frequently do not correlate with improved ventricular function. Recently, however, immune globulin was shown to increase ejection fraction dramatically in a small controlled trial. Because all patients with peripartum cardiomyopathy are relatively young, usually do not have other diseases, and frequently fail to respond to standard therapy for heart failure, early evaluation for cardiac transplantation is indicated.

The present patient developed intractable heart failure and subsequently underwent cardiac transplantation with a successful clinical outcome.

Clinical Pearls

1. Peripartum cardiomyopathy typically occurs in black, multiparous women in the last trimester through 6 weeks of postpartum.

2. Peripartum cardiomyopathy may improve spontaneously, but this outcome is less likely in the United States than in Africa. If improvement does not occur, most patients are excellent candidates for cardiac transplantation.

3. A woman who recovers from peripartum cardiomyopathy is at high risk for recurrence during subsequent pregnancies.

REFERENCES

1. Demakis JG, Rahimtoola SH, Sutton GC, et al: Natural course of peripartum cardiomyopathy. Circulation 1971;44:1053–1061.
2. Homans DC: Peripartum cardiomyopathy. N Engl J Med 1985;312:1432–1437.
3. Carvalho A, Brandao A, Martinez EE, et al: Prognosis in peripartum cardiomyopathy. Am J Cardiol 1989;64:540–542.
4. Midei MG, DeMent SH, Feldman AM, et al: Peripartum myocarditis and cardiomyopathy. Circulation 1990;81:922–928.
5. Bozkurt B, Villaneuva FS, Holubkov R, et al: Intravenous immune globulin in the therapy of peripartum cardiomyopathy. J Am Coll Cardiol 1999;34(1)177–180.

PATIENT 94

An 18-year-old man with dyspnea and lower-extremity cyanosis

An 18-year-old man presents with progressive dyspnea on exertion. A heart murmur was noted at birth, but the patient was lost to follow-up. For the past several months he has noted easy fatigue and dyspnea after walking one city block. He also notes that his toes have become cyanotic.

Physical Examination: Vital signs: pulse 90 (regular); blood pressure 110/60. Cardiac: prominent venous "a" wave; right ventricular lift; narrowly split second heart sound with a loud P2 component; II/VI systolic ejection murmur; and a II/VI diastolic blowing murmur in the pulmonic area that increased in intensity with inspiration. Extremities: face and hands pink; lower extremities cyanotic; no clubbing.

Laboratory Findings: Hct 70%. Arterial blood gases: see below.

	Radial artery	Femoral artery
PO_2	75 mmHg	36 mmHg
PCO_2	40 mmHg	40 mmHg
pH	7.40	7.40
O_2 sat	93%	72%

Question: What cardiac abnormalities explain these blood gas values?

Diagnosis: Ductus arteriosus with Eisenmenger's syndrome.

Discussion: The ductus arteriosus admits right ventricular outflow into the aorta *in utero* at a time when the pulmonary vascular resistance in the unexpanded lungs is high. Following birth, pulmonary vascular resistance falls rapidly and increased oxygenation normally closes the ductus. Prostaglandins, particularly prostaglandin E, help to maintain ductus patency, whereas prostaglandin inhibitors may pharmacologically close a patent ductus.

Failure of the ductus to close following birth causes a left-to-right shunt from the aorta to the pulmonary artery usually at the level of the left subclavian artery. If the shunt is large, pulmonary hypertension may develop. The mechanisms for increased pulmonary vascular resistance leading to pulmonary hypertension include: pulmonary vasoconstriction, pulmonary artery and arteriolar medial hypertrophy, necrotizing arteritis, and the development of plexiform lesions of the small pulmonary vessels. These last two conditions are irreversible even after the left-to-right shunt is corrected. In some cases the volume overload that the shunt imposes on the left ventricle may lead to left ventricular failure prior to the development of severe pulmonary artery hypertension.

In the present patient, Eisenmenger's syndrome developed. Eisenmenger's syndrome is present when a large shunt causes pulmonary vascular resistance to increase to the degree that right-sided pressures equal or exceed left-sided pressures, leading to shunt reversal (right-to-left flow) and cyanosis. The chest radiograph usually shows the reduced pulmonary vasculature that occurs due to decreased pulmonary blood flow. Reversed shunts due to the development of pulmonary artery hypertension can occur at the atrial, ventricular, or distal level. The key to diagnosing the site of the right-to-left shunt in the present patient was the differential cyanosis. Because the right-to-left shunt in a patent ductus arteriosus occurs after the takeoff of the left subclavian artery, the vessels before the shunt transmit normally oxygenated blood to the upper extremities, which are free of cyanosis. The right-to-left shunt, however, delivers desaturated blood to the lower extremities, producing cyanosis. Distal cyanosis also triggers increased marrow production of red cells and the hematocrit may exceed 70%.

Standard therapy for a patent ductus arteriosus is to close it pharmacologically, by transcatheter techniques, or with surgery prior to the development of left ventricular failure and severe pulmonary artery hypertension. Once Eisenmenger's syndrome develops, surgery only results in greater right ventricular pressure overload because the right ventricle no longer has the "escape" valve of the shunt postoperatively. Surgery is usually not attempted if the pulmonary vascular resistance to systemic vasculature resistance ratio is greater than 0.7.

Anticoagulation is usually employed in Eisenmenger's syndrome because of the high rate of thromboembolism. Because blood viscosity increases sharply as the hematocrit exceeds 58%, phlebotomy to maintain the hematocrit below this level is recommended. However, little data support this therapy—which actually may increase the risk of hemoptysis, a sometimes fatal complication. In general, phlebotomy is reserved for patients in whom symptoms of hyperviscosity develop (headache, dizziness, thrombosis) or the hematocrit exceeds 65%. Such patients may be considered for heart-lung transplantation.

The present patient died suddenly while awaiting transplantation.

Clinical Pearls

1. Eisenmenger's syndrome associated with a patent ductus arteriosus produces differential cyanosis (hands pink, toes cyanotic), a clue to the diagnosis.

2. Once Eisenmenger's syndrome has developed, correction of the shunt is no longer possible.

3. Phlebotomy to reduce blood viscosity is a mainstay of therapy in patients with Eisenmenger's syndrome when hematocrit exceeds 65% or if symptoms of hyperviscosity occur.

REFERENCES

1. Campbell M: Natural history of persistent ductus arteriosus. Br Heart J 1968;30:4–13.
2. Fisher RG, Moodie DS, Serba R, et al: Patent ductus arteriosus in adults: Long-term follow-up: Nonsurgical versus surgical treatment. J Am Coll Cardiol 1986;8:280–285.
3. Daliento L, Somerville J, Presbitero P, et al: Eisenmenger syndrome. Factors relating to deterioration and death. Eur Heart J 1998;19:1845–1855.

PATIENT 95

A 71-year-old man with an acute myocardial infarction and a new heart murmur

A 71-year-old man is evaluated in the emergency department for severe substernal chest pain. He is started on intravenous nitroglycerin and admitted to the CCU. Seven years earlier, he underwent three-vessel coronary bypass grafting for unstable angina. At that time, the left internal mammary artery was grafted to the left anterior descending artery, and saphenous vein grafts were anastomosed to two obtuse marginal branches of the circumflex.

Physical Examination: Vital signs: weak, thready pulse; systolic blood pressure 60. Cardiac: prominent systolic murmur along the left sternal border at the fourth intercostal space, with some radiation to the right.

Laboratory Findings: Total CPK and MB fractions: 687, 12% MB. EKG: ST elevation in leads 2, 3, aVF, and V_4R.

Question: What is the probable cause of the patient's heart murmur?

Diagnosis: Myocardial infarction (MI) complicated by ventricular septal rupture.

Discussion: The most common causes of new heart murmurs in patients with acute MI are papillary muscle dysfunction or rupture, rupture of the interventricular septum, or, rarely, rupture of the chordae tendineae.

Papillary muscle rupture most commonly results in rupture of a single head of the papillary muscle rather than the papillary muscle belly. Often such patients develop acute pulmonary edema. Rupture is more often due to right coronary artery occlusion with acute infarction involving the posteromedial papillary muscle. The murmur is usually holosystolic and heard best at the apex. However, because of the high left atrial pressure, the murmur may be audible only in early systole.

Ventricular septal rupture occurs in 1–2% of all patients dying of an acute MI. This complication usually results within the first week after the infarction and may occur with an anterior or inferior MI. The murmur due to ventricular septal rupture is loudest at the left sternal border and may be associated with a thrill. Because the location of the rupture is often in the lower apical septum, however, it may be difficult at the bedside to distinguish a ventricular septal defect from the murmur of mitral insufficiency secondary to ruptured papillary muscle. Two-dimensional echocardiography and color Doppler readily establish the correct diagnosis. Confirmation is made with right heart catheterization. A step-up of oxygen saturation at the ventricular or pulmonary level establishes the diagnosis of a ventricular septal rupture and is used to quantitate the shunt magnitude by the formula:

$$\text{Shunt ratio} = \frac{\text{sys artery sat (\%)} - \text{mixed venous sat (\%)}}{\text{sys artery sat (\%)} - \text{pulmonary artery sat (\%)}}$$

A large V wave in the pulmonary capillary wedge and pulmonary artery tracings may be seen with either papillary muscle or ventricular septal rupture. In septal rupture, impairment of right ventricular function is an important marker for the development of shock and a poor prognosis. Best results are obtained if surgery is performed early because delay results in complications secondary to poor tissue perfusion. In patients with circulatory collapse, it is imperative that the circulation at first be supported by intra-aortic balloon counterpulsation, which reduces left ventricular afterload, thereby promoting increased aortic flow and preferentially decreasing the left-to-right shunt. At the same time, balloon counterpulsation supports the patient's systemic circulation.

Current operative mortality is 25%, and survival at 5 years is 65%. Debate continues regarding the efficacy of concomitant bypass surgery at the time of repair. In general, revascularization is provided to areas remote from the infarct when appropriate, but revascularization of the ruptured area itself is of questionable benefit.

The present patient was immediately placed on an aortic balloon pump and taken to the catheterization laboratory. A large septal rupture was found with a 3:1 left to right shunt. The vein grafts and the internal mammary artery were patent. All of his native vessels were occluded. The ventricular septal defect was repaired successfully.

Clinical Pearls

1. Papillary muscle dysfunction, papillary muscle rupture, and rupture of the ventricular septum are the commonest causes of a new heart murmur associated with an acute MI.

2. While two-D echocardiography and color Doppler can establish the diagnosis, a right heart catheter should be used to obtain oximetry data, which allow calculation of the shunt ratio to help gauge the success of initial medical therapy.

3. Although there may be a temptation to delay surgery in order to achieve greater patient stability, early surgery for a ruptured ventricular septum produces the best results.

REFERENCES

1. Wei JY, Hutchins GM, Bulkley BH: Papillary muscle rupture in fatal acute myocardial infarction: A potentially treatable form of cardiogenic shock. Ann Intern Med 1979;90:149–152.
2. Radford MJ, Johnson RA, Daggett WM, et al: Ventricular septal rupture: A review of clinical and physiologic features and an analysis of survival. Circulation 1981;64:545–553.
3. Pretre R, Ye Q, Grunenfelder J, et al: Operative results of "repair" of ventricular septal rupture after acute myocardial infarction. Am J Cardiol 1999;84:785–788.

PATIENT 96

A 46-year-old obese man with acute chest pain and dyspnea following surgery

An obese 46-year-old man with a past history of degenerative joint disease underwent a left total knee replacement without complications. Three days following surgery, he complains of acute onset of shortness of breath and right-sided chest pain. He is receiving aspirin 325 mg q.d. and took warfarin 15 mg daily for 2 days.

Physical Examination: Vital signs: temperature 98.8°; pulse 110; respirations 30; blood pressure 110/70. General: obese, in apparent distress. Chest: splinting on right side; minimal right-sided wheezes. Cardiac: no jugular venous distention; S_4 present; no S_3; no rub or murmur noted. Abdomen: obese; benign. Extremities: left knee with surgical bandage; no calf tenderness or inflammation noted.

Laboratory Findings: PT 13.8 sec; PTT 25 sec. ABGs (room air): pH 7.50; PCO_2 30 mmHg; PO_2 76 mmHg. Previous and current EKG: see below.

Question: What is the significance of the EKG pattern?

Previous EKG

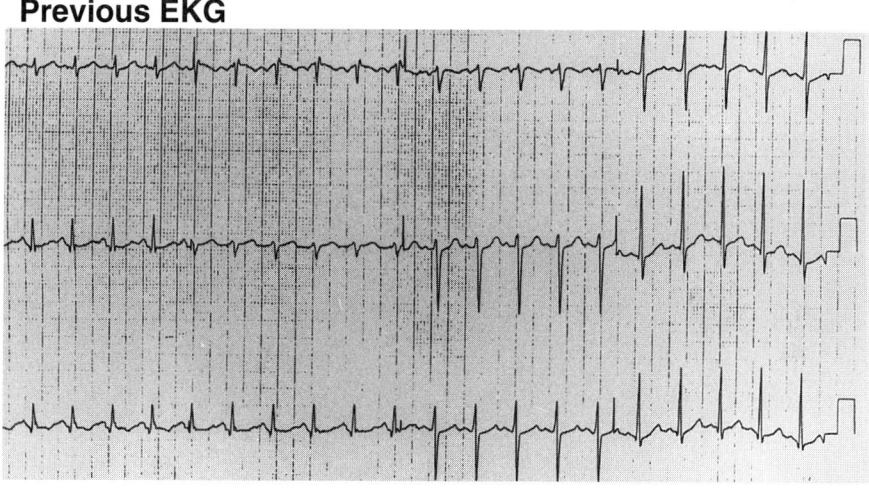

Current EKG

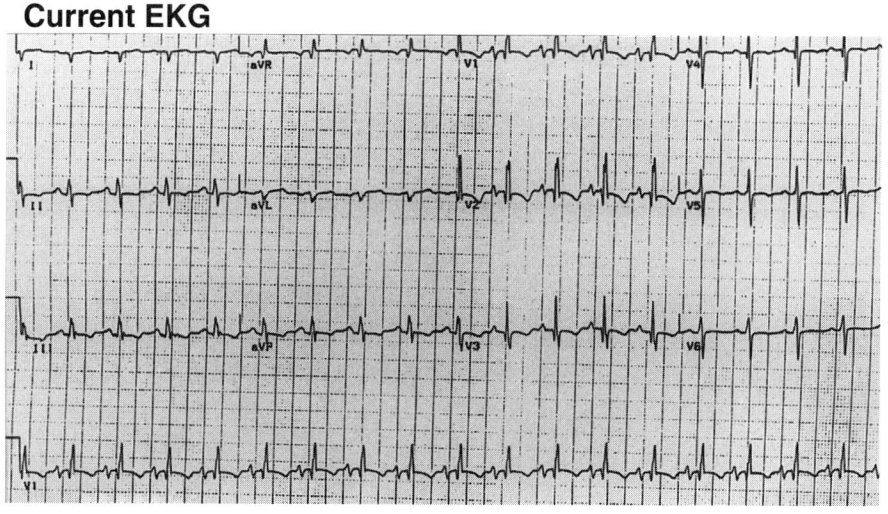

Diagnosis: Pulmonary embolism with pseudoinfarct pattern.

Discussion: The most typical EKG finding in pulmonary embolism is no change from the previous EKG. However, when the embolus has been large enough to occlude more than 50% of the pulmonary vasculature, acute pulmonary hypertension and right heart strain develop. These physiologic changes are manifested electrocardiographically as **acute right axis deviation** (manifested as the appearance of an S wave in lead I and often a Q wave in lead III), **clockwise rotation,** and **peaked P waves.** At times a dilated right ventricle can cause right precordial T-wave inversion. Right bundle branch block may also appear, with new Q waves in the right precordial leads produced by the axis shift. These latter findings may be misinterpreted as evidence for acute enteroseptal myocardial infarction.

The classic clinical picture is exemplified by the present patient. The most common complaints are the acute onset of chest pain and dyspnea. If pulmonary infarction develops, the chest pain may become pleuritic and be associated with hemoptysis. These symptoms usually occur with a background of factors that have predisposed the patient to venous thrombosis. These factors include immobility, surgery, congestive heart failure, previous lower-extremity venous disease, lower-extremity injury, and hypercoagulable states such as estrogen use.

In the area of the embolus, lung units are not perfused but ventilation is maintained, causing areas of increased ventilation to perfusion that can produce dyspnea and an increased dead space ventilation but not typically hypoxemia. The release of humoral factors, such as histamine, bradykinin, and other mediators, can lead to bronchoconstriction, which produces low ventilation-to-perfusion ratios in areas adjacent to the embolus. These ventilation-perfusion mismatches are the major cause of hypoxemia in pulmonary embolism and further contribute to the dyspnea.

On physical examination the respiratory rate is almost always in excess of 20 per minute. If the embolus is massive (>50% of pulmonary vascular bed) or the patient has underlying chronic obstructive pulmonary disease with loss of pulmonary vasculature, hypotension may occur. Low-grade fever and tachycardia are common. If the embolus has been large enough to cause right heart strain, jugular venous distention and increased loudness of the pulmonic component of the second heart sound are often present. Examination of the lungs rarely detects wheezing, unless the patient has underlying hyperreactive airways from asthma or smoking.

The chest radiograph may demonstrate areas of reduced pulmonary markings due to hypoperfusion. Elevation of the hemidiaphragm from atelectasis and pleural effusion (50%) are common. The arterial blood gases are almost always abnormal. Although often the PO_2 is less than 80 mmHg when the patient is breathing room air, this finding is not invariable and its absence should not be used to exclude the diagnosis. However, hypocarbia and a respiratory alkalosis are almost always seen.

When a pulmonary embolism is suspected, a D-dimer is ordered. This test is highly sensitive, so that a negative D-dimer nearly excludes pulmonary embolus. A positive test, however, is not specific. If the test is positive or suspicion is very high, a ventilation perfusion scan should be performed next. If the diagnosis remains uncertain, spiral CT scanning or pulmonary arteriography can conform the diagnosis.

Standard therapy for pulmonary embolus includes anticoagulation with heparin for 5 days followed by oral anticoagulation with warfarin, which should be started with the heparin. With refractory hypotension or hypoxemia, thrombolytic therapy should be given promptly. In massive pulmonary embolism that has led to shock and is refractory to thrombolytics, pulmonary embolectomy may be lifesaving.

The EKG in the present patient showed a new right bundle branch block and possible Q waves in leads V_1–V_3 and right axis deviation. Pulmonary embolism was confirmed by a ventilation-perfusion scan that demonstrated multiple segmental areas of ventilation-perfusion mismatch. He was treated with heparin followed by warfarin without recurrence of pulmonary embolism.

Clinical Pearls

1. Although the EKG changes little in most cases of pulmonary embolism, with right ventricular overload the EKG changes may be striking. In the patient with acute chest pain and dyspnea, new Q waves or deeply inverted T waves in leads V_1–V_3 may be misinterpreted as acute myocardial infarction.

2. Over 90% of patients with acute pulmonary embolism have a respiratory rate of greater than 20 per minute.

3. The hypoxemia of pulmonary embolism is not due to the areas of the lung obstructed by the emboli, but rather to the neurohumoral consequences of the event that limit ventilation elsewhere in the lung, causing areas of low ventilation-perfusion ratios.

REFERENCES

1. Stein PD, Dalen JE, McIntyre KM, et al: The electrocardiogram in acute pulmonary embolism. Prog Cardiovas Dis 1975;17:247–257.
2. Kelly MA, Carson JL, Palevsky HI, et al: Diagnosing pulmonary embolism: New facts and strategies. Ann Intern Med 1991;114:300–306.
3. Goldhaber SZ: Pulomary embolism. N Engl J Med 1998;339:93–104.

PATIENT 97

A 52-old man with increasing abdominal girth and peripheral edema 10 years following a motor vehicle accident

A 52-year-old man is admitted to the hospital because of increasing abdominal girth and peripheral edema. Several years ago, he experienced paroxysmal nocturnal dyspnea, orthopnea, and exertional dyspnea, which cleared intermittently with diuretic therapy. However, as his abdominal girth and peripheral edema have increased, his dyspnea has lessened. He gives no personal or family history of tuberculosis or heart disease. Ten years previously, he was hospitalized for a fractured femur from an automobile accident; he cannot recollect if he sustained chest trauma. At times, he drinks alcohol excessively.

Physical Examination: Vital signs: pulse 80; blood pressure 90/70. Neck: jugular venous distention with minimal deep jugular pulsations and prominent external jugular veins; during inspiration the neck veins became more distended. Cardiac: slightly enlarged; prominent third sound in early diastole; no murmurs. Chest: evidence of a right pleural effusion. Abdomen: distended because of ascites, making it difficult to detect organ enlargement. Extremities: peripheral edema to above the ankles.

Laboratory Findings: CBC and urinalysis: normal. Renal studies: normal. Bilirubin 4.5 mg/dl; AST 46 units/L. Prothrombin time 15.4 sec. Chest radiograph: slightly enlarged cardiac silhouette; no cardiac calcification; right pleural effusion. EKG: right axis deviation; a pattern resembling right ventricular hypertrophy. No cardiac calcifications noted. Cardiac catherization: see data below.

	Pressures (mmHg)	
	Inspiration	Expiration
Right atrium	27	15
Right ventricle	47/25	
Pulmonary capillary wedge	25	
Pulmonary artery	47/26	
Left ventricle	90/26	
Aorta	90/60	

Question: What is the cause of this patient's congestive heart failure?

Diagnosis: Constrictive pericarditis.

Discussion: The present patient demonstrated many of the clinical features of constrictive pericarditis, including an inspiratory increase in systemic venous pressure (Kussmaul's sign), third heart sound (diastolic knock), and a narrow pulse pressure. Right-sided heart findings usually are more prominent than those of left heart failure. At times, the patient may have atrial fibrillation, the diastolic knock is misinterpreted as an opening snap, and the diagnosis of mitral stenosis is entertained. If the neck veins are not observed carefully, hepatic enlargement and edema lead to the misdiagnosis of cirrhosis of the liver.

The EKG usually shows low QRS voltage with inverted T waves. About 30% of patients have atrial flutter or fibrillation. The present patient had an unusual EKG that simulated right ventricular hypertrophy (RVH). This pattern has previously been reported in 6 of 122 cases of constriction, and only one had fibrotic annular subpulmonic constriction as a possible explanation for the RVH pattern.

The echocardiogram is of limited diagnostic value, but it will exclude significant systolic dysfunction as the cause of the congestive failure. As noted in Case 85, marked respiratory variation of Doppler mitral valve in-flow velocity is very suggestive of constriction. Restrictive cardiomyopathy (amyloidosis, hemochromatosis, and others) can have a clinical and hemodynamic presentation similar to that of constrictive pericarditis. If left ventricular end-diastolic pressure is considerably higher than that in the right ventricle, then restrictive cardiomyopathy is more likely. The left ventricular filling rate measured echocardiographically or by MUGA is slower in cardiomyopathy during the first half diastole than in constrictive pericarditis, in which early filling is rapid. MRI or CT scan, both of which can image the pericardium and measure its thickness, may be important aids in the diagnosis. If the diagnosis is still uncertain, a subxiphoid thoracotomy may be necessary to explore the pericardium.

Cardiac catheterization in the present patient showed equalization of the mean right atrial, pulmonary artery, diastolic, pulmonary capillary wedge, and right and left ventricular end-diastolic pressures. In addition, the ventricular pressures showed early diastolic dips. The right atrial and capillary wedge pressure pulses had an "M" configuration.

The EKG taken after the accident 10 years previously showed acute pericarditis. This traumatic pericarditis probably resulted in subsequent constriction. Initially, he may have had effusoconstriction in which the presence of a pericardial effusion produced the tamponade-like symptoms of dyspnea and orthopnea. As the effusion resolved, more typical findings of constriction ensued, producing primarily right-sided findings. Fibrous pericarditis with minimal pockets of fluid were found at pericardiectomy. He improved markedly after surgery.

Clinical Pearls

1. A patient with signs and symptoms of congestive heart failure for many years should be reevaluated for constrictive pericarditis, especially when the findings of right-sided failure are more prominent than those of left-sided failure.

2. Patients with constrictive pericarditis often have atrial fibrillation and a pericardial knock, which may lead to the mistaken diagnosis of mitral stenosis.

3. Kussmaul's sign may be overlooked if the neck veins are extremely distended.

4. Restrictive cardiomyopathy may simulate constrictive pericarditis clinically and hemodynamically, but restriction usually produces a left ventricular end-diastolic pressure that is significantly higher than that of the right ventricle.

REFERENCES

1. Chesler F, Mitha AS, Matisonn RE: The ECG of constrictive pericarditis—pattern resembling right ventricular hypertrophy. Am Heart J 1976;91:420–424
2. Tyberg TI, Goodyear AVN, Hurst VW III, et al: Left ventricular filling in differentiating restrictive amyloid cardiomyopathy and constrictive pericarditis. Am J Cardiol 1981;47:791–796.
3. Boltwood CM Jr, Shah PM: The pericardium in health and disease. Curr Probi Cardiol 1984;9:1–70.

PATIENT 98

A 72-year-old woman with hyperpyrexia on beta-blocker therapy

A 72-year-old woman was begun on a beta blocker for hypertension in March. In July she is brought to the emergency department after being found unconscious at home.

Physical Examination: Vital signs: pulse 110; blood pressure 70/40; temperature 42°C. Skin: dry and hot to the touch. Chest: clear. Cardiac: normal. Neurologic: responds only to deep pain.

Laboratory Findings: ABGs (room air): pH 7.19; PCO_2 26 mmHg; PO_2 96 mmHg.

Questions: What is the likely cause of the patient's clinical presentation? What is the phase of the underlying process?

Diagnosis: Heat stroke.

Discussion: Heat stroke typically occurs in elderly patients or those with underlying infirmities, most commonly 3 days or longer after the onset of particularly hot and humid weather. The risk of developing heat stroke increases when drugs that inhibit sweating are prescribed, such as beta blockers, phenothiazines, or antihistamines. Young, healthy subjects also can develop the disease when they pursue rigorous physical activity in extremely hot weather.

Patients with heat stroke usually present with only mild degrees of dehydration because the underlying pathophysiology of the disease depends on intense vasoconstriction and the absence of sweating. Hypotension develops, therefore, from direct myocardial depression and/or myocardial necrosis from effects of the hyperpyrexia rather than from intravascular volume depletion.

Patients initially present with a respiratory alkalosis and attendant hypokalemia. As hypotension ensues, lactic acid is generated, leading to metabolic acidosis, as seen in the present patient, which is an ominous sign. Complications of heat stroke include disseminated intravascular coagulation with subsequent damage to visceral organs, rhabdomyolysis, hepatic damage, and renal failure. Hypophosphatemia commonly occurs. The overall mortality is approximately 20%, but is higher in the elderly patient with underlying comorbid conditions.

When ordering arterial blood gases, it is important to note the patient's temperature to the laboratory. PO_2 must be corrected upward by 6% for each degree centigrade the patient's temperature is above 37°. PCO_2 must be corrected upward by 4.4%, while pH is corrected downwardly 0.015 per degree.

The mainstay of therapy for heat stroke is **rapid cooling** of the patient. Debate exists as to whether the patient should be immersed in ice water or whether immersion in somewhat warmer water (10°C) is preferable. Ice water may induce shivering and convulsions, which might be avoided by the somewhat warmer immersion temperature. Hypotension is initially treated with volume repletion, although, as noted above, aggressive volume repletion is generally not indicated. If administration of 500–1000 cc of normal saline fails to restore blood pressure, a Swan-Ganz catheter should be placed to guide fluid management. Acidosis may worsen as the circulation improves and lactate is removed from the tissues. Although sodium bicarbonate therapy for acidosis is often recommended, this point is debatable in light of recent evidence that bicarbonate administration in lactic acidosis is deleterious. Acute cooling with immersion in ice water may be discontinued once the temperature has fallen to 38°C. Following initial resuscitation, patients must be monitored carefully for the appearance of disseminated intravascular coagulation, cardiac arrhythmias, myocardial infarction, and bacterial infections.

Despite vigorous attempts to reduce her temperature and support her blood pressure, the patient died with intractable hypotension.

Clinical Pearls

1. The only satisfactory therapy for heat stroke is immediate cooling of the patient by immersion in cold water.

2. The initial acid base disturbance is a respiratory alkalosis, which is followed by a metabolic acidosis if significant lactic acid is produced.

3. Myocardial damage is common, may worsen shock, and may lead to congestive heart failure.

4. Arterial blood gases must be corrected for the patient's temperature.

REFERENCES

1. Hart GR, Anderson RJ, Crumpler CP, et al: Epidemic classical heat stroke: Clinical characteristics and course of 28 patients. Medicine 1982;61:189–197.
2. Zahger D, Moses A, Weiss AT: Evidence of prolonged myocardial dysfunction in heat stroke. Chest 1989;95:1089–1091.
3. Vassallo SU, Delaney KA. Pharmacologic effects on thermoregulation: Mechanisms of drug-related heatstroke. J Toxicol 1999;27:199–224.
4. Simon HB: Hyperthermia. N Engl J Med 1993;329:483–487.

PATIENT 99

A 53-year-old woman with mitral stenosis and left upper- and lower-extremity weakness

A 53-year-old woman with mitral stenosis presents with the new onset of left upper- and lower-extremity weakness. The patient has previously noted only mild dyspnea on exertion. She has been in atrial fibrillation for the past 2 years. Medications include dogoxin and an aspirin a day.

Physical Examination: Vital signs: pulse 85, irregularly irregular; blood pressure 120/75. Chest: clear. Cardiac: irregularly irregular rhythm; opening snap; II/VI systolic murmur at the apex. Abdomen: benign. Extremities: left-sided hemiparesis.

Laboratory Findings: Head CT: bland infarct in the region of right middle cerebral artery. Echocardiogram: see below.

Question: What is the source of the patient's neurologic problem?

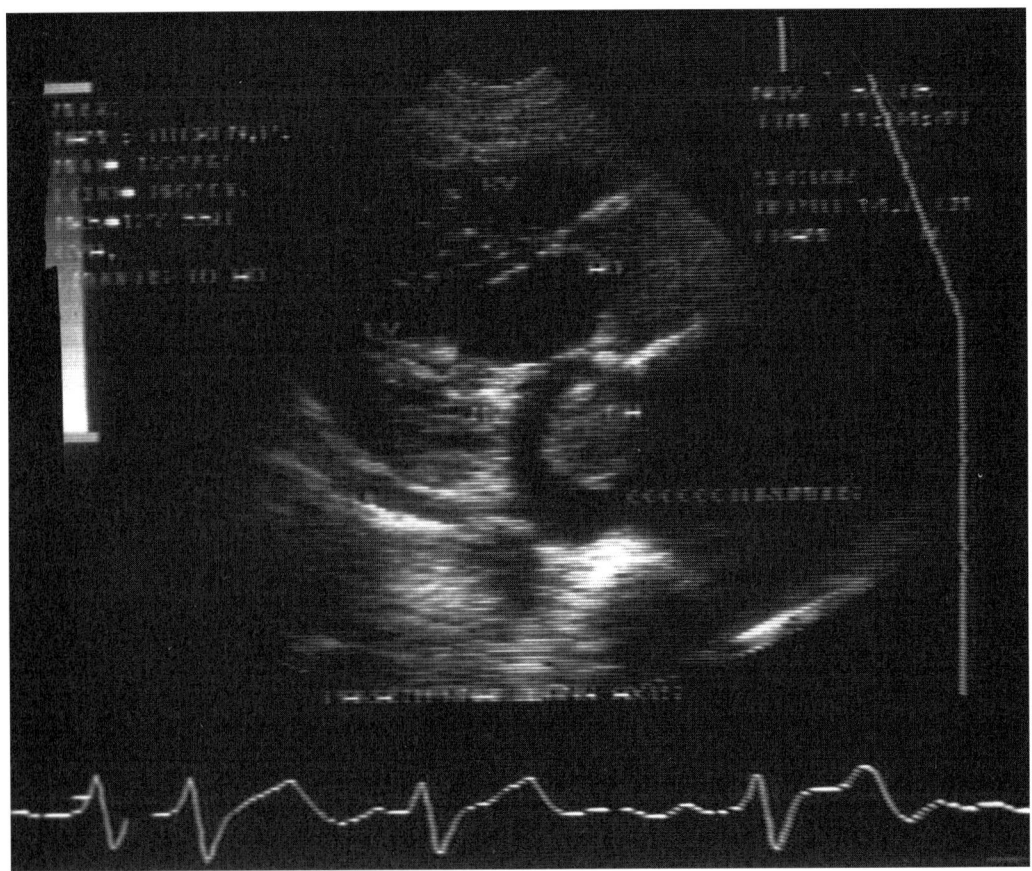

Diagnosis: Systemic embolism secondary to mitral stenosis.

Discussion: When atrial fibrillation coincides with mitral stenosis, the two pathologic conditions are additive in producing left atrial stasis and thrombosis, making the risk of systemic embolization high. The risk of embolic stroke may be as high as 75 per patient/year. Although aspirin may have some efficacy in reducing the incidence of embolic stroke, it is not a substitute for systemic anticoagulation. Previous recommendations had been to administer enough warfarin to prolong the prothrombin time to 1.5 to 2 times control. Now, however, the **international normalized radio** (INR) is used. INR is the ratio of the patient's prothrombin time (PT) to control PT raised to the power of the reagent (r) used in the study — $[PT_{PT}/PT_{CON}]^r$. INR accounts for the fact that different laboratories use different reagents. Thus, while a patient's PT may vary from laboratory to laboratory, INR does not. An INR of 3 should be utilized in patients with rheumatic valve disease in atrial fibrillation, a higher value than for nonrheumatic atrial fibrillation, in which an INR of 2 is recommended.

In some patients with mitral stenosis, the first presenting manifestation of the disease is systemic embolism. Previous data suggested that such patients had a high likelihood of having a second embolus unless the mitral stenosis was corrected. Currently, however, it is thought that anticoagulation is usually adequate to prevent a second embolism. Thus, systemic embolism without other symptoms related to mitral stenosis probably does not justify mechanical intervention if effective anticoagulation can be initiated. If a systemic embolism occurs in the setting of heart failure, then the mitral stenosis should be mechanically corrected.

The presence of a large left atrial thrombus precludes mechanical correction by mitral valvotomy because catheter manipulation might dislodge the thrombus. Thus, open commissurotomy or mitral valve replacement during which the atrial thrombus can be safely removed would be the only mechanical options for correcting the mitral stenosis. Emboli frequently arise from a thrombus in the left atrial appendage, which is not visualized by transthoracic echocardiography. When there is a suspicion of a cardiac source for an embolus, transesophageal echocardiography should be employed to exclude a thrombus in the left atrial appendage. Following surgery, if the patient is restored to normal sinus rhythm and left atrial size diminishes, anticoagulation can be safely discontinued after a few months of therapy. However, if atrial fibrillation remains and there is some degree of residual mitral stenosis, lifelong anticoagulation is indicated.

In the present patient, the echocardiogram demonstrated a large left atrial thrombus. She underwent open commissurotomy during which the thrombus was removed.

Clinical Pearls

1. Systemic embolism may be the presenting clinical manifestation of mitral stenosis.
2. Anticoagulation to at least 1.5 times control prothrombin time is recommended in patients with mitral stenosis and atrial fibrillation.
3. Transesophageal but not transthoracic echocardiography visualizes the left atrial appendage—a potential source for emboli.

REFERENCES

1. Rowe JC, Bland EF, Sprague HB, et al: The course of mitral stenosis without surgery: Ten- and twenty-year perspectives. Ann Intern Med 1960;52:741–749.
2. Seward JB: Cardiac tumors and thrombus: Transesophageal echocardiographic experience. In Erbel R et al (eds): Transesophageal Echocardiography: A New Window to the Heart. New York, Springer Verlag, 1989.
3. The Boston Area Anticoagulation Trial for Atrial Fibrillation Investigators: The effect of low-dose warfarin on the risk of stroke in patients with nonrheumatic atrial fibrillation. N Engl J Med 1990;323:1505–1511.
4. Cannegieter SC, Rosendaal FR, Wintzen AR, et al: Optimal oral anticoagulant therapy in patients with mechanical heart valves. N Engl J Med 1995;333:11–17.

PATIENT 100

A 76-year-old man with a mitral valve prosthesis and on anticoagulation who requires rectal polypectomy

A 76-year-old man had his mitral valve replaced with a St. Jude prosthesis 8 years previously for severe mitral insufficiency with heart failure. Following surgery he had persistent left atrial enlargement and chronic atrial fibrillation and was maintained on warfarin. Recently, he began having bleeding during defecation. Flexible sigmoidoscopy demonstrates a 2.5-cm rectal polyp. A gastroenterologist advises colonoscopy and endoscopic polypectomy. Besides the warfarin, the patient is taking digoxin and verapamil. He is allergic to penicillin.

Physical Examination: Vital signs: irregularly irregular rhythm; blood pressure 140/70. Cardiac: no jugular venous distention; prosthetic sounds crisp; a faint murmur of aortic insufficiency noted along left sternal border.

Laboratory Findings: Hct 45%; prothrombin time 20 sec. EKG: atrial fibrillation with a satisfactory ventricular response; left ventricular hypertrophy; digitalis effect.

Question: How should this patient's preparation for colonoscopy and polypectomy be managed?

Answer: The patient requires careful management of perioperative anticoagulation. and endocarditis prophylaxis.

Discussion: This patient has two important problems that need management prior to colonoscopy and polypectomy—anticoagulation for his mechanical valve and bacterial endocarditis prophylaxis. Stopping **anticoagulation** could lead to prosthetic valve thrombosis and systemic embolization. In such patients, warfarin should be discontinued at least 3 days before the procedure to allow the prothrombin time to decrease to within 20% of normal; concomitantly an intravenous heparin infusion should be started to maintain partial thromboplastin time about twice control value. The effect of heparin can be reversed immediately before the procedure by giving protamine sulfate intravenously. After the polypectomy, when there is no evidence of bleeding, heparin and warfarin should be restarted, and once the prothrombin time is at a therapeutic level, heparin should be discontinued and warfarin maintained.

In a study of 159 patients with prosthetic valves undergoing noncardiac surgery, no thromboembolic complications occurred when anticoagulation was discontinued an average of 2.9 days preoperatively and restarted an average of 2.7 days postoperatively. Although this study suggests that a short period off of anticoagulants is safe, we do not consider this management optimal for the high-risk patient with a mitral valve prosthesis, large left atrium, and chronic atrial fibrillation.

The second issue is **prevention of bacterial endocarditis.** Remarkably, many patients at high risk, such as the present patient, fail to receive any prophylaxis. The following regimen has recently been recommended for gastrointestinal procedures: intravenous or intramuscular ampicillin 2.0 gm, plus gentamicin 1.5 mg/kg (not to exceed 80 mg) 30 minutes before the procedure followed by amoxicillin 1.5 gm orally 6 hours after the initial dose; alternatively, the parenteral regimen may be repeated once, 8 hours after the initial dose. Because the present patient had a history of penicillin allergy, intravenous vancomycin 1.0 gm given over 1 hour plus IV or IM gentamicin 1.5 mg/kg (not to exceed 80 mg) should be given 1 hour before the procedure; this may be repeated once, 8 hours after the initial dose.

The present patient was anticoagulated with heparin and received antibiotic prophylaxis. The heparin was stopped 6 hours prior to polypectomy. There were no postoperative complications.

Clinical Pearls

1. In the patient with a mechanical valve prosthesis, total withdrawal of anticoagulation perioperatively should not occur for any extended period of time, as there is potential for thrombotic valvular dysfunction and secondary embolization.

2. Discontinue warfarin and start heparin before surgery. The heparin can be neutralized just prior to the procedure and restarted together with warfarin postoperatively when there is no evidence of bleeding.

3. A remarkable underutilization of endocarditis prophylaxis in patients at high risk for endocarditis is one of the leading causes of endocarditis today.

REFERENCES

1. Tinker JH, Tarham S: Discontinuing anticoagulant therapy in surgical patients with cardiac valve prostheses. Observations in 180 operations. JAMA 1978;239:738–739.
2. Katholi RE, Nolan SP, McGuire LB: The management of anticoagulation during noncardiac operations in patients with prosthetic heart valves: A prospective study. Am Heart J 1978;96:163–165.
3. Dajani AS, Bisno AL, Chung KJ, et al: Prevention of bacterial endocarditis: Recommendations by the American Heart Association, JAMA 1990;264:2919–2922.
4. Kearon C, Hirsh J: Management of anticoagulation before and after elective surgery. N Engl J Med 1997;336:1506–1511.

PATIENT 101

A 45-year-old man with improved ventricular function after coronary bypass surgery

A 45-year-old man reports a 1-month history of progressive chest pain typical of angina pectoris, mild dyspnea on exertion, and two-pillow orthopnea. There is no history of a myocardial infarction. The patient's EKG is normal, but his coronary arteriograms show severe three-vessel disease. An internal mammary graft to his left anterior descending artery and two saphenous vein bypass grafts to his right and circumflex coronaries are inserted in an uncomplicated operative procedure. He develops pain atypical of ischemia 2 months after surgery.

Physical Examination: Vital signs: pulse 80 (regular); blood pressure 120/70. Neck veins: flat. Chest: clear. Cardiac: summation gallop. Extremities: no peripheral edema.

Laboratory Findings: EKG: normal. Postoperative repeat coronary arteriograms: all grafts widely patent; ejection fraction increased from 0.44 to 0.64.

Question: What accounts for these ventriculographic changes?

Diagnosis: Previously hibernating myocardium.

Discussion: As recently as a decade ago, it was believed that cardiac ischemia was either transient with full recovery following a typical anginal attack or persistent with progression to myocardial infarction—no middle ground was thought to exist. It is now clear, however, that persistently ischemic but viable myocardium can persist in a "hibernating" state. Preoperative catheterization evidence of wall motion abnormalities suggestive of infarcted myocardium can be restored to normal function with a successful revascularization procedure.

The biologic mechanisms of hibernation are poorly understood. It has been assumed that blood flow to hibernating areas is chronically reduced, but recent studies challenge this concept by finding normal coronary blood flow in some patients in the areas of hibernation. In light of these data, hibernation may reflect **repeated episodes of stunning,** at least in some patients. In any case, it is likely that the absence of contraction in these areas is protective because it reduces oxygen consumption and maintains myocardial viability. Once blood flow is restored, contraction improves, although full myocardial recovery may require several days or weeks.

It is important to distinguish hibernating from infarcted myocardial tissue during preoperative assessments. Patients with infarcted hypokinetic myocardial regions will not benefit from revascularization and should not undergo surgery. **Thallium imaging** assists in this distinction because thallium is taken up by hibernating but not by infarcted myocardial tissue. During cardiac catheterization, **augmentation ventriculography**—in which a ventricular extrasystole is interposed between normal beats—also aids in the differential diagnosis. In this test, there is a 50% chance that myocardial contractility will be restored after effective revascularization when the beat following an extrasystole demonstrates improved wall motion in areas suspected to be hibernating. However, when extrasystolic potentiation fails to induce enhanced myocardial contraction, it is highly unlikely that any improvement will be gained by revascularization. Thus, the test is particularly helpful in directing therapy when no post-extrasystolic accentuation occurs. Importantly, patients with depressed ejection fractions preoperatively who demonstrate improvement with augmentation ventriculography have an improved prognosis compared with patients with similar ejection fractions whose wall motion does not improve with post-extrasystolic potentiation.

Positron emission tomography (PET) scanning is also useful in distinguishing hibernating from infarcted tissue. Hibernating myocardial tissue takes up fluorodeoxyglucose in contrast to infarcted tissue. Unfortunately, PET scanning is extremely expensive and currently cannot be used to screen the large number of patients with wall motion abnormalities undergoing bypass surgery.

The present patient's chest pain was considered nonischemic in nature. It resolved with administration of ibuprofen therapy. The improvement in the postoperative ventriculogram was considered to be due to a region of previously hibernating myocardium.

Clinical Pearls

1. There clearly exists a chronic physiologic state in which ischemia can lead to myocardial dysfunction but not true infarction. This condition is referred to as "hibernating" myocardium.
2. Thallium imaging, post-extrasystolic potentiation during ventriculography, and PET scanning are ways to distinguish hibernating from infarcted myocardium.
3. Some hibernation may reflect repeated episodes of stunning.

REFERENCES

1. Topol EJ, Weiss JL, Guzman PA, et al: Immediate improvement of dysfunctional myocardial segments after coronary revascularization: Detection by intraoperative transesophageal echocardiography. J Am Coll Cardiol 1984:4:1123–1134.
2. Rankin JS, Newman GE, Muhlbaier LH, et al: The effects of coronary revascularization on left ventricular function in ischemic heart disease. J Thorac Cardiovasc Surg 1985;90:818–832.
3. Rahimtoola SH: The hibernating myocardium. Am Heart J 1989;117:211–221.
4. Gerber BL, Vanoverschelde J-L, Bol A, et al: Myocardial blood flow, glucose uptake, and recruitment of inotropic reserve in chronic left ventricular ischemic dysfunction. Circulation 1996;94:651–659.
5. Kloner RA, Bolli R, Marban E, et al: Medical and cellular implications of stunning, hibernation, and preconditioning: An NHLBI Workshop. Circulation 1998;97:1848–1867.

PATIENT 102

A 53-year-old man with dyspnea on exertion and a heart murmur following an episode of acute chest pain

A 53-year-old man is seen on several occasions over a 2-month period for progressive dyspnea on exertion. He reports an episode of acute chest pain while carrying firewood 2 months before admission; the pain resolved over the ensuing 12-24 hours, but dyspnea began following this episode. A previous outpatient evaluation included a normal EKG and radiographic evidence of mild cardiomegaly and pulmonary vascular congestion. A transthoracic echocardiogram is technically difficult, but reveals normal systolic global and regional left ventricular function. The patient denies a prior history of cardiac disease, hypertension, familial heart disease, or elevated cholesterol.

Physical Examination: Vital signs: pulse 100; respirations 24; blood pressure 140/85. Chest: bibasilar rales over lower third of lung fields. Cardiac: no gallops; I/VI holosystolic apical murmur. Extremities: 1+ edema.

Laboratory Findings: Transesophageal echocardiogram: see below.

Question: What is the cause of the patient's murmur and heart failure?

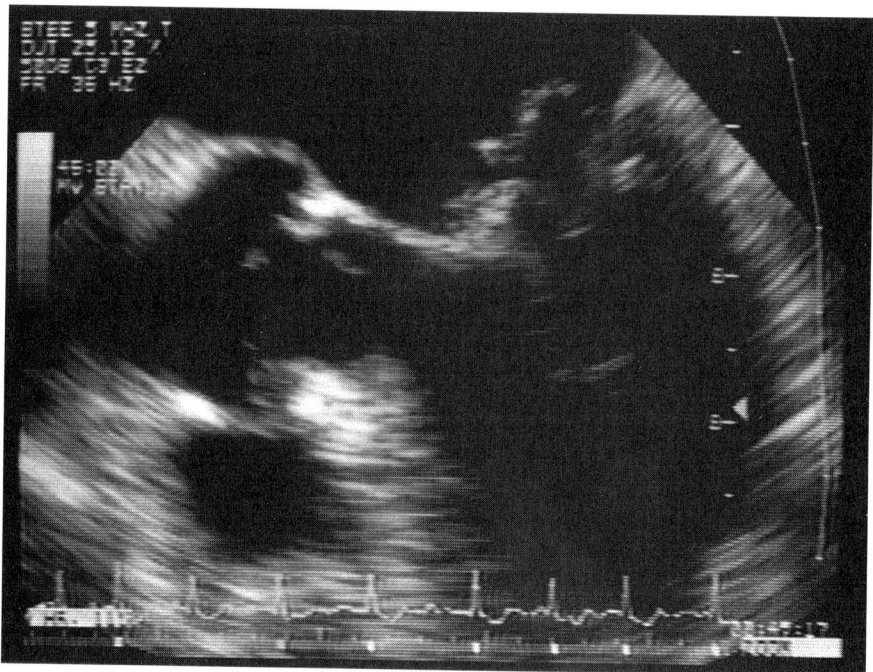

Diagnosis: Acute mitral regurgitation secondary to spontaneous rupture of a chorda tendinea.

Discussion: The common causes of acute mitral regurgitation include rupture of a chorda tendinea, bacterial endocarditis, and papillary muscle ischemia or infarction. In the present patient, the acute mitral regurgitation was due to rupture of a chorda tendinea. Although normal chordae tendineae have tensile strength greater than steel, some rupture spontaneously without apparent cause. In other cases, infection, myxomatous degeneration, or the mitral valve prolapse syndrome may contribute to chordal rupture. Usually chordal rupture produces no primary symptoms but, as in this case, can occasionally be associated with acute chest pain.

Although acute mitral regurgitation is usually associated with the typical loud holosystolic murmur, in some instances the murmur may be soft. This may be due in part to the fact that the regurgitant orifice is so large that minimal turbulence and, thus, little sound is generated from the valvular regurgitation. The murmur may also be short in duration because the pressure gradient between the left ventricle and atrium declines at the end of systole if the atrial V wave is large.

Decompensation in acute mitral regurgitation results from two hemodynamic factors. First, the volume regurgitated into an unprepared small and noncompliant left atrium produces high left atrial pressure that is referred to the lungs, producing pulmonary edema. Second, the fall in forward stroke volume may produce systemic hypoperfusion and/or shock.

The present patient serves to demonstrate the utility of **transesophageal echocardiography** in diagnosing acute mitral regurgitation. For reasons that are not clear, transthoracic color flow Doppler studies often underestimate the degree of mitral regurgitation when the process is acute. The close proximity of the esophagus to the mitral valve produces an excellent echocardiographic view of the mitral valve. In the present patient, it demonstrated a flail mitral leaflet.

Medical therapy for acute mitral regurgitation is aimed at lowering left ventricular afterload. By reducing resistance to flow in the aorta, blood is preferentially expelled forward into that vessel while less is regurgitated back into the left atrium. These hemodynamic changes both increase forward output and reduce left atrial pressure, two obvious goals of therapy. At the same time, afterload reduction may reduce left ventricular annular size and partially restore mitral valve competence. **Nitroprusside** offers excellent acute afterload reduction. However, if the patient is in shock, nitroprusside is contraindicated. **Intra-aortic balloon counterpulsation** should be used for the patient in shock, as it lowers afterload and helps restore systemic blood pressure. While chronic vasodilator therapy has been demonstrated to be beneficial in *aortic* regurgitation, it is unproven in *mitral* regurgitation.

Definitive therapy requires mitral valve repair or replacement. It is now accepted that repair is superior to replacement because it avoids the risks of prosthetic valves and provides better postoperative left ventricular function.

The present patient underwent successful mitral valve repair with resolution of his heart failure.

Clinical Pearls

1. Transesophageal echocardiography is helpful in making the diagnosis of acute mitral regurgitation, whereas transthoracic echocardiography often underestimates the severity of the lesion.

2. Afterload reduction is the initial treatment of choice for acute mitral regurgitation, but chronic vasodilator therapy is still unproven therapy.

3. Mitral valve repair is preferable to mitral valve replacement in many cases of acute mitral regurgitation. Repair obviates the need for anticoagulation and usually leads to better ventricular function than does mitral valve replacement with chordal transection.

REFERENCES

1. Yoran C, Yellin EL, Becker RM, et al: Mechanism of reduction of mitral regurgitation with vasodilator therapy. Am J Cardiol 1979;43:773–77.
2. Carabello BA: Mitral regurgitation: Proper timing of mitral valve replacement. II. Mod Concepts Cardiovasc Dis 1988;57:59–64.
3. Horstkotte D, Schulte HD, Bircks W, et al: The effect of chordal preservation on late outcome after mitral valve replacement: A randomized study. J Heart Valve Dis 1993;2(2):150–158.
4. Horstkotte D, Schulte HD, Niehues R, et al: Diagnostic and therapeutic considerations in acute, severe mitral regurgitation: Experience in 42 consecutive patients entering the intensive care unit with pulmonary edema. J Heart Valve Dis 1993;2(5):512–522.
5. Ling LH, Enriquez-Sarano M, Seward JB, et al: Clinical outcome of mitral regurgitation due to flail leaflet. N Engl J Med 1996;335(19):1417–1423.

PATIENT 103

A 19-year-old woman with cyanosis and a heart murmur

A 19-year-old woman was known to have cyanosis and a heart murmur since birth. In childhood, she had frequent upper respiratory tract infections and episodic dyspnea that was relieved by squatting. While in high school, she avoided sports. She is admitted to the hospital for further studies.

Physical Examination: Vital signs: pulse 80; blood pressure 100/60. Cardiac: right ventricular lift; pulmonary artery pulsation not palpable; S_2 loud and single; harsh; systolic ejection murmur at second and third intercostal spaces to left of sternum. Extremities: clubbing, cyanosis of fingers and toes.

Laboratory Findings: Hct 60%. EKG: right ventricular hypertrophy. Chest radiograph: right ventricular enlargement; lung fields oligemic. Two-dimensional echocardiogram: see below.

Question: What is the diagnosis?

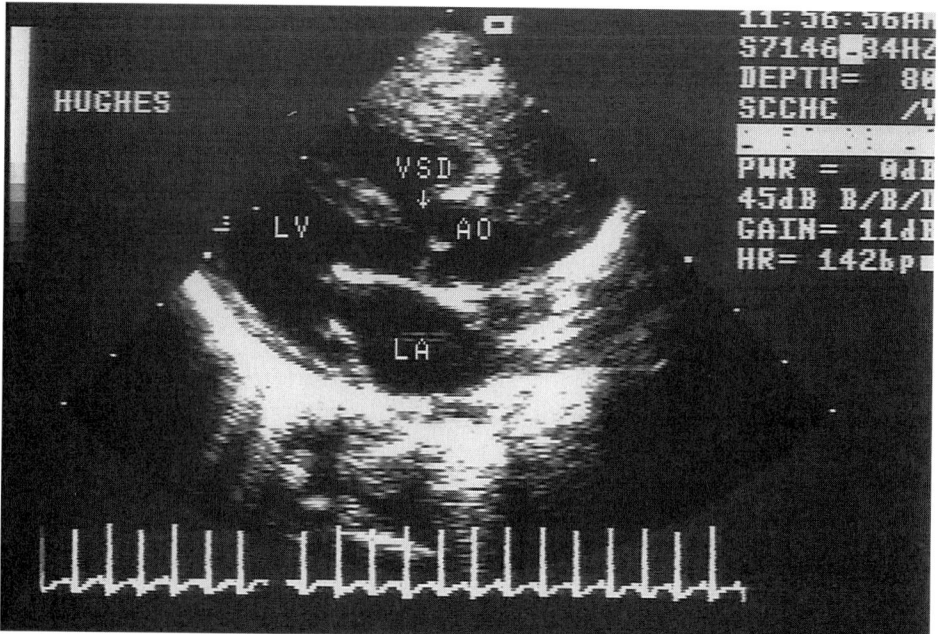

Diagnosis: Tetralogy of Fallot.

Discussion: Tetralogy of Fallot is the most common cyanotic congenital heart disease seen after 1 year of age. It consists of a ventricular septal defect (VSD), infundibular or pulmonary valve stenosis, right ventricular hypertrophy, and an aorta that overrides the ventricular septum. About 25% of patients with tetralogy of Fallot have a right aortic arch. Clinical findings vary depending on the size of the VSD and the degree of the right ventricular outflow tract obstruction. If the right ventricular outflow obstruction is mild, a left-to-right shunt may be present even though the ventricular pressures are equal. Thus, the patient will not be cyanotic. At the other extreme, there is severe cyanosis associated with severe pulmonary outflow tract obstruction.

Patients with both tetralogy of Fallot and **Eisenmenger's syndrome** from any lesion can reach adulthood and present as having cyanotic congenital heart disease. The distinction can usually be made at the bedside. Eisenmenger's syndrome is defined as any shunt between the right and left circulations in which the pulmonary vascular resistance has become equal to or greater than the systematic resistance producing a right-to-left shunt. Patients with Eisenmenger's syndrome will have a prominent A wave in the jugular venous pulse and a palpable pulmonary artery pulsation. These findings are not noted in patients with tetralogy of Fallot where the pulmonary artery is protected from high pressure by the outflow tract obstruction. It is this protection that allows surgical correction of the syndrome well into adulthood.

Eisenmenger's syndrome also produces a right ventricular lift, a loud second heart sound in the pulmonic area, and pulmonary insufficiency (Graham Steele murmur). The VSD of tetralogy usually does not produce a murmur since the ventricular pressures are equal. The systolic ejection murmur of tetralogy is caused by and varies with the degree of right ventricular outflow obstruction.

The 2-D echocardiogram in the present patient showed a VSD and an overriding aorta (Ao). Right ventricular hypertrophy was noted, and Doppler studies demonstrated right ventricular outflow tract stenosis and confirmed the presence of the VSD. Heart catheterization revealed the systolic pressure in the right ventricular infundibulum and pulmonary artery to be 20 mmHg, while the right ventricular systolic pressure was 90 and the left ventricular pressure was 95. Right atrial oxygen saturation was 57.5%, and femoral artery saturation was 82%. A biplane right ventricular cineangiocardiogram showed marked infundibular stenosis of the right ventricular outflow tract. The VSD was also noted and there was right-to-left shunting and filling of the transposed aorta. The right-to-left shunt was calculated to be 1.4:1.

At surgery, a Teflon patch was used to close the VSD and a pericardial graft was used to increase the size of the right ventricular outflow tract. Repeat heart catheterization 12 years later showed normal pressures, a small VSD, and mild pulmonary stenosis with some pulmonary insufficiency, and an aneurysmal dilatation of the right ventricular outflow tract. Subsequently the patient has done well, and her only complaint has been an occasional "skipping of her heart." Holter monitoring revealed many premature ventricular beats. Recent echo Doppler studies showed a small residual VSD, a 14 mmHg gradient across the pulmonic valve, mild pulmonary insufficiency, and right ventricular dilatation. These findings of postsurgical pulmonary insufficiency and arrhythmias are not unusual. Infective endocarditis may also occur and standard prophylaxis should be employed.

Clinical Pearls

1. Patients with tetralogy of Fallot can live to adulthood and still have a successful total surgical repair because the pulmonary outflow obstruction protects the pulmonary vasculature.

2. Tetralogy of Fallot has to be differentiated from Eisenmenger's syndrome, which also may present in adulthood as cyanotic congenital heart disease. In Eisenmenger's syndrome, signs of pulmonary hypertension predominate.

3. Because the ventricular pressures are equal in patients with tetralogy of Fallot, the VSD does not produce a murmur. The typical systolic murmur is due to right ventricular outflow tract obstruction.

4. Even after total surgical repair, patients with tetralogy of Fallot still have residual findings such as pulmonary insufficiency. Arrhythmias and bacterial endocarditis also may develop.

REFERENCES

1. Wood P: The Eisenmenger syndrome or pulmonary hypertension with reverse central shunt. Br Med J 1958;2:701.
2. Guntheroth WG, Mortan BC, Mullins GL, et al: Venous return with knee-chest position and squatting in tetralogy of Fallot. Am Heart J 1968;75:313–318.
3. Hu DC, Seward JB, Puga FJ, et al: Total correction of tetralogy of Fallot at age 40 years and older: Long-term follow-up. J Am Coll Cardiol 1985;5:40–44.
4. Hughes CF, Lim YC, Cartmill TB, et al: Total intracardiac repair for tetralogy of Fallot in adults. Ann Thorac Surg 1987;43:634–638.

PATIENT 104

A 42-year-old morbidly obese woman with dyspnea

A 42-year-old obese woman is admitted with dyspnea on exertion and orthopnea. She has noted gradually decreasing exercise tolerance over the 2 months before admission. The patient recently began sleeping on three pillows, but denies paroxysmal nocturnal dyspnea or chest pain. She also has noted ankle swelling in the previous 2 months.

Physical Examination: Height 5′3″; weight 440 pounds. Vital signs: pulse 100 and regular; blood pressure 140/90. Neck: jugular veins not discerned. Chest: bibasilar rales. Cardiac: difficult examination; S_1 and S_2 barely audible. Extremities: 2+ peripheral edema.

Laboratory Findings: EKG: low-voltage and nonspecific ST- and T-wave abnormalities. Chest radiograph: poor study but suggestive of vascular congestion. Transthoracic echocardiogram: attempted but impossible to perform. Pulmonary function studies: mild restrictive abnormality. Gated blood pool scan: left ventricular ejection fraction of 40%.

Question: What is the probable cause of the patient's left ventricular dysfunction?

Diagnosis: Left ventricular dysfunction due to obesity.

Discussion: Morbid obesity profoundly affects the cardiovascular system. Cardiac output is abnormally high in the setting of obesity, even after normalizing it for body surface area. Increased output is provided by increased end-diastolic volume that enlarges both from the development of eccentric hypertrophy as well as from use of the Frank-Starling mechanism. Afterload as estimated by systolic wall stress is also usually increased in obesity and may lead to the development of concentric hypertrophy. Systolic stress is almost always increased when hypertension coexists with obesity but systolic stress also may be increased in normotensive obese patients.

Obesity is also a risk factor for the development of hypertension, diabetes, and lipid abnormalities. These in turn may lead to the development of coronary disease. Additionally, obesity was recently recognized by the American Heart Association as an **independent risk factor** for heart disease.

Management of cardiovascular function in the particularly obese patient is often difficult, as it was in the present patient. Blood pressure must be taken with a cuff of appropriate dimensions to fit the arm so that pseudohypertension is not recorded. The rest of the cardiac examination may be entirely obscured because of the inability to see the neck veins or hear cardiac sounds through the chest wall. Roentgenography and echocardiography are often rendered difficult if not impossible, although transesophageal echocardiography may be a good alternative imaging technique.

In the present patient the history of gradually worsening dyspnea, a chest radiograph suggestive of venous congestion, a reduced ejection fraction, and relatively normal pulmonary function studies suggested cardiac dysfunction as a cause for the patient's symptoms. Many such patients also have chest pain, which raises the issue of coronary artery disease. Pursuing this diagnosis is complicated by the difficulties presented by obesity in performing an exercise test. Additionally, some extremely obese patients exceed the safety limits for cardiac catheterization equipment. In such cases, a dobutamine thallium stress test or a dobutamine transesophageal echo stress test can be employed to detect regional perfusion or wall motion abnormalities suggestive of ischemia.

Initial management for patients with congestive heart failure and obesity includes diuretics and control of hypertension if present. The key to therapy, however, is weight reduction. Left ventricular function may improve markedly with complete resolution of congestive heart failure after only modest weight reduction.

The present patient's congestive heart failure was complicated by bacterial pneumonia. She died of respiratory failure after prolonged hospitalization.

Clinical Pearls

1. Obesity itself can cause severe cardiac overload and left ventricular dysfunction.
2. Overload in obesity is both a volume overload and a "pressure" overload, even in normotensive subjects.
3. Even moderate weight loss is often enough to significantly improve cardiac function and relieve the symptoms of congestive heart failure.

REFERENCES

1. Messerli FH, Sundgaard-Riise K, Reisin ED, et al: Dimorphic cardiac adaptation to obesity and arterial hypertension. Ann Intern Med 1983;99:757–761.
2. Nakajimi T, Fujioka S, Tokunaga K, et al: Noninvasive study of left ventricular performance in obese patients: Influence of duration of obesity. Circulation 1985;71:481–486.
3. Alpert MA, Terry BE, Kelly DL: Effect of weight loss on cardiac chamber size, wall thickness and left ventricular function in morbid obesity. Am J Cardiol 1985;55:783–786.
4. Carabello BA, Gittens L: Cardiac mechanics and function in obese normotensive persons with normal coronary arteries. Am J Cardiol 1987;59:469–473.

PATIENT 105

A 44-year-old man with a heart murmur and hypertension

A 44-year-old man is referred for treatment of hypertension. He complains of easy fatigability and mild dyspnea on exertion, but denies other cardiac symptoms.

Physical Examination: Vital signs: pulse 90; blood pressure 170/100. Cardiac: PMI forceful in the fifth interspace 2 cm to the left of the mid-clavicular line; II/VI short systolic ejection murmur to the left of the sternum. Extremities: femoral pulses present, but diminished in strength.

Laboratory Findings: Chest radiograph: see below.

Question: What is the likely cause of the patient's hypertension and easy fatigability?

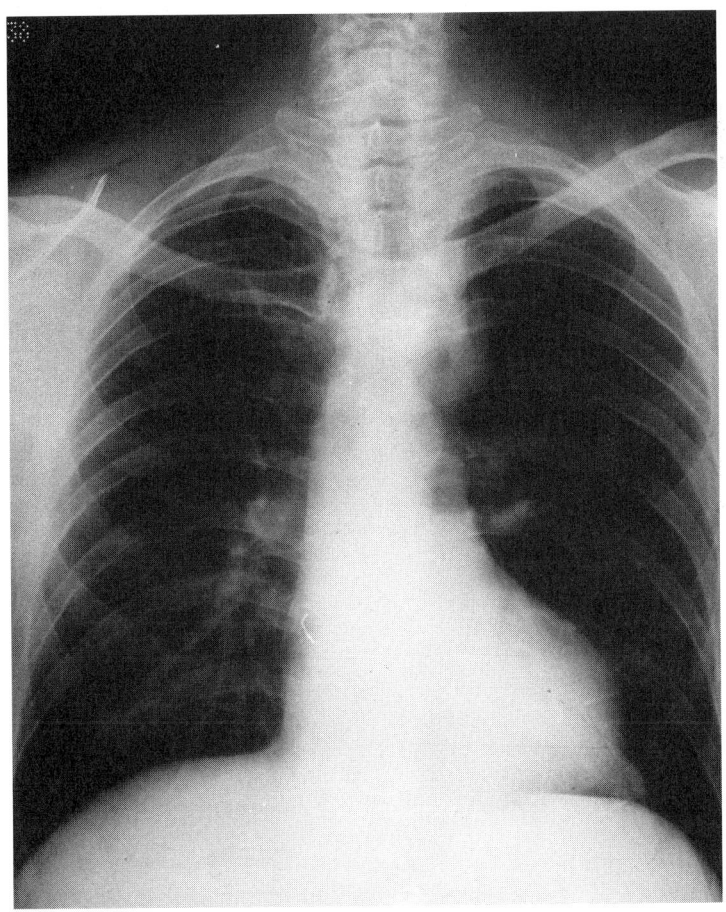

Diagnosis: Coarctation of the aorta.

Discussion: Although most aortic coarctations are detected and corrected in childhood, some are recognized for the first time in adulthood during evaluation of hypertension. Collateral circulation around the coarctation is usually adequate to provide lower-extremity perfusion; thus, claudication is unusual. Occasionally the extremities develop disproportionately, with normal upper extremities and atrophic lower extremities.

On physical examination, a systolic ejection murmur from the coarctation is heard along the left sternal border, and may also be heard over the back. Continuous murmurs from high flow in collateral vessels may be heard posteriorly. Coarctation of the aorta is often associated with a congenitally bicuspid aortic valve that may be suspected when an ejection click is heard. These findings, together with brachial hypertension and reduced or absent lower-extremity pulses, usually lead to the diagnosis.

The chest radiograph is often pathognomonic. It demonstrates notching of the ribs produced by the large collateral vessels and the indentation of the aorta made by the coarctation. This indentation, along with dilatation on either side of it, produces a **figure "3" sign**. Doppler interrogation of the coarctation demonstrates increased flow velocity, which can be used to quantify the gradient across the stenosis. If all findings are consistent with a coarctation distal to the left subclavian artery (a coarctation's usual site), and there is no concern that coronary artery disease is present, cardiac catheterization is usually unnecessary. However, if the site of the coarctation is uncertain or if there is evidence of valvular aortic stenosis or insufficiency, catheterization should be performed to angiographically define the coarctation and to measure gradients at both sites.

The major sequelae of coarctation in adults include **aortic dissection** and **left ventricular failure due to long-standing hypertension.** The etiology of the hypertension is not entirely certain. Despite the coarctation, there is usually adequate renal blood flow from collaterals, which maintains normal renal function. Yet, in some patients, the reninangiotensin system is activated; in others it is not. Following surgery, hypertension may persist despite successful correction. Because the likelihood of postoperative hypertension increases directly with age at surgery, early correction (approximately at age 5) is advocated. In adults, postoperative hypertension may be severe and lead to mesenteric arteritis. Fortunately, this complication has become rare because today the hypertension can usually be controlled pharmacologically. Hypertension may be only transient or may recur later even after normotension has been established. Thus, lifelong surveillance of blood pressure is mandatory. Balloon dilatation for coarctation in adults causes substantial improvement, but with a modest risk of aneurysm formation at the site of dilatation. Thus, it remains debatable whether balloon dilatation or surgery is the preferred therapy. While repair of the coarctation may reduce the incidence of endocarditis, long-term prophylaxis for bacteremic procedures is advisable. Apart from the coarctation itself, aortic stenosis of the frequently associated bicuspid aortic valve and rupture of associated berry aneurysms produce additional morbidity or mortality.

The present patient underwent successful repair of his coarctation. He is currently normotensive on antihypertensive medication.

Clinical Pearls

1. Coarctation of the aorta must be included in the differential diagnosis of any patient with hypertension.
2. The finding of decreased or absent bilateral femoral pulses should lead to further work-up for coarctation.
3. Bicuspid aortic valve, a condition likely to lead to aortic stenosis or aortic regurgitation, commonly coexists with coarctation.
4. Hypertension may recur after a successful coarctation repair has initially produced normotension; thus, careful surveillance is advised.

REFERENCES

1. Simon AB, Zloto AE: Coarctation of the aorta: Longitudinal assessment of operated patients. Circulation 1974;50:456–464.
2. Daniels SR, James FW, Loggie JMH, et al: Correlates of resting and maximal exercise systolic blood pressure after repair of coarctation of the aorta: A multivariable analysis. Am Heart J 1987;113:349–353.
3. Cohen M, Fuster V, Steele PM, et al: Coarctation of the aorta: Long-term follow-up and prediction of outcome after surgical correction. Circulation 1987;80:840–845.
4. Brickner ME, Hillis LD, Lange RA: Congenital heart disease in adults. New Engl J Med 2000;342:256–263.

PATIENT 106

A 55-year-old man with an abnormal thallium scan 2 years after heart transplantation

A 55-year-old man with idiopathic cardiomyopathy presented with intractable heart failure. He underwent orthotopic cardiac transplantation without difficulty and did well postoperatively. Two years after surgery, the patient has developed fatigue and dyspnea on exertion. A routine follow-up stress thallium test reveals reversible posterior wall ischemia.

Physical Examination: Vital signs: pulse 72; blood pressure 132/86. Chest: clear. Cardiac: no murmurs or gallops.

Laboratory Findings: Coronary angiogram: see below.

Question: What is the basis of the patient's thallium scan and angiographic abnormalities?

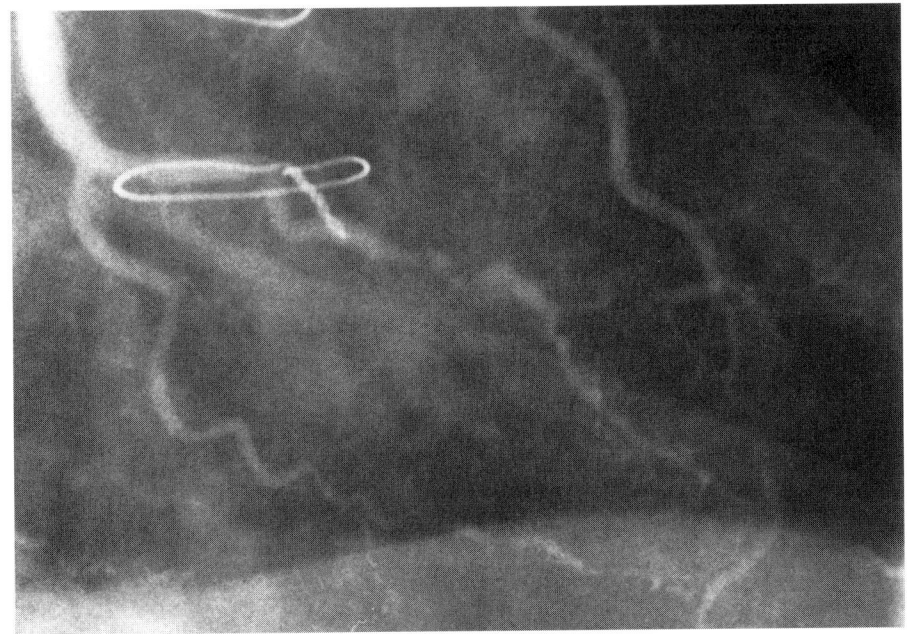

Diagnosis: Coronary artery disease following cardiac transplantation.

Discussion: New-onset coronary artery disease is a frequent complication of cardiac transplantation, occurring as early as 12 months after surgery. In a recent study, vasculopathy was present in 25%, 35%, and 61% of patients, 1, 2, and 5 years after transplantation. The arteriosclerosis of the transplanted heart differs from native disease in being more diffuse, more distally located, and more cellular with less lipid accumulation. The classic risk factors associated with native atherosclerosis such as smoking, hyperlipidemia, and hypertension have not correlated well with the appearance of arteriosclerosis following transplantation. Donor age is also not a significant factor. A history of **early cardiac rejection, two or more episodes of rejection,** and **cytomegalovirus (CMV) infection** increase the risk of developing graft coronary disease. However, it has been difficult to detect CMV in transplanted hearts at autopsy.

Coronary disease following transplantation is believed to be an immunologic reaction against the foreign coronary endothelium of the transplanted heart. While many patients have typical atherosclerotic coronary artery disease as the cause of heart failure prior to transplantation, the occurrence of coronary disease following transplantation is not specifically related to the pretransplantation disease.

The diagnosis of transplant coronary disease may be problematic. Cardiac denervation, which occurs at the time of transplantation, makes it unlikely that the patient will report angina even when significant cardiac ischemia develops. Occasionally, reinnervation occurs and allows patients to experience chest discomfort, but the angina is frequently different in quality from that reported preoperatively.

Currently, a reasonable surveillance strategy consists of yearly stress thallium scintigraphy because of the unreliability of chest symptoms in monitoring for new coronary disease. A new thallium defect suggests the development of arteriosclerosis and determines the need for coronary arteriography. The prevention and treatment of coronary disease in the transplanted heart are controversial. Prophylactically, coronary arteriography is performed on the donor heart prior to transplantation to ensure the absence of antecedent coronary disease. Although it makes sense to alter risk factors known to cause classic atherosclerosis, there is no evidence that risk factor intervention is useful in post-transplant coronary disease prevention. Because symptoms cannot adequately gauge therapy, medical management is difficult to regulate. Currently, the most rational approach is to perform coronary angioplasty on significant lesions that have produced a thallium defect. These lesions appear to respond to angioplasty as well as those of native coronary artery disease.

The present patient's coronary angiograms showed diffuse irregularities and significant restenoses of the circumflex obtuse marginal artery and distal anterior descending artery. He underwent successful angioplasty of his left circumflex obtuse marginal artery.

Clinical Pearls

1. New-onset coronary arteriosclerosis is one of the most common complications that limits the success of cardiac transplantation for the management of heart failure.

2. The coronary artery lesions are presumably immunologic in origin and do not correspond to the typical coronary risk factors.

3. Following transplantation and cardiac denervation, the inability to sense angina limits the value of monitoring symptoms in the detection of post-transplant coronary disease.

REFERENCES

1. Grattan MT, Moreno-Cabral CE, Starnes VA, et al: Cytomegalovirus infection is associated with cardiac allograrft rejection and atherosclerosis. J Am Med Assoc 1989;261:3561–3566.
2. Johnson DE, Alderman EL, Schroeder JS, et al: Transplant coronary artery disease: Histopathologic correlations with angiographic morphology. J Am Coll Cardio 1991;17:449–457.
3. Julius BK, Attenhofer Jost CH, Sutsch G, et al: Incidence, progression, and functional significance of cardiac allograft vasculopathy after heart transplantation. Transplantation 2000;68(5):847–853.
4. Sambiase NV, Higuchi ML, Nuovo G, et al: CMV and transplant-related coronary atherosclerosis: An immunohistochemical, in situ hybridization, and polymerase ch reaction in situ study. Mod Pathol 2000;13(2):173–179.

PATIENT 107

A 30-year-old intravenous drug user with fever and acute pulmonary edema

A 30-year-old intravenous drug user is admitted to the hospital with a 1-week history of fever, chills, weakness, and mild dyspnea. His past medical history is otherwise unremarkable. Two consecutive sets of blood cultures are positive for *Staphylococcus epidermidis,* methicillin-sensitive, and diphtheroids.

An echocardiogram reveals aortic valve vegetations and moderate to severe aortic insufficiency with normal chamber dimensions, normal mitral valve closure, and an ejection fraction greater than 60%. He is placed on intravenous vancomycin and gentamicin and monitored in the ICU. Twenty-four hours later the patient is acutely short of breath.

Physical Examination: Vital signs: pulse 120; respirations 30; blood pressure 100/60. General: diaphoretic, in obvious distress. Chest: rales at both bases up to mid-lung fields. Cardiac: II/VI systolic murmur and a II/VI diastolic murmur along the right sternal border.

Laboratory Findings: Repeat echocardiogram: see below.

Question: What therapy is indicated for this echocardiographic finding?

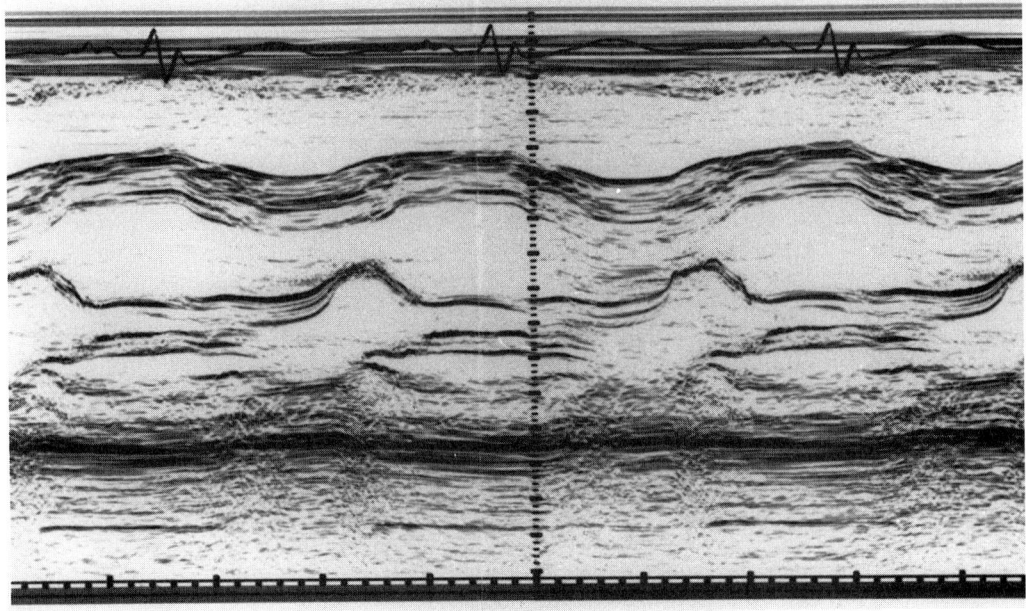

Diagnosis: Severe acute aortic insufficiency.

Discussion: The echocardiogram shows **early mitral valve closure**, which virtually always indicates severe acute aortic insufficiency and a need for surgical management. Normally the mitral valve is closed at the beginning of systole by the difference in pressure between the contracting left ventricle and the left atrium. In severe aortic insufficiency, the mitral valve closes before systole begins because the regurgitant flow and diastolic flow across the aortic valve generate enough pressure inside the ventricle to close the mitral valve without requiring muscular contraction. While this feature is protective because the closed mitral valve isolates the lungs from this severe increase in diastolic pressure, it also limits forward flow across the mitral valve (since the valve closes before the end of diastole) and, therefore, limits cardiac output.

In the present patient, it is likely that further deterioration of the aortic valve caused by the infection led to a sudden worsening in aortic insufficiency and the new finding of mitral valve preclosure. Other causes of severe acute aortic insufficiency include **aortic dissection, leaflet rupture,** and **ruptured sinus of Valsalva**. The only evidence that acute aortic insufficiency is present may be congestive heart failure, a diastolic murmur, and echocardiographic findings. The traditional findings of chronic aortic insufficiency, such as widened pulse pressure, Corrigan's pulse, and de Musset's sign, are not seen in acute aortic insufficiency because these signs are predicated upon a large increase in left ventricular stroke volume that does not occur until the ventricle has time to dilate due to eccentric cardiac hypertrophy. In acute aortic insufficiency, end-diastolic volume does not increase greatly and, therefore, does not produce the increase in stroke volume. Thus, in patients with acute aortic insufficiency, *careful examination for subtle evidence of congestive heart failure is mandatory*. Repeat echocardiography is useful to confirm progression of the lesion. Cardiac catheterization is not usually necessary prior to surgery if the diagnosis is obvious and the patient has no risk for coronary artery disease to warrant coronary arteriography.

In the present patient, although vasodilator therapy with an agent such as nitroprusside might be of some temporizing benefit, immediate surgery is the only tenable definitive therapy. Even though the institution of antibiotics in the present case had been relatively recent, the chance of infecting a new prosthetic valve is relatively low (approximately 10%). It may be even lower if an aortic homograft is inserted. Even with mild heart failure in conjunction with mitral valve preclosure, the mortality for acute aortic insufficiency is approximately 75% with medical treatment in comparison to 25% for patients treated surgically. The high medical mortality may accrue from the high diastolic ventricular pressure and the low diastolic aortic pressure that together limit coronary blood flow, possibly leading to ventricle dysfunction secondary to ischemia.

The present patient underwent aortic valve replacement. Unfortunately, his drug abuse persisted, leading to reinfection of his prosthesis.

Clinical Pearls

1. Mitral valve preclosure is an ominous sign in acute aortic insufficiency, indicating high left ventricular filling pressure and imminent heart failure.

2. Once heart failure develops in acute aortic insufficiency, valve replacement is almost always required.

3. Valve replacement can usually be performed without infection of the prosthesis, even when antibiotic therapy has been initiated only recently.

REFERENCES

1. Mann T, McLaurin L, Grossman W, et al: Assessing the hemodynamic severity of acute aortic regurgitation due to infective endocarditis. N Engl J Med 1975;293:108–113.
2. Sareli P, Klein HO, Schamroth CL, et al: Contribution of echocardiography and immediate surgery to the management of severe aortic regurgitation from active infective endocarditis. Am J Cardiol 1986;57:413–418.
3. Jaffe WM, Morgan DE, Pearlman AS, et al: Infective endocarditis, 1983–1988: Echocardiographic findings and factors influencing morbidity and mortality. J Am Coll Cardiol 1990;15:1227–1233.
4. Petrou M, Wong K, Albertucci M, Brecker SJ, Yacoub MH: Evaluation of unstented aortic homografts for the treatment of prosthetic aortic valve endocarditis. Circulation 1994;90:II-198–II-204.
5. Yu VL, Fang GD, Keys TF, et al: Prosthetic valve endocarditis: Superiority of surgical valve replacement versus medical therapy only. Ann Thorac Surg 1994;58:1073–1077.

PATIENT 108

A 62-year-old man with a systolic ejection murmur and progressive dyspnea

A 62-year-old man presents with a 6-month history of progressive dyspnea. Ten months previously he had been told that he had a heart murmur. The patient also notes two-pillow orthopnea and one episode of paroxysmal nocturnal dyspnea. There is no history of syncope or angina.

Physical Examination: Vital signs: pulse 72 and regular; blood pressure 100/60. Neck: estimated central venous pressure 8 cm H_2O; carotid upstrokes mildly delayed. Chest: bibasilar rales. Cardiac: II/VI systolic ejection murmur radiating to the carotids; PMI left anterior axillary line in the sixth interspace. Extremities: 1+ edema.

Laboratory Findings: Echocardiogram: technically difficult study to perform and interpret. Cardiac catheterization results: see below.

	Baseline	Nitroprusside (0.5 µg/kg/min)
Cardiac output (L/min)	3.0	4.5
Left ventricular pressure (mmHg)	130/30	120/20
Aortic pressure (mmHg)	90/60	90/50
Aortic valve area (cm^2)	0.6	1.0
Valve resistance (dynes sec cm^{-5})	200	160

Questions: What is the explanation for the change in aortic valve area? Should this patient undergo aortic valve replacement?

Diagnosis: Aortic pseudostenosis.

Discussion: Patients with relatively mild aortic stenosis may initially appear to have severe disease at cardiac catheterization when valve area is calculated to be ≤ 0.7 cm^2 in the face of a low cardiac output. However, when cardiac output is increased by **infusion of a pressor agent** such as dobutamine **or a vasodilator** such as nitroprusside, the gradient may fail to increase or may even fall. These changes result in a large increase in calculated valve area. Increased calculated valve area could result from the increase in cardiac output, which physically opens the valve to a greater orifice area, or the increase could be due to flow dependence when the Gorlin formula is used to calculate the aortic valve orifice. Usually, when aortic stenosis is severe, increased flow does not increase the calculated area so much that it falls outside the critical range (>0.8 cm^2). Further, aortic valve resistance, another measure of stenosis severity, exceeds 250 dynes-sec-cm^{-5} in cases of severe disease.

Using the Gorlin formula, the mechanism by which the calculated valve area is flow-dependent is not clear. In the Gorlins' initial report, the investigators had no data regarding the aortic valve and thus did not try to calculate the empirical constant for the aortic valve. This constant was calculated only for the mitral valve where flow dependence is much less marked. Flow dependence is not generally a problem in the mid-range of flows (cardiac output 4.0–5.5 L/min) or when the gradient is greater than 50 mmHg. It does become a problem, however, in the low-output, low-gradient situation.

The use of any vasodilator in patients with true aortic stenosis may be hazardous and result in severe hypotension. If vasodilators are to be used diagnostically, a vasodilator with a very short half-life such as nitroprusside is the safest choice. The benefit of using the vasodilator in this fashion is that if the patient benefits from vasodilator therapy in the catheterization laboratory, he or she may benefit from chronic vasodilator therapy as an outpatient. An alternative to use of a vasodilator to increase forward output is the use of an inotropic agent such as dobutamine. While inotropic agents should be avoided in patients with coronary artery disease, they do not entail the potential hypotensive risk of vasodilators.

In the present patient, the initial calculated aortic valve area indicated "critical" severity, a degree of stenosis capable of causing death. Thus, the initial data (lefthand panel of the table) would suggest that the patient's severe aortic stenosis had led to left ventricular dysfunction, low cardiac output, and congestive heart failure. Because aortic valve replacement in such patients usually results in marked improvement in left ventricular function and improvement in symptoms, this initial data would have favored aortic valve replacement. However, the infusion of nitroprusside increased forward output, paradoxically lowered the aortic valve gradient, and caused the new calculated valve area to be greatly increased. The patient was begun on an ACE inhibitor, with improvement in his heart failure.

Clinical Pearls

1. A severely stenotic aortic valve orifice area can be calculated in patients with only mild aortic stenosis when the cardiac output and gradient are both low.

2. Maneuvers to increase cardiac output allow recalculation of the orifice area at a higher cardiac output. While increasing forward output almost always increases calculated area, the increase in truly severe aortic stenosis is usually small. In milder disease, however, the calculated area can increase dramatically, indicating that the stenosis is mild and that surgery will not be beneficial.

3. Valve resistance may be a useful adjunct to the Gorlin formula in assessing stenosis severity.

REFERENCES

1. Carabello BA: Do all patients with aortic stenosis and left ventricular dysfunction benefit from aortic valve replacement? (editorial). Cathet Cardiovasc Diagn 1989;17:131–132.
2. Carabello BA, Grossman W: Calculation of stenotic valve orifice area. In Grossman W (ed): Cardiac Catheterization and Angiography, 4th ed. Philadelphia, Lea and Febiger, 1990, pp. 152–165.
3. Cannon JD Jr, Zile MR, Crawford FA Jr, Carabello BA: Aortic valve resistance as an adjunct to the Gorlin formula in assessing the severity of aortic stenosis in symptomatic patients. J Am Coll Cardiol 1992;20:1517–1523.
4. deFilippi CR, Willett DL, Brickner ME, et al: Usefulness of dobutamine echocardiography in distinguishing severe from nonsevere valvular aortic stenosis in patients with depressed left ventricular function and low transvalvular gradients. Am J Cardiol 1995;75(2):191–194.

PATIENT 109

A 38-year-old man with a chronic murmur and rapidly progressive congestive heart failure

A 38-year-old man presents with dyspnea on exertion. At the age of 15, a soft diastolic murmur was noted, after which he was lost to follow-up. Recently, he developed progressive shortness of breath over a 3-month period and noted three-pillow orthopnea. On the day of admission, he is markedly dyspneic and in atrial fibrillation, with a ventricular response of 140. Digoxin, furosemide, and quinidine sulfate are administered, and he reverts to sinus rhythm.

Physical Examination: Vital signs: pulse 80 and regular; respirations 30; blood pressure left arm 136/38, right arm 130/30; left and right thighs equal at 160/45. General: tall, slender, and with head and upper torso bobbing with his heart beat. Eyes: grossly normal. Mouth: high-arched palate. Chest: bibasilar rales. Cardiac: carotid pulsations brisk and full with rapid descent; diffuse PMI sixth intercostal space anterior axillary line; I/VI systolic ejection murmur at the upper left sternal border; III/VI diastolic blowing murmur lower left sternal border.

Laboratory Findings: Echocardiogram: see below.

Questions: What valve lesion caused the patient's symptoms? What caused the lesion?

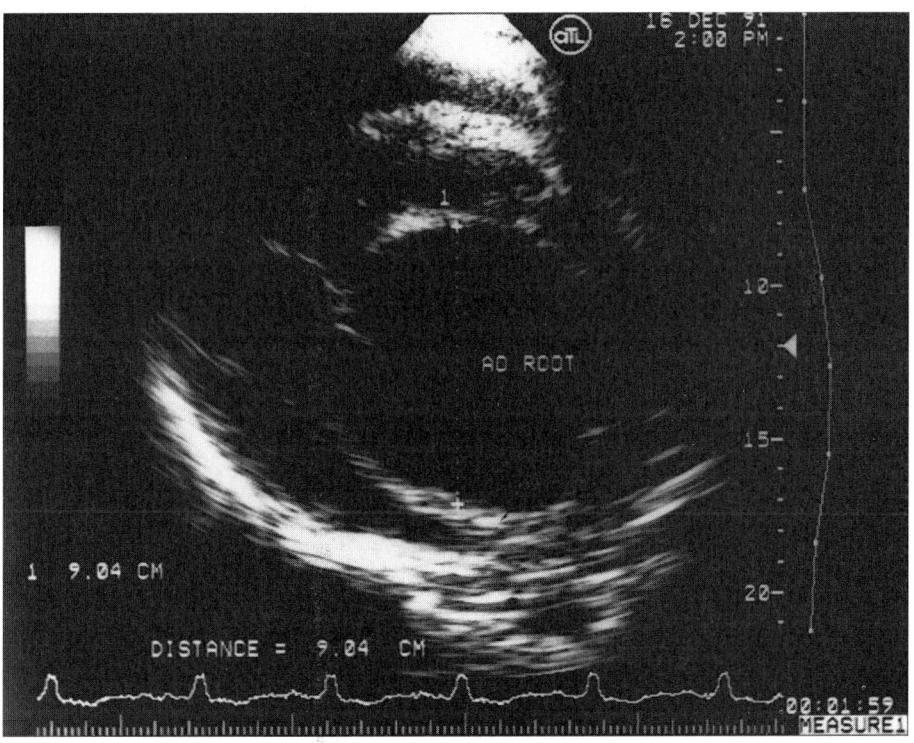

Diagnosis: Marfan syndrome.

Discussion: Marfan syndrome is a connective tissue disease that is usually inherited as an autosomal dominant trait; however, spontaneous mutation can cause the disease, in which case a positive family history is absent. The latter results from inherited mutations in the genes coding for fibrillin-1, a major component of the elastic fibers in connective tissue. Features include arachnodactyly, increased joint mobility, a tall stature with the pubis-to-heel dimension exceeding the crown-to-pubis dimension, dislocation of the lenses of the eye (ectopia lentis), a high-arched palate, pectus carinatum, and a history of inguinal hernias or inguinal herniorrhaphy. The most important clinical manifestations of the disease, however, involve the heart and aorta.

The major cardiovascular complications of Marfan syndrome are initiated by **accelerated aortic cystic medial necrosis,** which leads to dilatation of the proximal aorta. As in the present patient, the aortic pathology usually produces aortic insufficiency, causing morbidity and even mortality from left ventricular volume and pressure overload. Aortic root involvement also can lead to catastrophic proximal aortic dissection, which is the usual cause of death. Without therapy, the average age of death is 45 years. As the diameter of the aorta approaches 6 cm, the risk of dissection increases dramatically. Mitral valve prolapse is also common.

The diagnosis is suggested when physical examination demonstrates the aforementioned skeletal or ophthalmologic abnormalities. The physical finding of aortic insufficiency in a young patient without other obvious cause for that lesion or the finding of mitral valve prolapse in a patient with the typical body habitus should also raise the suspicion of the diagnosis. On the other hand, a tall and lanky appearance without other concomitant findings should not be cause for concern. For instance, echocardiographic surveys of basketball players rarely have detected the disease.

Echocardiography confirms the diagnosis when aortic root dilatation is found in a young person without hypertension. Typically, dilatation of the aortic root begins at the sinuses of Valsalva, whereas in patients with annuloaortic ectasia, dilatation occurs above the sinuses, producing a pear-shaped aorta. No specific confirmatory laboratory test for Marfan syndrome exists.

The major focus of management is to prevent catastrophic aortic dissection and to correct aortic regurgitation before it produces extreme cardiac dilatation and left ventricular dysfunction, as occurred in the present patient. Early institution of beta-adrenergic blockade, which reduces shearing forces in the aorta, has been demonstrated to be effective in slowing the progression of the aortic root disease. **Echocardiographic surveillance** of the left ventricle, aortic valve, and aortic root is essential. As the aortic root diameter approaches 5.5 cm in size, prophylactic proximal aortic root replacement should be strongly considered. Antibiotic prophylaxis against endocarditis is employed in patients with murmurs of mitral or aortic insufficiency.

The present patient's echocardiogram showed a severely dilated aortic root. He refused surgery and subsequently died of aortic root dissection.

Clinical Pearls

1. Unrecognized and untreated Marfan syndrome leads to death from aortic dissection at an early age.

2. While a tall, lanky appearance is not a cause for concern, the presence of any of the other skeletal, ophthalmologic, or cardiac abnormalities should prompt performance of an echocardiogram.

4. Once the syndrome is identified, echocardiographic surveillance of aortic root diameter and of aortic insufficiency is indicated.

REFERENCES

1. Gott VL, Pyeritz RE, Magovern GJ Jr, et al: Surgical treatment of aneurysms of the ascending aorta in the Marfan syndrome: Results of composite-graft repair in 50 patients. N Engl J Med 1986;314:1070–1074.
2. Pyeritz RE: Heritable disorders of connective tissue. In Pierpont ME, Miller JH (eds): The Genetics of Cardiovascular Disease. Boston, Martinus Nijhoff Publishing, 1987, p. 265.
3. Shores J, Berger KR, Murphy EA, Pyeritz RE: Chronic β-adrenergic blockade protects the aorta in the Marfan syndrome: A prospective, randomized trial of propranolol. N Engl J Med 1994;330:1335–1341. (The first randomized trial concluding that medication can reduce the risk of dissection and delay aortic dilatation.)
4. Dietz HC, Pyeritz RE: Mutations in the human gene for fibrillin-1 (*FBN1*) in the Marfan syndrome and related disorders. Hum Mol Genet; 1995;4:1799–1809.

PATIENT 110

A 49-year-old man with congestive heart failure and weight loss

A 49-year-old man with long-standing, poorly controlled hypertension presents with a 3-day history of paroxysmal nocturnal dyspnea, two-pillow orthopnea, and dyspnea on exertion. The patient was well until 2 months prior to admission when he noted a gradual 20-pound weight loss, occasional episodes of diarrhea, and diaphoresis. He presently takes no medications and previously had complied poorly with his beta-blocker antihypertensive regimen. There is no history of angina or myocardial infarction.

Physical Examination: Vital signs: pulse 120; blood pressure 180/100; temperature 99.6°. Neck: estimated central venous pressure 10 cm H_2O; brisk carotid upstrokes. Thyroid: slight enlargement. Chest: bibasilar rales. Cardiac: summation gallop; II/VI systolic murmur over the pulmonic area. Abdomen: 13-cm liver span. Extremities: 1+ peripheral edema.

Laboratory Findings: EKG: sinus tachycardia, nonspecific ST- and T-wave abnormalities. Echocardiogram: mildly dilated left ventricle; normal ejection fraction; 12-mm left ventricular wall thickness. Right heart catheterization: see below.

	Measured Values
Right atrium	
O_2 saturation	66%
Pressure	8 mmHg
Right ventricle	
O_2 saturation	65%
Pressure	40/8 mmHg
Pulmonary wedge	
O_2 saturation	96%
Pressure	19 mmHg
Cardiac index	4.5 L/min/m^2
Arterial-venous O_2 difference	50 ml/L

Question: What is the explanation for the high cardiac output occurring with an increased arterial-venous O_2 difference?

Diagnosis: High output failure secondary to thyrotoxicosis.

Discussion: The presence of increased left- and right-sided filling pressures, a high cardiac index, and a slightly widened arteriovenous oxygen difference indicates the presence of high output cardiac failure. In this condition, an inadequate oxygen supply despite a high cardiac output forces tissues to increase oxygen extraction. The increased right and left ventricular filling pressures probably indicate use of the **Frank-Starling mechanism** to help maintain a high cardiac output. Because systolic ejection performance was normal (normal ejection fraction), an alternative diagnosis to high output failure is primary diastolic dysfunction. While the thickened left ventricular wall secondary to the long-standing hypertension in this case is probably playing a role in increasing left ventricular filling pressure, the high cardiac index is not typical of pure diastolic dysfunction, in which cardiac output is usually reduced.

Anemia, thyrotoxicosis, beriberi heart disease, and **arteriovenous fistulas or malformations** are the most common causes of high output failure. The presence of weight loss, diaphoresis, and diarrhea, combined with a mildly enlarged thyroid gland and tachycardia, strongly suggests thyrotoxicosis as the cause of high output failure. Thyrotoxicosis usually does not precipitate congestive heart failure unless another heart disease, such as long-standing hypertension, is present.

A pathophysiologic feature common to all forms of high output failure is arterial vasodilatation. Arteriolar dilatation precipitated by the metabolic demands of a high output state facilitates left ventricular emptying and thus increases forward output. Increased venous return maximizes use of the Frank-Starling mechanism, further increasing forward output.

On physical examination, tachycardia, wide pulse pressure consistent with increased stroke volume, full carotid upstrokes, and flow murmurs are common.

In thyrotoxic high output failure, increased thyroid hormone itself increases myocardial inotropy and cardiac output. However, the tachycardia, tremor, and diaphoresis also suggest increased activation of the sympathetic nervous system (or increased sensitivity to catecholamines) as a second mechanism by which thyrotoxicosis increases cardiac output. Enhanced sympathetic nervous system activity is further suggested by the success with which beta blockade temporarily treats the condition. Beta-blockade in patients with thyrotoxicosis and high output failure may be beneficial by slowing heart rate or may worsen the failure by reducing inotropic state. If beta blockade is to be employed in such patients, a short-acting drug such as esmolol should be used initially so that it can be easily reversed if heart failure worsens.

The present patient had elevated thyroid function tests, which confirmed the presence of thyrotoxicosis. He improved with the initiation of propylthiouracil.

Clinical Pearls

1. Arterial vasodilation is the common pathway of all high output states.
2. High output failure usually occurs when a high output condition coexists with another form of heart disease.
3. In thyrotoxic heart failure, beta blockade may be a double-edged sword and should be initiated with short-acting agents.

REFERENCES

1. Skelton CL: The heart and hyperthyroidism. N Engl J Med 1982;307:1206–1208.
2. Feldman T, Borrow KM, Sarne DH, et al: Myocardial mechanics in hyperthyroidism: Importance of left ventricular loading conditions, heart rate and contractile state. J Am Coll Cardiol 1986;7:967–974.
3. Abreo G, Lenihan DJ, Nguyen P, Runge MS: High-output heart failure resulting from a remote traumatic aorto-caval fistula echocardiography. Clin Cardiol 2000;23(4):304–306.

PATIENT 111

A 54-year-old man with arthralgias and dyspnea

A 54-year-old man is referred to a cardiologist for evaluation of dyspnea. He has noted gradually worsening exercise tolerance over the previous 6 months and two-pillow orthopnea over the previous 4 weeks. He also complains of nocturia, decreased libido, and low back pain.

Physical Examination: Vital signs: pulse 110 and regular; blood pressure 90/60. Skin: appears well tanned. Chest: bibasilar rales. Cardiac: S_4; no murmurs. Joints: mild swelling and tenderness bilaterally over the metacarpophalangeal joints.

Laboratory Findings: Hematocrit: 35%. Blood sugar: 265 mg/dl. EKG: normal sinus rhythm; low voltage. Chest radiograph: slightly enlarged heart with interstitial pulmonary edema.

Question: What study would you order next?

Answer: Serum ferritin, in pursuit of the diagnosis of hemochromatosis.

Discussion: Hemochromatosis is a disorder in regulation of iron storage that results in abnormal deposition of iron in virtually every organ system. Inherited through an abnormality on the HLA locus, hemochromatosis is a genetic disease that usually affects only homozygotes.

Clinically, patients typically present with **bronze discoloration** and **diabetes** due to iron deposition in the skin and pancreas. This combination of findings gives hemochromatosis its nickname "bronze diabetes." Some of the earliest manifestations of the disease, however, occur when deposition of iron occurs in the gonads and in the joints, producing **loss of libido, arthralgias,** and **arthritis.** Abnormal iron stores deposited in the liver may lead to hepatic failure.

Cardiac dysfunction may be a major manifestation of hemochromatosis. Deposition of iron in the heart produces thickening of the cardiac walls and subsequent diastolic dysfunction. Eventually systolic dysfunction develops and contributes to congestive heart failure, which is a common cause of death in patients with hemochromatosis. The EKG and echocardiogram together may suggest the diagnosis by demonstrating the features of an infiltrative restrictive cardiomyopathy. The typical EKG shows low voltage and the echocardiogram reveals a relatively small heart with thick walls.

Once the diagnosis is considered, hemochromatosis may be substantiated by serum iron studies. Transferrin saturation is often in excess of 75%. Ferritin levels usually exceed 750 μg/L and may be as high as 10,000 μg/L. If the diagnostic data are not entirely consistent but suspicion of the diagnosis remains, a liver biopsy will be confirmatory.

The mainstay of treatment of patients with congestive heart failure due to hemochromatosis is diuretic therapy with furosemide. As for other forms of restrictive cardiomyopathy, vasodilators should be avoided because they often cause hypotension. Some clinical improvement in cardiac function has been reported in patients treated with phlebotomy or iron chelation with deferoxamine to decrease the tissue iron overload.

The present patient's serum iron was 250 μg/dl, iron-binding capacity was 300 μg/dl, and serum transferrin level was 2150 μg/L. He was begun on diuretics and managed with repeated phlebotomy, with some improvement in his congestive heart failure symptoms.

Clinical Pearls

1. Although rare, hemochromatosis should not be overlooked because it is one of the few cardiomyopathies that is reversible. Phlebotomy and iron chelation therapy are the mainstays of therapy.

2. Bronze skin pigmentation and diabetes may be relatively late manifestations of hemochromatosis. Arthralgias and loss of libido may precede these classic findings by several years.

3. The disease is a genetic disorder due to an abnormality in the HLA locus.

REFERENCES
1. Milder MS, Cook JD, Stray S, et al: Idiopathic hemochromatosis: An interim report. Medicine 1980;59:34–49.
2. Edwards CQ, Dadone MM, Skolnick MH, et al: Hereditary haemochromatosis. Clin Haematol 1982;11:411–435.
3. Niederau C, Fischer R, Sonnenberg A, et al: Survival and causes of death in cirrhotic and in noncirrhotic patients with primary hemochromatosis. N Engl J Med 1985;313:1256–1262.
4. Alizad A, Seward JB: Echocardiographic features of genetic diseases: Part 2. Storage disease. J Am Soc Echocardiogr 2000;13(2):164–170.

PATIENT 112

A 49-year-old man with congestive heart failure and acute left hemiparesis

A 49-year-old physician is admitted for management of an acute onset of left hemiparesis. The patient has a 2-year history of exertional dyspnea, orthopnea, and episodes of paroxysmal dyspnea. He denies chest pain, diabetes, and hypertension. He smokes two packs of cigarettes per day and consumes 4-8 oz of alcohol daily—and has for many years.

Physical Examination: Vital signs: pulse 87; blood pressure 120/70. Neck: no jugular venous distention. Cardiac: S_3 gallop. Chest: bibasilar rales.

Laboratory Findings: CBC, urinalysis, and blood chemistry: normal. EKG: regular sinus rhythm; intraventricular conduction delay; nonspecific T-wave inversion; and left atrial enlargement. Chest radiograph: cardiomegaly with pulmonary venous congestion.

Question: What is a likely working diagnosis?

Diagnosis: Congestive (dilated) alcoholic cardiomyopathy with mural thrombus and cerebral embolism.

Discussion: Dilated cardiomyopathies encompass a large group of diseases in which ventricular systolic function is severely compromised in the absence of hypertension, coronary artery disease, or valvular disease. The absence of these factors identifies the presence of primary myocardial dysfunction and excludes the possibility that damage has resulted from myocardial infarction or external hemodynamic overload.

In the majority of patients, an etiology of the dilated cardiomyopathy despite extensive evaluation is never found. Although a vital etiology is often suspected, it is rarely proved. Alcoholic cardiomyopathy represents the most commonly **reversible form** of dilated cardiomyopathy. Patients may partially or entirely reverse the observed degree of myocardial dysfunction following the cessation of alcohol consumption. Other potentially reversible dilated cardiomyopathies include thiamine deficiency (beriberi), hypophosphatemia, myopathy due to persistent tachycardia, and hemochromatosis. Some cardiomyopathies demonstrate remarkable spontaneous improvement in the absence of the above causes.

The mechanism by which alcohol damages the heart is unclear. Acute alcohol consumption universally depresses left ventricular contractility in all patients. This myocardial depression, however, rapidly improves with metabolic elimination of circulating alcohol. In chronic alcoholism, depressed contractile function persists after alcohol leaves the system. It has been considered that alcohol affects cardiac performance by causing abnormalities in calcium handling, in the mitochondria and in contractile proteins.

Standard medical therapy for dilated cardiomyopathy consists of **removal of any potential myocardial toxin** and **treatment with digoxin, a diuretic, and an ACE inhibitor.** This combination of drugs has been shown to definitely reduce mortality from the disease. Anticoagulation is advisable in all patients with cardiomyopathy who do not have a specific contraindication. The attractiveness of anticoagulation has been enhanced by knowledge that relatively low levels of anticoagulation (INR 1.7–2.0) are effective. Overall, the risk of stroke in patients with dilated cardiomyopathy and sinus rhythm is 2–3% per year. This risk increases as the ejection fraction falls. The need for anticoagulation increases when a clot is obvious in one of the cardiac chambers, as in the present patient, or when atrial fibrillation coexists.

Approximately 50% of patients with cardiomyopathy die suddenly, implicating malignant ventricular arrhythmias as a cause of death. To date, however, there is no convincing evidence that prophylactic therapy with antiarrhythmic drugs substantially reduces overall mortality. However, in patients who manifest sustained ventricular tachycardia or who have survived an episode of sudden death, aggressive antiarrhythmic therapy guided by electrophysiologic testing is indicated.

The present patient's echocardiogram revealed marked global hypokinesis with an ejection fraction of approximately 20%. A large mobile thrombus was noted in the left ventricle and a smaller laminar clot at the apex. A brain CT scan showed evidence of infarction involving the right posterior parietal region. The patient became abstinent from alcohol. He was anticoagulated and begun on digoxin, furosemide, and captopril. Left ventricular ejection fraction by MUGA increased to 66% 8 months later.

Clinical Pearls

1. Cardiomyopathy due to ethanol is the most common reversible cardiomyopathy.
2. Anticoagulation constitutes an important part of the therapeutic regimen in patients with atrial fibrillation.
3. Although 50% of patients with dilated cardiomyopathy die suddenly, nonselective use of prophylactic antiarrhythmic drugs has not yet been proved to be effective.

REFERENCES

1. Regan TJ: Alcoholic cardiomyopathy. Prog Cardiovasc Dis 1984;27:141–152.
2. Urbano-Marquez A, Estruch R, Navarro-Lopez F, et al: The effects of alcoholism on skeletal and cardiac muscle. N Engl J Med 1989;320:409–415.
3. Cohn JN, Johnson G, Ziesche S, et al: A comparison of enalapril with hydralazine-isosorbide dinitrate in the treatment of chronic congestive heart failure. N Engl J Med 1991;325:303–310.
4. The SOLVD Investigators: Effect of enalapril on survival in patients with reduced left ventricular ejection fractions and congestive heart failure. N Engl J Med 1991;325:293–302.
5. Dries DL, Rosenberg YD, Waclawiw MA, Domanski MJ: Ejection fraction and risk of thromboembolic events in patients with systolic dysfunction and sinus rhythm: Evidence for general differences in the studies of left ventricular dysfunction trails. J Am Coll Cardiol 1997;29:1074–1080.
6. Loh E, St John Sutton M, Wun CCC, et al: Ventricular dysfunction and the risk of stroke after myocardial infarction. N Engl J Med 1997;336:251–257.

PATIENT 113

A 28-year-old woman with chest pain and a positive stress test

A 28-year-old woman complains of episodes of chest pain that occur unpredictably both during activity and rest. The pain is left-sided substernal pressure that lasts anywhere from 5 minutes to several hours without associated radiation, diaphoresis, nausea, or vomiting. It has no predictable method of relief. The patient has experienced normal menses since age 13, denies diabetes, and has never had her serum cholesterol measured. There is no family history of coronary artery disease.

Physical Examination: Vital signs: pulse 72 and regular; blood pressure 110/72. Skin: no cutaneous manifestations of hyperlipidemia. Chest: clear. Cardiac: normal.

Laboratory Findings: Resting EKG: normal. Exercise stress test: exercised into stage IV of the Bruce protocol; achieved blood pressure 180/80; peak heart rate 165; no symptoms; exercise stopped because of fatigue. Peak exercise EKG: see below.

Questions: How should the exercise stress test be interpreted in light of the clinical presentation? What would be the next step in management?

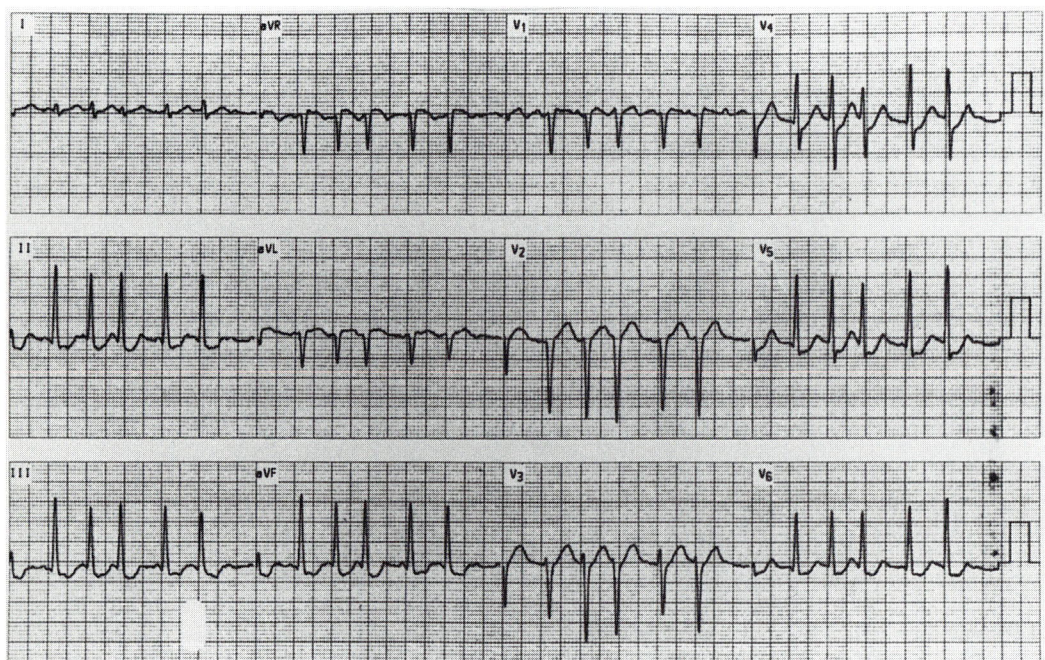

Diagnosis: False-positive stress test.

Discussion: Because coronary artery disease is still the leading cause of death in the United States, major concern always exists for the patient who presents with the acute onset of chest pain. The effort to exclude cardiac ischemia in these patients is complicated by the lack of a simple, reproducible, and accurate test to evaluate the coronary circulation. Coronary arteriography is the most reliable way of diagnosing coronary disease, but it is invasive and too costly to be applied to every patient with chest pain. At the other end of the spectrum, resting electrocardiography is safe and inexpensive, but provides little diagnostic benefit because it is normal or nondiagnostic in most patients with coronary disease.

Stress testing, which increases cardiac oxygen demand, should provoke ischemia in patients with coronary disease. Detection of this ischemia is usually inferred from changes in the EKG during or following exercise, by abnormalities in thallium perfusion scanning, or by new wall motion abnormalities detected by radionuclide ventriculography or echocardiography. Accurate interpretation of stress testing results, however, requires an understanding of **Bayes theorem** and **pretest probabilities.**

Bayes theorem states that the accuracy of a test is predicted in part upon the pretest probability that patients have the disease for which they are being tested. In women, sensitivity and specificity of the electrocardiographic response to exercise for detecting ischemia are approximately 0.7 and 0.7 respectively. The sensitivity (SEN) of a test is defined as the true positives in the population (TP) detected by the test divided by the true positives plus the false negatives (FN):

$$\text{SEN} = \frac{\text{TP}}{\text{TP} + \text{FN}}$$

Specificity (SPEC) is defined as the true negatives (TN) detected by the test divided by the true negatives plus the false positives (FP):

$$\text{SPEC} = \frac{\text{TN}}{\text{TN} + \text{FP}}$$

Accuracy (ACC) of a positive test is defined as:

$$\text{ACC} = \frac{\text{TP}}{\text{TP} + \text{FP}}$$

The patient described here has atypical chest pain and no risk factors for coronary disease. If, for example, the prevalence of coronary disease in such a population of 28-year-old women were 10%, then in a thousand such patients, 900 would be free of coronary disease and 100 would have coronary disease. The sensitivity (0.7) would equal the true positives (70) divided by the true positives (70) plus the false negatives (30):

$$0.7 = \frac{70}{70 + 30}$$

Specificity would equal the true negatives (630) divided by the true negatives (630) plus the false positives (270):

$$0.7 = \frac{630}{630 + 270}$$

The accuracy of a positive test would equal the true positives (70) divided by the true positives (70) plus the false positives (270):

$$\frac{70}{70 + 270} = 0.22$$

The accuracy of a positive test in this situation is only 22%. Thus, we have increased the probability that the patient has coronary disease from only 10% to 22% and, even though she has a positive test, it is still unlikely that she has coronary disease. The accuracy of a negative test is:

$$\frac{\text{TN}}{\text{TN} + \text{FN}} = \frac{630}{630 + 30} = 0.96$$

Thus, if the test is negative, we have lowered the probability of coronary artery disease from only 10% to 4%. In either case, the cost and benefit to the patient could clearly be questioned as ineffective.

Both **stress thallium scintigraphy** and **stress echocardiography,** which have sensitivities and specificities of 0.9 and 0.9, would provide increased accuracy in testing the present patient. Although her EKG during exercise demonstrated ST-segment depression "diagnostic of ischemia," subsequent cardiac catheterization demonstrated normal coronary arteries.

Clinical Pearls

1. EKG exercise testing is not useful in screening large populations of people for whom the probability of coronary disease is low.

2. Because the EKG response to exercise is often an inaccurate predictor of disease in women, thallium scintigraphy or stress echocardiography, both of which have a sensitivity of 0.9 and a specificity of 0.9, should be employed routinely.

REFERENCES

1. Detrano R, Leatherman J, Salcedo EE, et al: Bayesian analysis versus discriminant function analysis: Their relative utility in the diagnosis of coronary disease. Circulation 1986;73:970–977.
2. Schlant RC, Blomqvist CG, Brandenburg RO, et al: Guidelines for exercise testing. A report of the Joint American College of Cardiology/American Heart Association Task Force on Assessment of Cardiovascular Procedures (Subcommittee on Exercise Testing). Circulation 1986;74(Suppl III):653A–667A.
3. Patterson RE, Horowitz SF. Importance of epidemiology and biostatistics in deciding clinical strategies for using diagnostic tests: A simplified approach using examples from coronary artery disease. J Am Coll Cardiol 1989;13:1653–1655.
4. Ritchie JL, Bateman TM, Bonow RD, et al.: Guidelines for clinical use of cardiac radionuclide imaging. Report of the American College of Cardiology/American Heart Association Task Force on Assessment of Diagnostic and Therapeutic Cardiovascular Procedures (Committee on Radionuclide Imaging) developed in association with the American Society of Nuclear Cardiology. J Am Coll Cardiol 1995;25:521–547.

PATIENT 114

A 46-year-old woman with fever and a pericardial effusion

A 46-year-old woman reports increasing fatigue, night sweats, fever, poor appetite, exertional dyspnea, and orthopnea of several-month duration. She gives a history of heart murmur during a pregnancy 26 years previously. Five years previously she was diagnosed as having stage 1B cervical cancer and had a radical hysterectomy and radiation therapy (three positive pelvic nodes were noted at the time of surgery).

Physical Examination: Vital signs: temperature 100°; pulse 80; blood pressure 140/60. General: chronically ill. Cardiac: grade II/VI murmur of aortic insufficiency. Chest: bibasailar rales. Abdomen: no hepatomegaly. Extremities: ecchymotic areas on fingers and toes, but no clubbing.

Laboratory Findings: Hct 38.5%. WBC 11,500/μl. Liver function studies: normal. EKG: generalized ST elevation. Echocardiogram: moderate-sized pericardial effusion and thickening of the pericardium with heaped-up regions; moderate aortic insufficiency with normal left ventricular systolic function and dimensions; no valvular vegetations.

Question: What diagnosis should you consider?

Diagnosis: Metastatic disease secondary to cervical carcinoma, and aortic insufficiency.

Discussion: The pericardium is involved in approximately 10% of cancer patients. Lung cancer and breast cancer account for much of the secondary pericardial involvement because these tumors are common and lie in close proximity to the pericardium. Lymphoma, gastric carcinoma, cervical carcinoma, and ovarian carcinoma also frequently involve the pericardium. Rarely, primary mesotheliomas may arise from the pericardium in patients with asbestos exposure.

It is natural to assume that patients with known malignancy who develop a pericardial effusion have metastatic pericardial involvement. Interestingly, this frequently is not so, and other etiologies (infection, etc.) are responsible in about one-third to one-half of cases. Thus, a work-up to establish the cause of the pericardial effusion is usually warranted. Fractures that suggest metastatic involvement are (1) areas of focal pericardial thickening seen on echocardiogram, as in the present patient, and (2) new conduction disturbances on EKG, suggesting local myocardial involvement.

Pericardiocentesis is usually indicated to make the diagnosis of metastatic pericardial involvement. Typically, the effusion is bloody and is almost always an exudate. Besides standard chemistries and cultures, pericardial fluid should be examined cytologically and for various tumor markers such as carcinoembryonic antigen.

Survival following the diagnosis of malignant pericardial effusion is approximately 25% at 1 year. In general, the presence of a malignant effusion worsens the prognosis associated with most tumors. The one malignancy in which survival routinely exceeds 1 year despite a malignant effusion is breast cancer. Acute episodes of tamponade are treated with needle aspiration or surgical drainage. Radiation therapy may help to palliate the tumor locally to prevent recurrence of the effusion.

In the present patient, a transesophageal echocardiogram revealed a large pericardial effusion and heaped up-masses, suggesting metastatic disease to the visceral pericardium. Severe aortic insufficiency was noted without evidence of vegetations. Apparently this patient had prior aortic insufficiency that was not a factor in her present illness. A pericardial window was performed. The pericardial fluid (yellow serous) was negative for culture and cytology. Right open lung biopsy revealed undifferentiated squamous cell carcinoma with extensive vascular involvement metastatic from the previous cervical lesions.

Clinical Pearls

1. Patients with known malignancy and pericardial effusion frequently have a nonmalignant cause of the effusion; thus, a diagnostic work-up is almost always indicated.

2. Pulmonary and breast cancers are those that most frequently metastasize to the pericardium.

3. Breast cancer is one of few malignancies in which survival is expected to exceed 1 year in the face of a malignant effusion.

REFERENCES
1. Posner JB, Furneaux HM: Paraneoplastic syndrome. Res Publ Assoc Res Nerv Ment Dis 1990;68:187–219.
2. Malviya VK, Casselberry JM, Parekh N, et al: Pericardial metastases in squamous cell cancer of the cervix: A report of two cases. J Reprod Med 1990;35:49–52.

PATIENT 115

A 65-year-old man with electrocardiographic changes following abdominal surgery

A 65-year-old man with a history of hypertension and tobacco use is evaluated for the acute onset of diaphoresis and tachycardia 3 days after surgery for a 5.5-cm abdominal aortic aneurysm. His heart rate has increased from his postoperative baseline of 70 bpm to 100 bpm. Six months earlier, a Bruce protocol stress thallium test had been stopped after 3 minutes because of fatigue. His heart rate went from 50 to 85 and blood pressure from 120/70 to 170/90 during exercise. His EKG showed nonspecific ST-T wave changes at rest. A stress thallium imaging study was normal.

Physical Examination: Vital signs: pulse 100; respiration 20; blood pressure 140/90. General: diaphoresis without other complaints. Chest: clear. Cardiac: normal.

Laboratory Findings: EKG: see below.

Questions: What does the EKG show? Could this complication have been predicted and avoided?

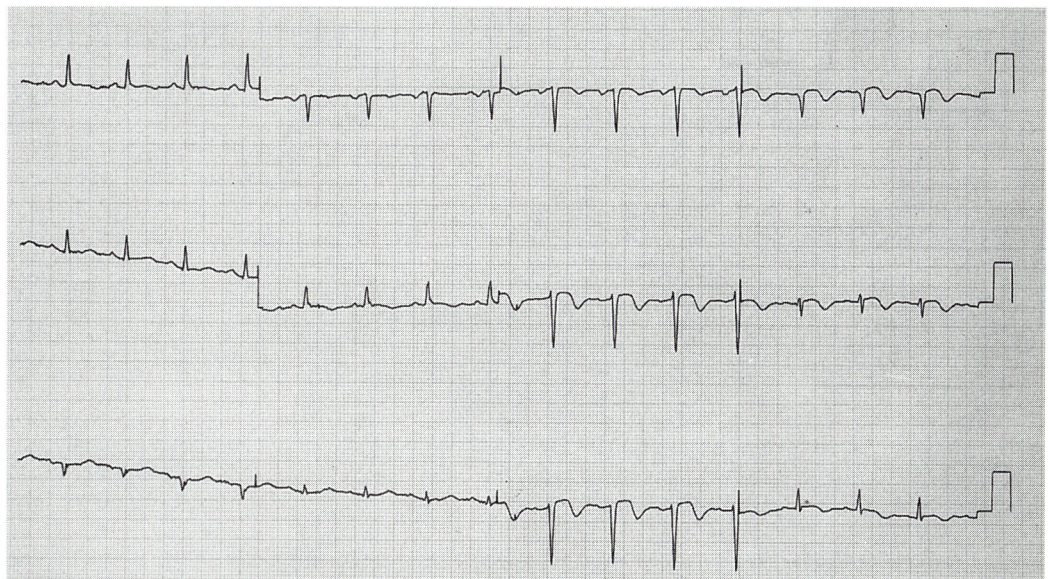

Diagnosis: Myocardial infarction following noncardiac surgery.

Discussion: The risk of a serious cardiac complication (death, myocardial infarction, or pulmonary edema) following noncardiac surgery is approximately 5%. An obvious goal of preoperative management in elective or semi-elective surgery is to identify patients who are likely to suffer a cardiac complication and to prevent such complications when possible. In the general population, several risk factors can help to identify such patients. **Major risk factors** include myocardial infarction within 1 month, unstable angina, decompensated heart failure, and symptomatic ventricular arrhythmias. The presence of any of these factors should postpone all but emergency surgery until the risk factor is ameliorated.

A special case is the patient undergoing noncardiac surgery involving **peripheral revascularization.** Patients with peripheral vascular disease have an increased incidence of coronary disease, and 40% of such patients have multi-vessel coronary disease. Patients with one or more of the following are at especially high risk: age ≥70 yrs, angina, Q wave on the EKG, arrythmia, diabetes, and compensated heart failure. Thallium scintigraphy may identify patients with peripheral vascular disease who are at increased risk for their revascularization. Patients with thallium redistribution following exercise or following the injection of dipyridamole have approximately a 35% risk of a cardiac complication. In such patients, cardiac catheterization before the noncardiac procedure may demonstrate remedial coronary disease. Although currently no data prove that coronary intervention will enhance the outcome of the noncardiac procedure, coronary revascularization seems prudent in patients with left main or severe three-vessel disease.

When patients at high risk have been identified, vigilance is required throughout the vulnerable postoperative period. Most cardiac complications of noncardiac surgery occur not in the operating room but rather on the **second or third postoperative day,** as in the present patient. Frequently, myocardial infarction does not cause chest pain in the immediate postoperative period. Patients identified with positive risk factors or because of a positive thallium test should be kept under close scrutiny during this high-risk period. Recent studies indicate that preoperative administration of beta blockers significantly reduces postoperative risk, probably by decreasing postoperative tachycardia and ischemia.

In the present patient, the thallium study was performed 6 months before surgery, and a low heart rate was achieved. Thus, the study should not have been particularly reassuring. On the other hand, he had none of the other risk factors for a cardiac complication. The outcome in this case was probably not predictable or preventable. He recovered from his surgery and inferior myocardial infarction.

Clinical Pearls

1. Patients with peripheral vascular disease are at especially high risk for a cardiac complication of noncardiac surgery.

2. Although elective surgery should be postponed after a recent myocardial infarction (MI), the risk for noncardiac surgery is considered to be present for 1 month following MI.

3. The most likely time for a patient to suffer a cardiac complication from noncardiac surgery is on the second or third postoperative day.

4. Frequently, ischemic events occurring postoperatively do *not* cause chest pain and are detected only by changes in clinical condition, changes in the EKG, or new segmental wall motion abnormalities on the echocardiogram.

REFERENCES

1. Golgman L, Caldera DL, Nussbaum SR, et al: A multifactorial index of cardiac risk in noncardiac surgery. N Engl J Med 1977;297:845–850.
2. Leppo J, Plaja J, Gionet M, et al: Noninvasive evaluation of cardiac risk before elective vascular surgery. J Am Coll Cardiol 1987;9:269–276.
3. Mangano DT, Wong MG, London MJ, et al: Perioperative myocardial ischemia in patients undergoing noncardiac surgery. II. Incidence and severity during the first week after surgery. J Am Coll Cardiol 1991;17:851–857.
4. American College of Cardiology/American Heart Association Task Force on Practice Guidelines (Committee on Perioperative Cardiovascular Evaluation for Noncardiac Surgery): Guidelines for perioperative cardiovascular evaluation for noncardiac surgery. J Am Coll Cardiol 1996;27(4):910–948.
5. Poldermans D, Boersma E, Bax JJ, et al: The effect of bisoprolol on perioperative mortality and myocardial infarction in high-risk patients undergoing vascular surgery. N Engl J Med 1999;341(24):1789–1794.

PATIENT 116

A 62-year-old man with arrhythmias, heart failure, and increasing dyspnea

A 62-year-old man presents with increasing dyspnea over the previous 1 month. Two years earlier, he suffered a large anterior myocardial infarction, followed 6 months later by symptoms of dyspnea on exertion and orthopnea compatible with congestive heart failure. He improved with digoxin, furosemide, and captopril therapy until 8 months before admission, when he suffered two episodes of syncope. After electrophysiologic studies demonstrated inducibility of sustained monomorphic ventricular tachycardia, he was placed on amiodarone at an initial dose of 1600 mg per day, which was gradually decreased to a maintenance dose of 400 mg per day. A radionuclide ventriculogram demonstrates a left ventricular ejection fraction of 32%.

Physical Examination: Vital signs: temperature 100.5°; pulse 100 (regular); respirations 24; blood pressure 100/60. Neck veins: flat. Chest: bilateral diffuse rales. Cardiac: S_4 gallop; no third heart sound; II/VI holosystolic apical murmur.

Laboratory Findings: Hct 39%; WBC 11,000/μl. Chest radiograph: see below.

Question: What is the likely cause of worsening dyspnea in this patient with heart failure?

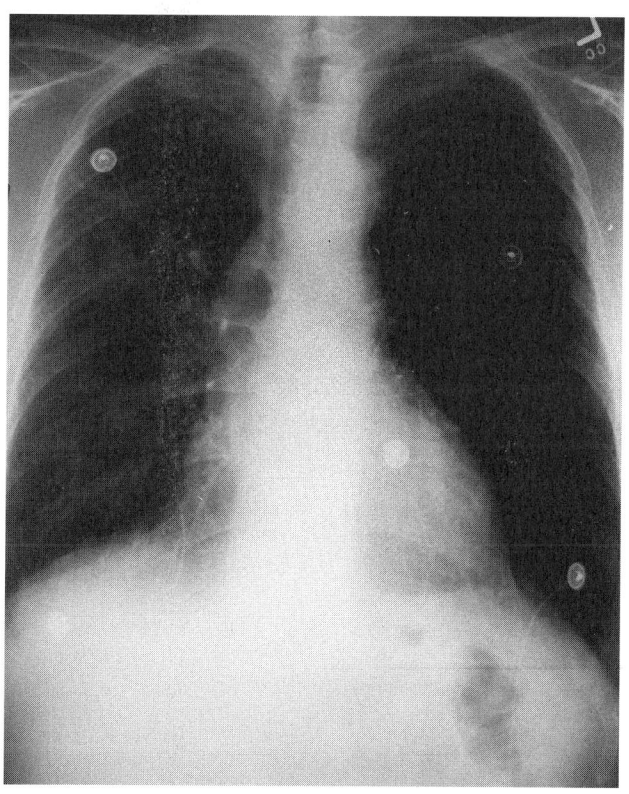

Diagnosis: Amiodarone-induced acute pneumonitis.

Discussion: Amiodarone is currently one of the most effective drugs for the treatment of life-threatening ventricular arrhythmias. Unfortunately, its use is attended by many side effects, affecting almost every organ system in the body. The most serious side effect other than proarrhythmia is the development of **pulmonary toxicity.** Initially the drug causes pneumonitis, which can progress rapidly to pulmonary fibrosis, pulmonary insufficiency, and death. Pulmonary toxicity occurs in 5–10% of patients receiving the drug. Typically, pulmonary complications arise when the dose exceeds 300 mg per day. Because almost all patients with life-threatening arrhythmias also have significant left ventricular dysfunction and heart failure, as in the present patient, worsening dyspnea may often be attributed to the underlying cardiac disease. Dry cough, fever, and absence of other signs suggestive of heart failure are clues that the patient is suffering from amiodarone toxicity rather than worsening congestive failure. A pulmonary gallium scan is often positive, indicating pulmonary inflammation, which further helps in make the diagnosis.

The chest radiograph in amiodarone-induced pulmonary disease typically shows **diffuse patchy infiltrates,** differing from the more diffuse classic pattern of acute pulmonary edema or congestive heart failure. Reports also exist of localized infiltrates that simulate bacterial pneumonia and pulmonary cavitation. Chest CT scans in patients with localized disease may demonstrate increased lung density because of pulmonary concentration of the iodine-containing drug. Pulmonary function studies show restrictions observed in patients with congestive failure. Diffusing capacity is reduced in patients with pulmonary intoxication from amiodarone, as opposed to patients with heart failure, who may have an increased lung diffusion. Bronchoalveolar lavage demonstrates **phospholipidosis** (foamy macrophages) in most patients with pulmonary intoxication. However, patients on amiodarone without pulmonary intoxication may also demonstrate this finding.

The only definitive therapy for amiodarone lung disease is discontinuation of the drug or significant reduction in dosage. Steroids may also be given, but definitive proof of effectiveness is currently lacking. When pulmonary toxicity occurs, the mortality is approximately 10%. Unfortunately, because the drug is almost always initiated because of life-threatening arrhythmias, its discontinuance may impose risks of lethal cardiac events and requires initiation of alternative effective antiarrhythmic therapy.

Other side effects of amiodarone include corneal deposits that usually do not interfere with vision, slate-gray discoloration of the skin, hypo- and hyperthyroidism, hepatocellular necrosis, hypotension, proarrhythmia, and worsening of congestive heart failure. Amiodarone usually increases the serum digoxin level, requiring a reduction in digoxin dosage.

The present patient's pulmonary status improved after discontinuation of amiodarone. An automatic implantable defibrillator was placed to manage his arrhythmias.

Clinical Pearls

1. Pulmonary toxicity is the most serious and life-threatening complication of amiodarone administration. The only effective therapy is to discontinue the drug or decrease its dosage.
2. The potential of amiodarone to cause pulmonary toxicity in patients who almost always have coexisting congestive heart failure complicates the differential diagnosis of dyspnea in amiodarone-treated patients. Pulmonary function studies should always accompany institution of the drug for later comparison to aid in making the diagnosis.
3. Digoxin dosage must routinely be decreased in patients receiving amiodarone.
4. Patients with amiodarone pulmonary toxicity may have bilateral patchy infiltrates or localized segmental or lobar infiltrates with or without cavitation.

REFERENCES

1. Morady F, Suave MJ, Malone P, et al: Long-term efficacy and toxicity of high-dose amiodarone therapy for ventricular tachycardia or ventricular fibrillation. Am J Cardiol 1983;52:975–979.
2. Fogoros RN, Anderson KP, Winkle RA, et al: Amiodarone: Clinical efficacy and toxicity in 96 patients with recurrent, drug-refractory arrhythmias. Circulation 1983;68:88–94.
3. Dusman RE, Stanton MS, Miles WM, et al: Clinical features of amiodarone-induced pulmonary toxicity. Circulation 1990;82:51–59.
4. Jessurun GA, Boersma WG, Crijns HJ: Amiodarone-induced pulmonary toxicity. Predisposing factors, clinical symptoms and treatment. Drug Saf 1998;18(5):339–344.

PATIENT 117

A previously healthy 25-year-old man with pneumonia and shock

A previously healthy 25-year-old man presents to the emergency department with fever, chills, a productive cough for 3 days, and pleuritic chest pain. He denies intravenous drug abuse and recently tested HIV negative when he applied for an insurance policy.
Physical Examination: Vital signs: temperature 101.2°; pulse 120; respirations 32; blood pressure 80/60. Mouth: dry mucous membranes; no pharyngeal lesions. Neck: no adenopathy. Chest: right basilar ronchi with egophony and dullness to percussion. Cardiac: II/VI systolic ejection murmur. Extremities: cold and clammy.
Laboratory Findings: WBC 25,000/μl with 70% polys and 10% bands; toxic granulations. Swan-Ganz catheter data: see below.

Right atrial pressure	8 mmHg
Pulmonary artery pressure	28/10/14 mmHg
Pulmonary wedge pressure	11 mmHg
Cardiac index	3.8/L/min/m²

Question: What is the hemodynamic mechanism of this patient's shock?

Diagnosis: Endotoxic shock.

Discussion: Shock occurs when there is inadequate blood pressure or inadequate cardiac output to maintain tissue perfusion. Blood pressure is equal to the product of cardiac output and total peripheral resistance. In hypovolemic and cardiogenic shock, blood pressure falls because cardiac output is inadequate and only partially compensated by vasoconstriction, which increases total peripheral resistance. In contradistinction, in the early phase of endotoxic shock, hypotension results from abnormally low systemic vascular resistance while cardiac output is actually elevated. These alterations in normal hemodynamics result in **distributive shock,** which is a maldistribution of blood flow to various tissues.

Endotoxin, a lipopolysaccharide (LPS) contained in gram-negative organisms, by itself can produce most of the features of endotoxic shock. In turn, LPS activates other humoral substances, including tissue necrosis factor, the interleukins, the kinins, myocardial depressant substance, histamine, and the coagulation cascade, all of which probably play a role in mediating the hemodynamic pattern seen in this form of shock.

Although initially the hemodynamic pattern is one of vasodilatation with a high cardiac output as seen here, the heart itself in endotoxic shock rapidly develops **myocardial depression.** Myocardial function during this phase of sepsis is characterized by a normal stroke volume, decreased ejection fraction, and increased end-diastolic volume. As endotoxic shock progresses, the clinical picture may look more typical of other types of shock, with depressed cardiac output and increased total peripheral resistance. Although terminally, coronary perfusion pressure may fail to provide adequate myocardial perfusion, at least initially coronary blood flow is increased. Despite adequate myocardial oxygen consumption and supply, significant changes occur in the substrates used for fuel. Free fatty acid consumption falls, while lactate utilization increases. These changes may ultimately be responsible for the fall in myocardial performance that occurs.

Although initially total peripheral resistance is reduced and cardiac output is increased, shunting deprives some tissues of adequate perfusion. **Inadequate perfusion** in turn is compounded by activation of the clotting system, producing microthrombi, which further impair tissue perfusion. Thus, in endotoxic shock, **lactic acidosis** can occur despite globally adequate total oxygen consumption—presumably due to local failure of adequate tissue perfusion.

Therapy for endotoxic shock must focus on eradicating the source of the infection. Because the vasodilation present reduces intravascular volume, volume expansion is appropriate. If these measures are ineffective, vasopressor agents seem indicated, although none has been demonstrated to significantly improve survival. In view of the known myocardial depression that occurs, pressor agents such as dopamine, which promote both an increase in contractile function as well as vasoconstriction, are useful. Dobutamine may be indicated in patients with myocardial depression to improve cardiac output. High-dose corticosteroids have also been advocated in the treatment of this syndrome, but most studies have failed to demonstrate any benefit.

Inhibitors of toxic mediators of sepsis are presently undergoing intensive evaluation, but most trials have been unsuccessful. Lack of benefit probably accrues from the fact that mediators of shock, which in high quality are deleterious, are actually beneficial in smaller amounts. Benefit from cytokines probably stems from augmentation of the immune response. Thus, mediator inhibitors blunt not only toxic effects of the mediator, but also the beneficial effects.

The present patient received high-dose intravenous nafcillin and gentamicin. Urine and blood culture grew enterococcus. The patient rapidly improved over the ensuing 24 hours.

Clinical Pearls

1. Although endotoxic shock is associated initially with high cardiac output and reduced total peripheral resistance, myocardial depression is a prominent feature in the later stages of the syndrome.
2. Currently the only effective measure of therapy is eradication of the bacterial source of infection. Pressor agents and corticosteroids have not altered mortality.
3. Despite high cardiac output, some tissues may actually suffer ischemic damage.

REFERENCES

1. Michie HR, Manogue KR, Spriggs DR, et al: Detection of circulating tumor necrosis factor after endotoxin administration. N Engl J Med 1988;318:1481–1486.
2. Suffredini AF, Fromm RE, Parker MM, et al: The cardiovascular response of normal humans to the administration of endotoxin. N Engl J Med 1989;321:280–287.
3. Parillo JE, Parker MM, Natanson C, et al: Septic shock in humans. Ann Intern Med 1990;113:227–242.
4. Parillo JE: Pathogenetic mechanisms of septic shock. N Engl J Med 1993;328:1471–1477.
5. Fisher CJ Jr, Agosti JM, Opal SM, et al: Treatment of septic shock with the tumor necrosis factor receptor: Fc fusion protein. N Engl J Med 1996;334:1697.

PATIENT 118

A 55-year-old man with a Starr-Edwards aortic valve and progressive dyspnea

A 55-year-old man underwent a Starr-Edwards aortic valve replacement for aortic stenosis 10 years ago. He was well until 6 months prior to admission when he noted progressive dyspnea on exertion and occasional exertional chest pain. There is no history of coronary artery disease. He takes warfarin as directed.

Physical Examination: Vital signs: pulse 90 and regular; blood pressure 160/80. Chest: clear. Cardiac: regular rate and rhythm; PMI fifth intercostal space midclavicular line; mechanical valve sounds noted; II/VI systolic murmur at the second intercostal space left sternal border; III/VI diastolic murmur at the second intercostal space. Extremities: no edema.

Laboratory Findings: EKG: sinus rhythm; left atrial enlargement; left ventricular hypertrophy. PT 14.2 seconds. Doppler interrogation: see below.

Question: Could this complication have been avoided?

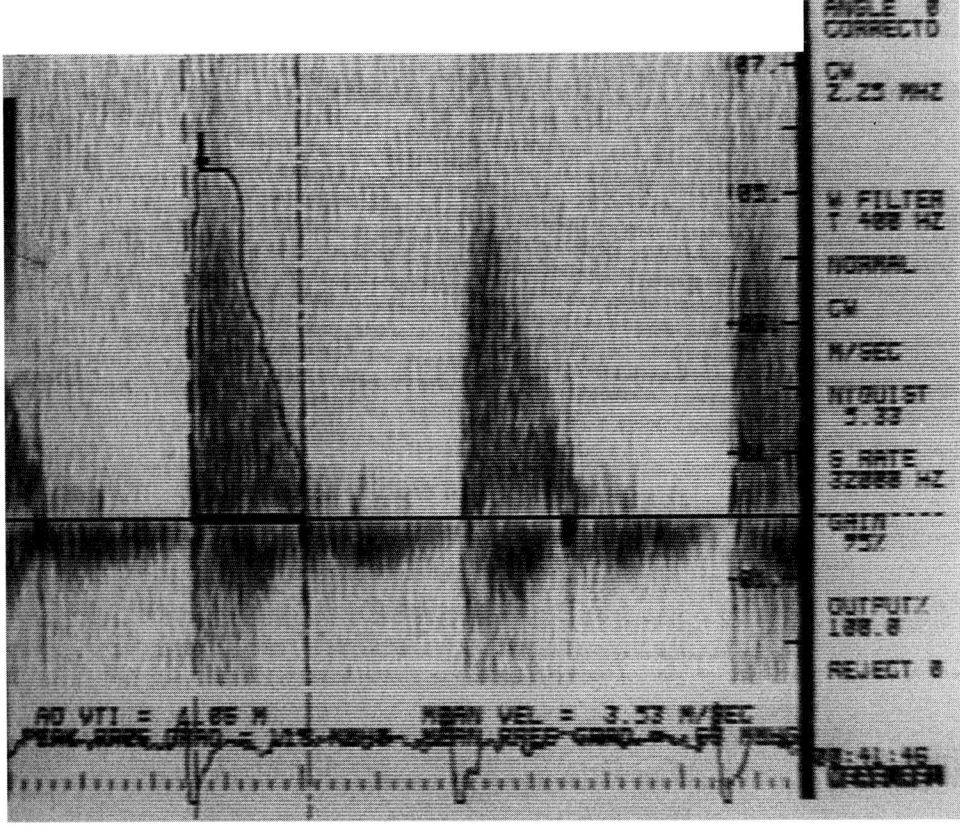

Diagnosis: Prosthetic valvular stenosis. The ingrowth of pannus demonstrated at surgery could not have been prevented.

Discussion: Although a valvular prosthesis improves the hemodynamics in patients with severe native valvular disease, complications inherent to the prosthesis may develop, including thromboembolism, prosthetic endocarditis, primary valve failure, stenosis relative to the normal native valve, and perivalvular leak. Bioprostheses and mechanical valves are the two categories of implants currently used. **Bioprostheses** are further subdivided into heterografts and hemografts. Bioprostheses have the advantage of not requiring anticoagulation to prevent thromboembolism. However, the durability of heterografts is limited, and after 10 years primary valve failure begins to occur as the leaflets degenerate either by becoming calcified or by developing perforations and tears. Human cryopreserved aortic homografts appear to have a longer survival than heterografts, but more experience is needed to fully evaluate homograft durability.

Mechanical prostheses may also primarily fail, and the type of failure tends to be characteristic for the individual prostheses. Caged ball valves may develop pannus ingrowth into the valve orifice, causing restriction of flow and mimicking valvular stenosis, as in the present patient. Pannus also may limit normal valve closure, causing insufficiency. These complications are usually not related to adequacy of anticoagulation therapy. The most common valve failure with Björk-Shiley tilting disk valves is fracture of either or both of the valve struts. Fracture of one strut places more stress on the second strut, making it more likely to fail. To date, the St. Jude valve seems to be most free of primary valvular failure. The most common form of dysfunction with the St. Jude valve is incorporation of thrombus into the pivot points of the valve, reducing leaflet mobility and causing stenosis, regurgitation, or both.

Mechanical prostheses require lifelong anticoagulation to reduce the risk of thrombotic valve dysfunction and thromboembolism. Frequently, complications of mechanical prostheses arise from poor patient compliance in taking anticoagulants.

The diagnosis of prosthetic dysfunction may be problematic. Echocardiographic and Doppler examination of prosthetic valves is difficult because of acoustic shadowing (sound clutter from valve obscures leaflet motion and orific area), particularly in the mitral position. **Transesophageal echocardiography** reduces this problem and affords a much clearer picture of prosthetic mitral valves. Each valve has its typically normal Doppler profile that must be considered in assessing whether the function of that individual valve is normal or abnormal. Doppler profiles from prosthetic valves cannot be compared with those of normal native valves. While cardiac catheterization and angiography may be useful, especially for assessing mitral valve prostheses, retrograde catheterization of aortic prosthetic valves may be hazardous. Such attempts may lead to artifactual inhibition of normal valve motion, catheter entrapment, or damage to the valve itself.

Problems inherent in mechanical valves and older bioprostheses have led to an exciting new era in the field of substitute valves. Human homografts, stentless heterografts, and pulmonary autograts (Ross procedure) are all undergoing intensive clinical trials. As a group, these biologic valves have excellent hemodynamics, avoid the need for anticoagulents, and hopefully will have extended durability.

The present patient's Doppler studies showed a high velocity jet across the prosthetic aortic valve consistent with a gradient in excess of 100 mmHg. He underwent successful reimplantation of a St. Jude medical valve. At surgery, pannus ingrowth was found to be the cause of the prosthetic valvular obstruction. It is unlikely that this complication could have been prevented.

Clinical Pearls

1. Echocardiographic evaluation of a prosthetic valve is most difficult in the mitral position. Transesophageal studies help to obviate the problem.

2. There is no exception to the need for anticoagulation for mechanical prostheses.

3. Heterograft bioprostheses have limited durability; homografts may have better longevity.

REFERENCES

1. Bloomfield P, Kitchin AH, Wheatley DJ, et al: A prospective evaluation of the Bjork-Shiley, Hancock, and Carpentier-Edwards heart valve prostheses. Circulation 1986;73:1213–1222.
2. Angell WW, Angell JD, Oury JH, et al: Long-term follow-up of viable frozen aortic homografts. J Thorac Cardiovasc Surg 1987;93:815–822.
3. Hammermeister KE, Henderson WG, Burchfiel CM, et al: Comparison of outcome after valve replacement with a bioprosthesis versus a mechanical prosthesis: Initial 5-year results of a randomized trial. J Am Coll Cardiol 1987;10:719–732.
4. Rothbart RM, Castriz JL, Harding LV, et al: Determination of aortic valve area by two-dimensional and Doppler echocardiography in patients with normal and stenotic bioprosthetic valves. J Am Coll Cardiol 1990;15:817–824.
5. Carabello BA, Stewart WJ, Crawford FA Jr: Aortic valve disease. In Topol EJ, (ed): Textbook of Cardiovascular Medicine. Lippincott-Raven Publishers, Philadelphia, 1998, pp 533–555.

PATIENT 119

A 28-year-old pregnant patient with heart failure in the second trimester

A 28-year-old patient complains of increasing dyspnea on exertion, orthopnea, and paroxysmal nocturnal dyspnea. She suffered an episode of acute rheumatic fever at age 8 and a second episode at age 10. A school physical examination disclosed a heart murmur. Prior to her pregnancy, the patient noted dyspnea after walking two flights of stairs or carrying groceries from the store to her car, but denied orthopnea or paroxysmal nocturnal dyspnea. There is no history of chest pain. She was in the 25th week of her first pregnancy when the symptoms of increased dyspnea, orthopnea, and paroxysmal nocturnal dyspnea appeared.

Physical Examination: Vital signs: pulse 110 (regular); blood pressure 100/60. Chest: occasional rales at both bases. Cardiac: neck veins not distended; increased intensity of the first heart sound; opening snap followed by the second heart sound by approximately 80 msec; II/VI diastolic rumble heard best at the apex. Extremities: no peripheral edema.

Laboratory Findings: EKG: normal sinus rhythm and right axis deviation. Echocardiogram: see below.

Question: What is the diagnosis?

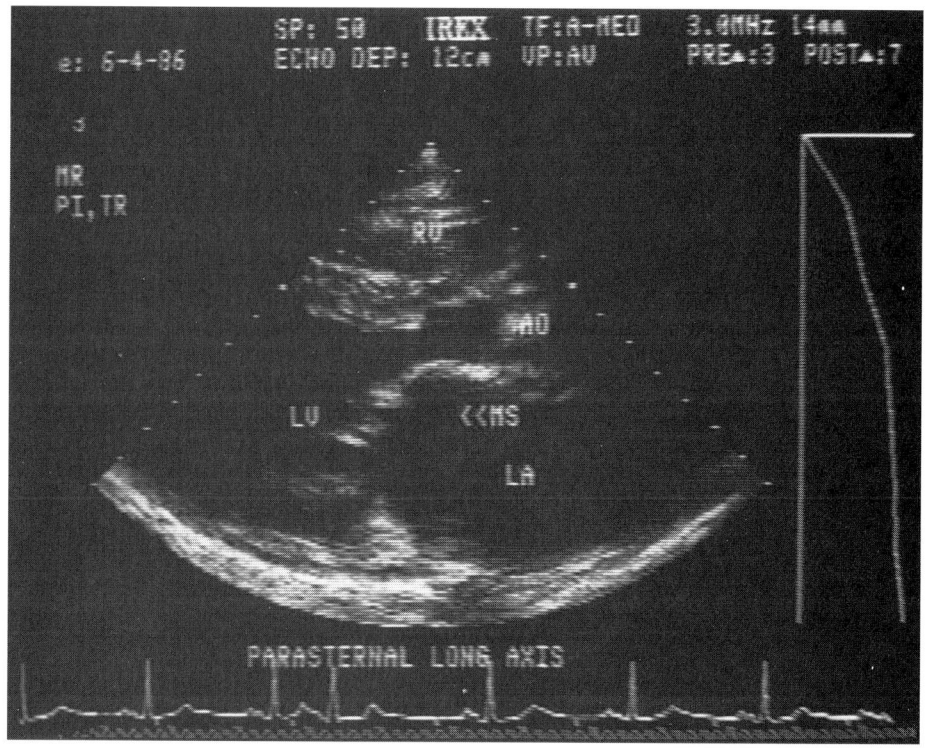

Diagnosis: Mitral stenosis complicated by pregnancy.

Discussion: During normal pregnancy, blood volume and cardiac output increase, peaking toward the end of the second trimester. Increased cardiac output is maintained by increased left ventricular stroke volume and increased heart rate. Left ventricular stroke volume is increased both by an increase in end-diastolic volume due to volume expansion and by a decrease in end-systolic volume caused by reduced total peripheral resistance to left ventricular emptying. The **increased cardiac demands of pregnancy** are likely to complicate any antecedent heart disease.

Mitral stenosis is the most common acquired heart disease to complicate pregnancy. Although congenital heart disease is usually detected and corrected prior to pregnancy, occasionally it is not. Most commonly, an atrial septal defect that was not diagnosed previously is diagnosed under the scrutiny of prepartum care; this defect is tolerated well. Ventricular septal defect, patent ductus arteriosus, congenital heart block, and congenital aortic valve disease may be less well tolerated. Cyanotic congenital heart disease is poorly tolerated during pregnancy.

A good rule of thumb is that the patient's New York Heart Association classification will advance one class during pregnancy. Thus, most patients who are Class I or Class II will have increased symptoms, but usually will not require correction of their cardiac lesion during pregnancy.

Mitral stenosis may be recognized for the first time during pregnancy. The demand for increased flow through the stenotic valve combined with an increase in heart rate, which compromises the diastolic filling period, causes or exacerbates the patient's symptoms as the pregnancy progresses. For a patient who already manifests Class III or Class IV symptoms, pregnancy should be discouraged until the mitral stenosis is corrected. In patients with Class I or Class II symptoms, a safe pregnancy and delivery is usually accomplished with medical therapy. **Diuretics** to reduce left atrial and pulmonary venous filling pressures, and **beta blockers** to reduce heart rate and in turn improve diastolic transfer of blood from the left atrium to the left ventricle, are the mainstays of therapy. Beta blockers may occasionally depress respirations in the newborn at birth and also may cause newborn hypoglycemia and bradycardia. In patients young enough to become pregnant, atrial fibrillation is uncommon but should be controlled with digitalis if needed. Quinidine and procainamide usually are well tolerated without producing fetal side effects. If the patient is unstable or not responding well to drug therapy, electrical cardioversion can be performed safely.

Pregnant patients with mechanical prosthetic heart valves or with other needs for anticoagulation pose a major problem. Warfarin commonly causes fetal malformations and mortality (especially during the first trimester) and should be avoided. Heparin, which does not cross the placental barrier, is safer but more difficult to use, requiring constant intravenous infusion or daily subcutaneous injections.

If heart failure cannot be controlled medically during the pregnancy, surgical intervention may be required. Both open and closed surgical commissurotomy have been performed successfully and safely in the pregnant patient with mitral stenosis. Balloon mitral valvotomy has the obvious benefit of not requiring surgery but involves a radiation risk of unknown consequences to the fetus.

The present patient's symptoms were controlled with furosemide. Her delivery was uncomplicated.

Clinical Pearls

1. Pregnancy patients with heart disease usually advance one New York Heart Association classification grade during pregnancy.

2. Anticoagulation with warfarin during pregnancy entails high risk to the fetus. Strategies that avoid its use such as employment of porcine heterograft valves, which do not require anticoagulation, should be considered in women desiring to become pregnant.

3. Heart failure usually can be controlled with diuretics alone, which can be safely employed during pregnancy.

4. Except for in the presence of maternal cyanotic congenital heart disease, termination of the pregnancy is rarely required.

REFERENCES

1. Cohn LH: Anticoagulation in pregnant women with artificial heart valves. N Engl J Med 1987;316:1662–1663.
2. Robson SC, Hunter S, Boys RJ, et al: Serial study of factors influencing changes in cardiac output during human pregnancy. Am J Physiol 1989;256:H1060–H1065.
3. Elkayam U, Gleicher N: Hemodynamics and cardiac function during normal pregnancy and the puerperium. In Elkayam U, Gleicher N (eds): Cardiac Problems in Pregnancy: Diagnosis and Management of Maternal and Fetal Disease, 2nd ed. New York, Alan R. Liss, Inc., 1990, pp 5–24.
4. Patal JJ, Mitha AS, Hassen F, et al: Percutaneous balloon mitral valvotomy in pregnancy patients with tight pliable mitral stenosis. Am Heart J 1993;125:1106–1109.

PATIENT 120

A 34-year-old man with a 10-year history of a heart murmur

A 34-year-old athlete who was an all-American soccer player presents with paroxysmal nocturnal dyspnea. He denies a history of rheumatic fever. The patient was told of a heart murmur 10 years previously. Recently, he noted four to five episodes of paroxymal nocturnal dyspnea and was unable to continue his usual athletic activity due to fatigue and dyspnea on exertion.

Physical Examination: Vital signs: pulse 100; respirations 20; blood pressure 150/60. General: tall and thin, in mild respiratory distress. Chest: bibasilar rales. Cardiac: diffuse PMI at the sixth intercostal space anterior axillary line; S_3 gallop; III/VI decrescendo diastolic murmur along left sternal border; II/VI mid-diastolic rumble (Austin-Flint murmur). Extremities: arachnodactyly; 2+ edema.

Laboratory Findings: EKG: left atrial enlargement; left ventricular hypertrophy. Echocardiogram: dilated left ventricle (EDD—6.8, ESD—5.6, FS—19%); left ventricular ejection fraction 40% with global hypokinesis; dilated aortic root (3.9 cm). Color flow Doppler study: see below.

Question: What do these echocardiographic indices indicate regarding prognosis and management?

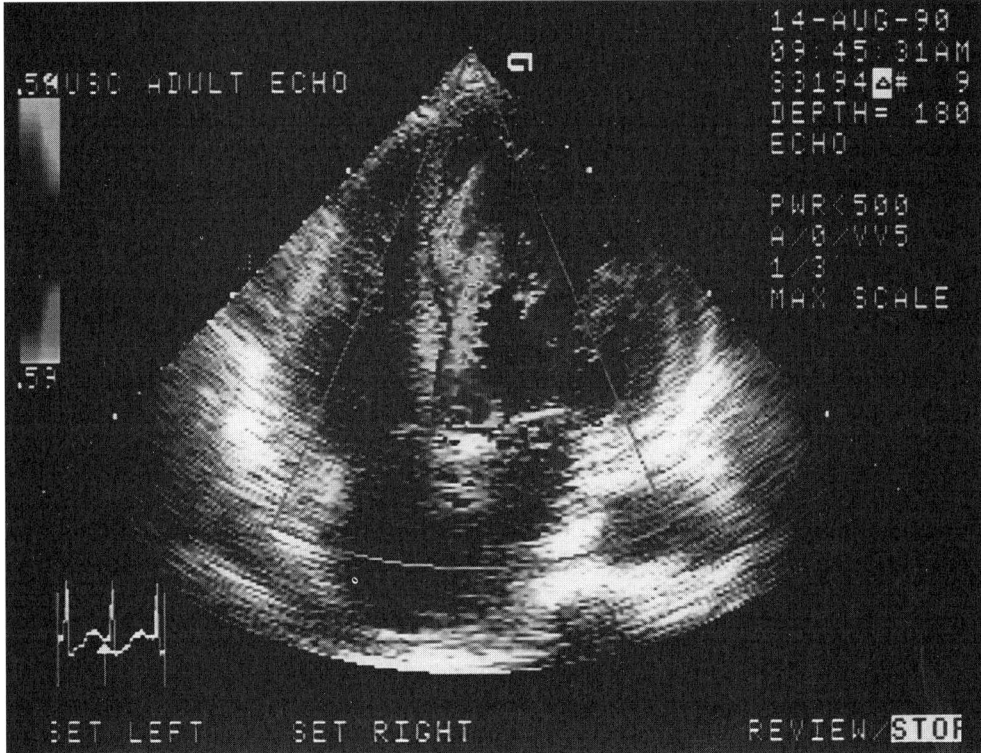

Diagnosis: Chronic aortic insufficiency with left ventricular dysfunction; probable Marfan syndrome.

Discussion: Common causes of chronic aortic insufficiency include healed endocarditis, rheumatic heart disease, syphilis, hypertension, collagen vascular disease, and Marfan syndrome with or without aortic root dissection. The physical description of the present patient suggests Marfan syndrome as the etiology of his aortic insufficiency.

Chronic aortic insufficiency imposes both a volume and pressure overload on the left ventricle. The excess volume regurgitated back into the left ventricle is pumped out as high stroke volume, producing a wide pulse pressure (e.g., 200/60 mmHg) and high systolic pressure. Thus, left ventricular systolic stress (a measure of afterload) in aortic regurgitation may approach that of aortic stenosis, an obvious pressure overload. While this overload may be compensated for by the development of hypertrophy and tolerated for years in many patients, eventually it leads to left ventricular dysfunction. If the left ventricular dysfunction is ignored, surgery, which is successful in restoring valvular competence, may not lead to restoration of ventricular function.

In the past decade, many investigators have established **echocardiographic and angiographic markers** to indicate that left ventricular dysfunction from aortic insufficiency is becoming severe and potentially irreversible. These markers are based on ventricular size and extent of shortening. Increased left ventricular volume (or echo dimension) at the end of systole can be due to an increase in afterload, a decrease in contractility, or both. However, end-systolic dimension is not affected by the increased preload of aortic insufficiency. Increased preload can augment ejection fraction (echo shortening fraction), causing ejection fraction to overestimate contractile function. When the echocardiographic end-systolic dimension approaches 55 mm or cineangiographic end-systolic volume index approaches 100 cc/m^2, it is likely that contractile dysfunction has developed, usually in tandem with increased afterload. An ejection fraction <0.55 is also worrisome. Correction of the aortic insufficiency before further deterioration occurs usually allows a return to normal ventricular size and function.

If these signs of left ventricular dysfunction are detected before they have been present chronically (longer than 18 months), improvement in left ventricular dysfunction following surgery almost always occurs. Occasionally, these echocardiographic or volumetric signs of left ventricular dysfunction precede the development of symptoms, creating the issue of whether to commit an asymptomatic patient to aortic valve replacement. While the physical examination is not helpful in making this decision, echocardiography is quite helpful. Although a decision should never be based on a single echocardiographic measurement, if repeated echocardiograms show a progressive increase in end-systolic dimension and a decline in shortening fraction, surgery should be contemplated. An exercise test performed at this point in the patient's course frequently demonstrates exercise intolerance, suggesting that the patient may be avoiding symptom-producing activities and confirming that surgery is indicated

Although this discussion has focused on the objective markers of left ventricular dysfunction, the **development of symptoms** is also an important negative prognosticator. Even if the thresholds for dysfunction have not been crossed, surgery should not be delayed if symptoms have developed.

The present patient underwent aortic valve replacement. Six months later his symptoms had disappeared and his ejection fraction by echocardiogram was >0.50.

Clinical Pearls

1. Careful echocardiographic follow-up of patients with chronic aortic insufficiency is required to detect the onset of significant left ventricular dysfunction.

2. Correction of the aortic insufficiency before left ventricular end-systolic dimension exceeds 55 mm usually leads to a good operative result, with improvement in ventricular function and a reduction in heart size.

3. Even if left ventricular dysfunction is present, surgery can restore function if dysfunction has been present for less than 18 months.

REFERENCES

1. Wisenbaugh T, Spann JF, Carabello BA: Differences in myocardial performance and load between patients with similar amounts of chronic aortic versus chronic mitral regurgitation. J Am Coll Cardiol 1984;3:916–923.
2. Bonow RO, Epstein SE: Is preoperative left ventricular function predictive of survival and functional results after aortic valve replacement for chronic aortic regurgitation. J Am Coll Cardiol 1987;10:713–716.
3. Bonow RO, Dodd JT, Maron BJ, et al: Long-term serial changes in left ventricular function and reversal of ventricular dilatation after valve replacement for chronic aortic regurgitation. Circulation 1988;78:1108–1120.
4. Taniguchi K, Nakano S, Kawashima Y, et al: Left ventricular ejection performance, wall stress, and contractile state in aortic regurgitation before and after valve replacement. Circulation 1990;82:798–807.
5. Klodas E, Enriquez-Sarano M, Tajik AJ, et al: Optimizing timing of surgical correction in patients with severe aortic regurgitation: Role of symptoms. J Am Coll Cardiol 1997;30(3):746–752.

PATIENT 121

A 65-year-old woman with mitral stenosis and right upper quadrant pain

A 65-year-old woman with mitral stenosis complains of insidious onset of progressive dyspnea on exertion, with occasional episodes of paroxysmal nocturnal dyspnea. Over the previous month, the patient also noted right upper quadrant pain and decreased appetite.

Physical Examination: Vital signs: pulse 90; respirations 22; blood pressure 125/80. General: thin; mild respiratory distress. Neck: jugular venous distention with estimated central venous pressure of 16 mm H_2O. Chest: bibasilar rales. Cardiac: PMI fifth intercostal space mid-clavicular line; irregularly irregular rhythm; prominent P_2 component of S_2; opening snap; II/VI diastolic murmur at the apex; II/VI systolic murmur in the tricuspid area that varies with respiration. Abdomen: liver span 16 cm and pulsatile. Extremities: 2+ pretibial edema.

Laboratory Findings: EKG: atrial fibrillation; right ventricular hypertrophy with strain. Doppler interrogation of the tricuspid valve: see below.

Question: What is the etiology of the right upper quadrant pain?

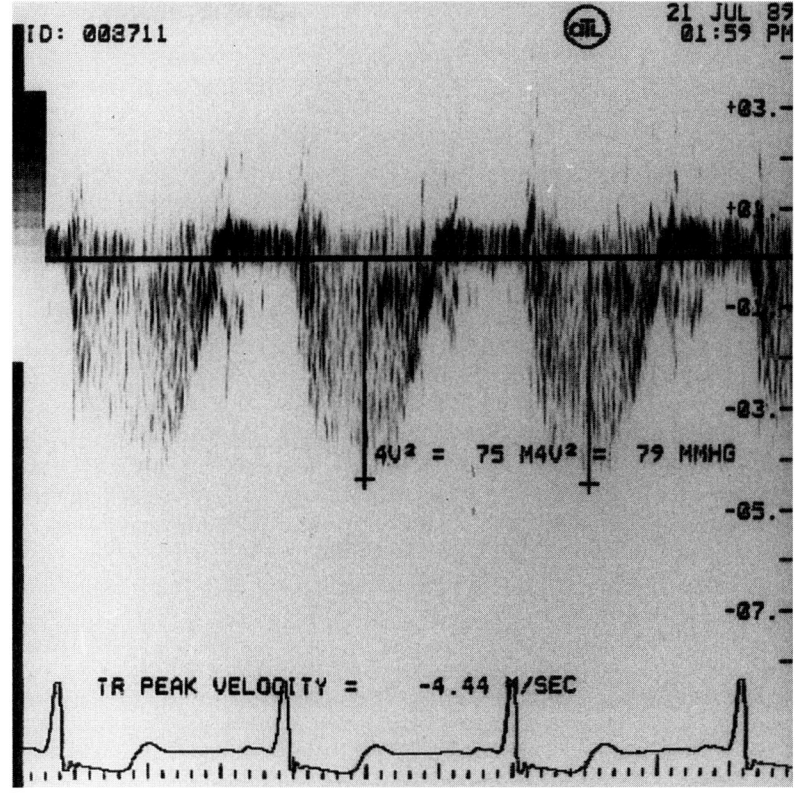

Diagnosis: Right heart failure from pulmonary hypertension due to mitral stenosis.

Discussion: The etiology of pulmonary hypertension in mitral stenosis is unclear. Because the primary function of the right ventricle is to fill the left ventricle, part of the increase in right ventricular pressure is needed to provide the extra force for driving blood across the stenotic mitral valve. Mitral stenosis per se, however, accounts for only a portion of the observed pulmonary hypertension; the remainder results from pulmonary vasoconstriction that occurs for unclear reasons. Right ventricular performance is determined by preload, afterload, and contractility. The increased right ventricular afterload produced by the pulmonary hypertension causes the right ventricle to utilize its preload reserve, increasing end-diastolic volume and also right ventricular filling pressure. In turn, these changes cause tricuspid regurgitation, peripheral edema, and ascites. Although the afterload excess may lead to a reduction in right ventricular ejection fraction, most studies indicate that right ventricular contractile function is normal in mitral stenosis.

The presence of pulmonary hypertension increases **operative mortality** threefold, from 3% to 9%, if mitral valve replacement becomes necessary. Although these data might not pertain to balloon valvotomy, success with the latter in patients with mitral stenosis is not guaranteed, and surgery may be required. Thus, optimal management of mitral stenosis depends on correcting the valvular stenosis either with balloon mitral valvotomy or surgical mitral valve repair or replacement *before* pulmonary hypertension develops.

Unlike congenital heart disease, in mitral stenosis, pulmonary hypertension usually improves dramatically after successful relief of the valvular obstruction. Thus, while the presence of pulmonary hypertension increases the risks of surgery, it does not contraindicate surgical repair because the pulmonary hypertension almost always improves postoperatively. When the mitral valve is relatively pliable and uncalcified and there is only mild mitral regurgitation, mitral valvotomy can provide a satisfactory result and avoid the need for valve replacement. Medical therapy, including the use of vasodilators, has not been successful in reversing the pulmonary hypertension of mitral stenosis. In fact, vasodilators are contraindicated because they lead to systemic hypotension.

The physical examination in the present patient was diagnostic of pulmonary hypertension and right ventricular failure. These signs included elevated neck veins, a loud P_2 component of the second heart sound, tricuspid regurgitation, and peripheral edema. The Doppler interrogation of the tricuspid valve demonstrated tricuspid regurgitation with a jet velocity of 4.4 mm/sec. Using the modified Bernoulli equation and adding 10 mmHg for right atrial pressure, the estimated right ventricular systolic pressure was $77 + 10 = 87$ mmHg. The patient underwent balloon mitral valvotomy with improvement in her symptoms, but they recurred 2 years later. After undergoing mitral valve replacement, her pulmonary artery pressure returned nearly to normal.

Clinical Pearls

1. The pulmonary hypertension of mitral stenosis adversely affects the outcome of surgery. Thus, surgery should be performed before pulmonary hypertension develops.

2. Pulmonary hypertension is not a contraindication to surgery, because the severity of pulmonary hypertension improves or resolves following valve replacement or mitral valvotomy.

3. Vasodilator therapy is not an effective measure preoperatively to reduce the degree of pulmonary hypertension and may cause systemic hypotension.

REFERENCES

1. Dalen JE, Matloff JM, Evans GL, et al: Early reduction of pulmonary vascular resistance after mitral-valve replacement. N Engl J Med 1967;277:387–394.
2. Kirklin JW, Hickey MSJ, Blackstone EH, et al: Outcome after closed and open surgical commissurotomy: Implications for balloon valvuloplasty [abstract]. Circulation 1989;80(Suppl II):II–359.
3. Palacios IF, Block PC, Wilkins GT, et al: Follow-up of patients undergoing percutaneous mitral balloon valvotomy: Analysis of factors determining restenosis. Circulation 1989;79:573–579.
4. Casale PN, Stewart WJ, Whitlow PL: Percutaneous balloon valvotomy for patients with mitral stenosis: Initial and follow-up results. Am Heart J 1991;121:476–479.
5. Vincens JJ, Temizer D, Post JR, et al: Long-term outcome of cardiac surgery in patients with mitral stenosis and severe pulmonary hypertension. Circulation 1995;92(Suppl 9):II–130—II–142.

PATIENT 122

A 54-year-old man in shock following a myocardial infarction

A 54-year-old man is admitted to the hospital 5 hours after the onset of severe substernal chest pain, nausea, and diaphoresis.

Physical Examination: Vital signs: pulse 120 and regular; blood pressure 80/40. Neck: veins not elevated. Chest: clear. Cardiac: no gallop rhythm.

Laboratory Findings: EKG: diagnostic of an acute anterior myocardial infarction. Chest radiograph: normal. Initial Swan-Ganz catheter values: see left column below.

Hospital Course: The patient is treated with dopamine 10 µg/kg/min, which increases his blood pressure to 100/60 and his urinary output to 50 cc/hr. He cannot, however, be weaned from the dopamine. The patient then inadvertently receives a liter of normal saline over an hour, after which he is easily weaned from dopamine. Repeat Swan-Ganz catheter values: see right column below.

	Initial values	Repeat values
Right atrial pressure	10 mmHg	10 mmHg
Pulmonary artery pressure	70/25/35 mmHg	70/25/35 mmHg
Pulmonary wedge pressure	33 mmHg	33 mmHg
Cardiac index	1.5 L/min/m^2	2.1 L/min/m^2
Pulmonary wedge O$_2$ saturation	—	65%

Question: How should these hemodynamic findings be interpreted?

Diagnosis: Anterior myocardial infarction with relative hypovolemia and misinterpretation of the hemodynamic data.

Discussion: Right heart catheterization is frequently employed to guide fluid management in difficult cases of nonhemorrhagic shock. Previous studies have demonstrated that following myocardial infarction, cardiac output reaches its maximum when the pulmonary wedge pressure (P_w) approaches 20–22 mmHg. Because a further increase in P_w leads to pulmonary edema, a reasonable goal of therapy in cardiogenic shock is to achieve a P_w of approximately 20 mmHg, which will maximize cardiac output and blood pressure safely. In shock following myocardial infarction when P_w is relatively low, volume infusion increases use of the Frank-Starling mechanism, producing increased force of contraction and an increase in forward output.

Because crucial fluid management decisions are often based on the P_w, accurate recording of this value is mandatory. A common error in management demonstrated in this case is improper wedging of the catheter. Proof of wedging includes the following: **(1)** the mean pulmonary artery pressure is ≥5 mmHg greater than the mean P_w, **(2)** the V wave of the wedge pressure tracing follows the T wave of the EKG when they are recorded simultaneously, **(3)** there are typical a and v waves if the patient is in sinus rhythm, and **(4)** oximetry confirms that the catheter is properly wedged by demonstrating high oxygenation consistent with blood withdrawn from the left atrium.

In the present patient, the presence of pulmonary hypertension made wedging difficult. Oximetric analysis of the blood sampled in the supposed P_w position was desaturated, indicating that it was not truly taken from the wedge position. Thus the previous determinations of the P_w were probably damped pulmonary artery tracings, significantly overestimating the true wedge pressure. When the patient received volume inadvertently, he got the correct management for a patient with a suboptimal filling pressure, which this patient had but which his catheter failed to record. Clues were the **absence of a gallop rhythm** and the **absence of findings of pulmonary congestion** on the chest radiograph. Following the oximetric determination, the catheter was repositioned and a confirmed wedge of 18 mmHg was obtained after the patient had received a liter of normal saline.

Other errors in hemodynamic monitoring include transducer failure and calibration errors. If such errors are suspected, calibration of the transducer with a mercury column is imperative.

The present patient recovered without further complications.

Clinical Pearls

1. Swan-Ganz catheter measurements are frequently made in error, thereby misdirecting therapy.
2. Whenever the hemodynamic and clinical data are disparate, oximetric confirmation of the wedge pressure is mandatory.
3. Internal transducer calibration devices frequently are inaccurate. When in doubt, employ mercury calibration.

REFERENCES

1. Crexells C, Chatterjee K, Forrester JS, et al: Optimal level of filling pressure in the left side of the heart in acute myocardial infarction. N Engl J Med 1973;289:1263–1266.
2. Forrester JS, Diamond GA, Swan HJC: Correlative classification of clinical and hemodynamic function after acute myocardial infarction. Am J Cardiol 1977;39:137–145.
3. Carabello BA, Grossman W: Bedside hemodynamic monitoring, cardiac catheterization and pulmonary angiography. In Cohn PF, Wynne J (eds): Diagnostic Methods in Clinical Cardiology. Boston, Little, Brown, 1982, pp 235–269.
4. Komadina KH, Schenk DA, LaVeau P, et al: Interobserver variability in the interpretation of pulmonary artery catheter pressure tracings. Chest 1991;100:1647–1654.

PATIENT 123

A 55-year-old renal transplant patient with hypertension, pulmonary edema, and tinnitus

A 55-year-old woman underwent renal transplantation 3 years previously for renal failure due to systemic lupus erythematosus. Her graft initially functioned well, but gradually deteriorated. On the night of admission, she is experiencing acute shortness of breath. There is no previous history of heart failure.

Physical Examination: Vital signs: pulse 100 (regular); respirations 32; blood pressure 240/140. General: severe dyspnea. Chest: rales throughout both lung fields. Cardiac: S_3 gallop.

Laboratory Findings: WBC 8000/µl; Hct 30%. Electrolytes normal. Cr 3.1 mg/dl. Chest x-ray: early pulmonary edema. EKG: sinus tachycardia.

Hospital Course: The patient is treated with intravenous furosemide 40 mg and a nitroprusside infusion titrated to control her blood pressure. She rapidly improves, but efforts to convert her to oral antihypertensive agents from nitroprusside are unsuccessful. On the fourth hospital day, the patient becomes confused, vomits, and complains of tinnitus.

Question: What is the cause of the patient's new difficulties?

Diagnosis: Thiocyanate toxicity.

Discussion: Sodium nitroprusside is a valuable agent in the management of severe hypertension because of its rapid onset, potency, and short duration of action. Unfortunately, nitroprusside therapy is associated with systemic toxicity because of its metabolism to cyanide ion, which combines with native thiosulfate to form thiocyanate. Both cyanide and thiocyanate toxicity can occur in patients who require **prolonged or high-dose infusions of sodium nitroprusside.** Thiocyanate toxicity is more common and is usually observed when doses greater than 2 μg/kg/min are employed for longer than 2 days. Because thiocyanate is excreted through the kidneys, however, renal failure causes a more rapid buildup of thiocyanate.

Tinnitus, nausea, vomiting, psychosis, delirium, convulsions, and muscle twitches are the signs of thiocyanate toxicity. The usual therapy is to slow or discontinue the use of the nitroprusside. If thiocyanate toxicity appears life threatening, thiocyanate levels can be reduced rapidly with dialysis. Thiocyanate intoxication can also lead to hypothyroidism because it temporarily blocks the organification of iodine.

Cyanide toxicity, which is usually more severe than thiocyanate toxicity, is fortunately much less common with nitroprusside use. It occurs only when the recommended dose of 10 μg/kg/min has been exceeded or when more than 2 μg/kg/min has been infused for several days. Cyanide ion binds to the cytochromes, where it inhibits phosphorylative oxidation, resulting in lactic acidosis, dyspnea, confusion, coma, and death. The classic evidence of cyanide intoxication is found in the venous blood gas determination. Because oxygen cannot be used, it is not extracted, and therefore the venous oxygen tension is abnormally high. At the same time there is evidence of metabolic acidosis. If cyanide intoxication is suspected, the nitroprusside infusion should be discontinued immediately. In life-threatening cases, sodium nitrate can be infused to create methemoglobinemia, which will bind to and neutralize the cyanide ion. Subsequent administration of sodium thiosulfate converts the bound cyanide ion to thiocyanate, which is then excreted by the kidneys.

Other side effects of sodium nitroprusside administration are methemoglobinemia and oxygen desaturation. Oxygen desaturation occurs as a consequence of the vasodilator properties of nitroprusside on the pulmonary vascular bed. In patients with acute lung disease, hypoxic vasoconstriction limits blood flow adjacent to nonfunctioning alveoli, which diminishes the severity of an intrapulmonary shunt. The infusion of nitroprusside reverses hypoxic vasoconstriction and increases capillary perfusion of nonfunctioning alveoli, thereby worsening shunt and decreasing oxygen saturation.

The present patient's thiocyanate level was 40 mg/L (nontoxic range 3–15 mg/L). She was begun on trimethaphan to control her blood pressure, which allowed the nitroprusside infusion to be discontinued and her symptoms to improve.

Clinical Pearls

1. Thiocyanate levels should be monitored in all patients receiving nitroprusside at a rate greater than 2 μg/kg/min for more than 24 hours.

2. Renal dysfunction increases the risk of thiocyanate intoxication.

3. Cyanide intoxication also can occur with nitroprusside use. A narrowed arteriovenous oxygen difference may herald the onset of cyanide intoxication.

4. PO_2 should be monitored in patients with borderline oxygenation who are begun on nitroprusside because of its effect on increasing intrapulmonary shunting.

REFERENCES

1. Schulz V: Clinical pharmacokinetics of nitroprusside, cyanide, thiosulfate and thiocyanate. Clin Pharmacokin 1984;9:239–251.
2. Calhoun DA, Oparil S: Treatment of hypertensive crisis. N Engl J Med 1990;323:1177–1183.
3. Smith TW, Braunwald E, Kelly RA: The management of heart failure. In Braunwald E (ed): Heart Disease, 4th ed. Philadelphia, W.B. Saunders, 1991, p 498.

PATIENT 124

A 62-year-old man with signs and symptoms of congestive heart failure and a large cardiac silhouette

A 62-year-old man is being followed for hypertension, chronic renal insufficiency secondary to nephrectomy for a hypernephroma, and congestive heart failure. He has been seen for several months as an outpatient for symptoms of dyspnea and peripheral edema. Treatment has included increasing doses of furosemide, hydralazine, and digoxin, but his symptoms are becoming progressively worse.

Physical Examination: Vital signs: pulse 90; blood pressure 180/100; no pulsus paradoxus. Cardiac: deep jugular neck veins pulsated to the angle of the jaw at 45°; apical impulse not visible or palpable; distant heart sounds. Chest: breath sounds decreased at the bases, with bronchial breathing noted mainly at the left base. Abdomen: hepatomegaly. Extremities: 3+ peripheral edema.

Laboratory Findings: CBC: normal. Creatinine: 2.8 mg/dl. EKG: low voltage and inverted T waves. Chest radiograph: marked cardiomegaly and bilateral pleural effusions. Echocardiogram: see below.

Questions: What is the most likely cardiac diagnosis? How would you establish it?

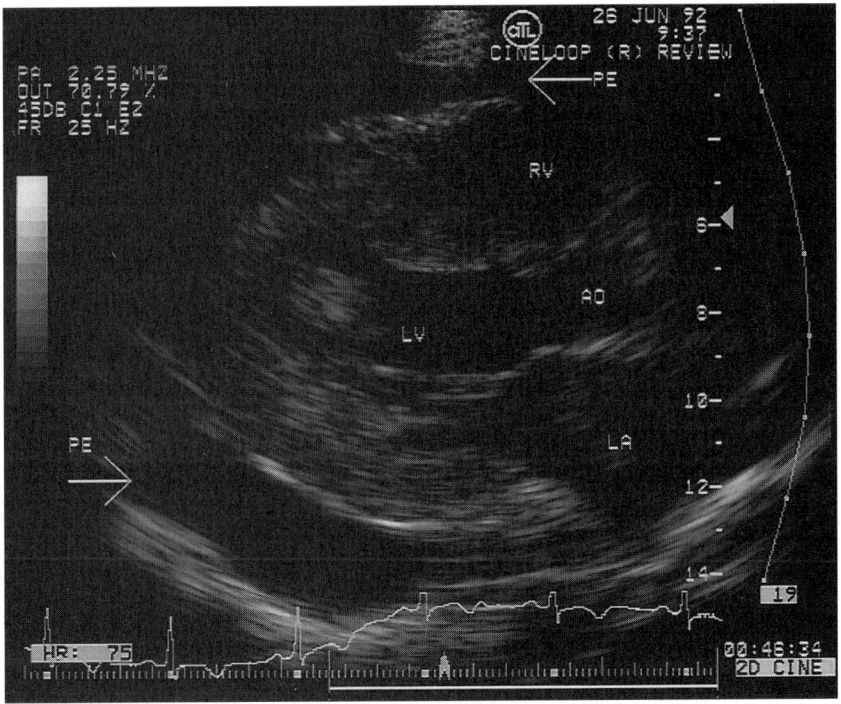

Diagnosis: Pericardial effusion with possible tamponade.

Discussion: The diagnosis of pericardial tamponade is usually made at the bedside, but proof rests on improvement in hemodynamics after pericardiocentesis. Signs of effusion include damped cardiac sounds, nonpalpable PMI, and bronchial breathing at the left base posteriorly below the angle of the scapula (Ewart's sign). Signs that the effusion is causing cardiac compromise (tamponade) include pulsus paradoxus, elevated neck veins, tachycardia, and narrowed pulse pressure. **Pulsus paradoxus** is generally viewed as the most reliable sign but is absent in 10% of cases of tamponade. In these cases, high antecedent left ventricular diastolic pressure or atrial septal defect prevent paradoxus from occurring.

New demonstration of low voltage on the EKG and enlargement of the cardiac silhouette on chest radiography support the diagnosis of pericardial effusion. The **echocardiogram** is a rapid method of establishing the diagnosis and may provide clues that cardiac tamponade is present. During cardiac diastole, right atrial and right ventricular collapse are often noted in tamponade, and the heart may show a pendular swinging motion that is often associated with electrical alternans.

In most cases of pericardial effusion and tamponade, **pericardiocentesis** is indicated. The risk of serious complications from the procedure is 1–5%. Complications include cardiac laceration, vasovagal episodes, and coronary artery laceration. Complications increase as the size of the effusion decreases, and, conversely, rarely occur when a large anterior effusion is present. In our view, nonemergent pericardiocentesis should be performed during hemodynamic monitoring, which is definitive proof that tamponade was or was not present. If the underlying diagnosis is one that makes recurrence of the effusion likely, balloon pericardiotomy is successful in providing permanent drainage.

In the present patient, the echocardiogram revealed a large pericardial effusion with normal systolic cardiac function. Hemodynamic measurements showed an arterial pressure of 180/100 mmHg, mean right atrial pressure of 12 mmHg, pulmonary capillary wedge pressure of 17 mmHg, and a pulmonary artery pressure of 44/16 mmHg. Because of the large effusion and the near equalization of pressures, diagnostic pericardiocentesis was done. The initial pericardial pressure was 13 mmHg, indicating tamponade. The increased pulmonary wedge pressure compared with the pericardial pressure was probably in part due to diastolic failure and hypertrophy from the renal disease; that wedge pressure was higher than the pericardial pressure probably explains the absence of a pulsus paradoxus. A thermodilution cardiac output was 6.4 L/min. The following day the hemodynamic pressures were normal, the cardiac output was 8.5 L/min, and the pericardial pressure was zero. Culture of the fluid was negative and a cell block did not show carcinoma, although carcinoma was considered likely because of the past history of hypernephroma.

Clinical Pearls

1. Bronchial breath sounds over the left posterior lung (Ewart's sign) are a frequently overlooked sign of pericardial effusion.
2. Ten percent of patients with tamponade do not have pulsus paradoxus.
3. The only definitive proof of a tamponade is increased intrapericardial pressure and reduced cardiac output that improves after pericardiocentesis.

REFERENCES

1. Feigenbaum H: Echocardiographic diagnosis of percardial effusion. Am J Cardiol 1970;26:475–479.
2. Kronzon I, Cohen MI, Winer HE: Diastolic atrial compression: A sensitive echocardiographic sign of cardiac tamponade. J Am Coll Cardiol 1983;2:770–775.
3. Bahl VK, Bhargava B, Chandra S: Percutaneous pericardiotomy using Inoue balloon catheter. Cathet Cardiovasc Diag 1995; 36:98–99.

PATIENT 125

A 28-year-old hunter with syncope

A 28-year-old man is well until the day of admission, when he felt lightheaded while driving his car. He pulled to the side of the road and lost consciousness for a few minutes. Three months previously he experienced flu-like symptoms that developed several days after a hunting trip. He denies rash, stiff neck, or arthritis.

Physical Examination: Vital signs: pulse 32 (regular); blood pressure 100/60. General: alert and oriented. Examination otherwise unremarkable.

Laboratory Findings: EKG: see below.

Question: What is the best explanation for his clinical presentation and EKG abnormality?

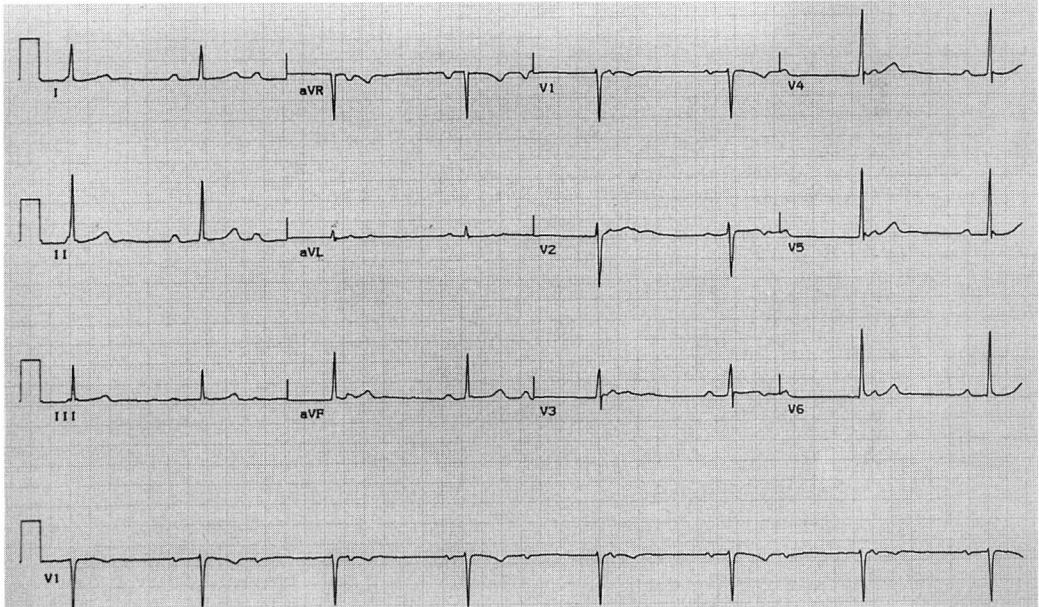

Diagnosis: Complete heart block, probably secondary to Lyme disease.

Discussion: Lyme disease is an infectious disease caused by the spirochete *Borrelia burgdorferi* and is passed to humans by the bite of the deer tick, *Ixodes dammini*. The course of the disease has been divided into three stages. Shortly after the initial bite, a characteristic rash, **erythema chronicum migrans,** develops. This erythematous, macular, papular rash spreads out from the site of the initial tick bite. As the rash enlarges, typically there is central clearing. It is painless and, remarkably, as in this case, the patient often fails to notice it. Coincident with the rash or shortly thereafter, approximately half of patients develop multiple **annular skin lesions.** There also may be flu-like symptoms such as headache, malaise, nuchal rigidity, arthralgias, and myalgias. Treatment with antibiotics at this stage of the disease is usually curative and prevents secondary manifestations.

If the disease is not treated, neurologic and/or cardiac manifestations may occur weeks to months later. The most common cardiac manifestation is **conducting system disease** involving the AV node. Thus, first-degree, second-degree, or, as in the present patient, complete heart block may develop. Syncope is common. The natural course following treatment with high-dose penicillin is resolution of the complete heart block without need for permanent pacing. However, temporary pacing may be required. Whether or not the heart block resolves without antibiotic therapy is unknown, but demonstration of the spirochete in cardiac tissue from patients with heart block suggests that the cardiac manifestations are due to local infection and, thus, antibiotic therapy is logical. Other cardiac manifestations include nonspecific ST- and T-wave abnormalities on EKG, increased myocardial gallium uptake indicating myocardial inflammation, and mildly to moderately reduced left ventricular function. Improvement in left ventricular function has been reported following successful antibiotic therapy.

Still later, in the third stage, arthritis may develop. Typically the large joints are affected, especially the knee. Joint effusions are common. It is presumed that the arthritis is also due to active infection, although the total spirochete load at this point in time is low. Antibiotic therapy is still recommended but its success is less certain than in the earlier stages of the disease.

If the classic rash is noted, the diagnosis can be made with certainty. This is fortunate because at this point in the course of the disease, antibody titers to *B. burgdorferi* are usually not increased and the spirochete is rarely demonstrated. Commonly in the second stage and almost always in the third stage, antibodies to the spirochete are present and aid in making the diagnosis.

The present patient underwent insertion of a temporary pacemaker and penicillin was administered. His heart block resolved 2 weeks later.

Clinical Pearls

1. Spontaneous complete heart block is unusual in young patients, and its occurrence should raise the suspicion of Lyme disease.
2. If the typical rash has been witnessed by the patient or the physician, the diagnosis can be made with certainty. However, many patients fail to notice the rash, which disappears by the time cardiac manifestations are present.
3. Heart block due to Lyme disease typically resolves following antibiotic therapy without need for permanent pacing.

REFERENCES

1. Malawista SE, Steere AC: Lyme disease: Infectious in origin, rheumatic in expression. Adv Intern Med 1986;31:147–166.
2. McAlister HF, Klementowicz PT, Andrews C, et al: Lyme carditis: An important cause of reversible heart block. Ann Intern Med 1989;110:339–345.
3. Stanek G, Klein J, Bittner R, et al: Isolation of *Borrelio burgdorferi* from the myocardium of a patient with longstanding cardiomyopathy. N Engl J Med 1990;322:249–252.
4. Dattwyler RJ, Luft BJ, Kunkel MJ, et al: Ceftriaxone compared with doxycycline for the treatment of acute disseminated Lyme disease. N Engl J Med 1997; 337:289.

INDEX

Acute coronary syndromes, 54
Adenosine
    supraventricular tachycardia with left bundle branch block management, 99
    tachycardia treatment, 11
Alcoholic cardiomyopathy
    congestive heart failure, 14, 15, 253, 254
    electrocardiography, 14, 15
    management, 254, 255
    pathophysiology, 254
    reversibility, 254
    sudden death in, 254, 255
Amiodarone
    acute pneumonitis induction, 263–264
    side effects, 264
Amyloid cardiomyopathy
    echocardiography, 196, 197
    electrocardiography, 196, 197
    fibril deposition, 197, 198
    findings, 196, 197
    management, 197, 198
Anemia
    congestive heart failure association, 52
    diagnosis, 52
Angina. *See* Prinzmetal's angina; Stable angina; Unstable angina
Angioplasty
    comparison with coronary artery bypass graft, 2
    comparison with medical therapy, 2
Anistreplase, clinical trials, 138
Aortic dissection
    classification, 85
    from coarctation of the aorta, 240
    diagnosis, 84–86
    epidemiology, 85
    imaging, 85
    treatment, 85, 86
Aortic insufficiency, acute
    causes of, 244
    early mitral valve closure with, 243, 244
    management, 244
Aortic insufficiency, chronic
    cardiac catheterization pressure tracing, 199, 200
    echocardiography, 274, 275, 276
    Hill's sign, 200
    left ventricular systolic stress, 275
    management, 275, 276
    in Marfan syndrome, 274–276
    metastasis as cause, 259–260
Aortic stenosis
    cardiac catheterization, 245, 246
    management, 178, 246
    murmur features, 178
    pressure tracing, 177, 178

Aortic stenosis (*Cont.*)
    prognosis, 178
    pseudostenosis, 245–246
    with recurrent heart failure, 177–178
Aortic trauma
    findings, 166, 167
    mortality, 167
    repair and management, 167
Aortic valve
    homografts
        degeneration with congestive heart failure, 51–52
        lifetime, 52
    murmur with supravalvular aortic lumen stenosis, 19–20
    prosthetic infective endocarditis, 205–206
    prosthetic valvular stenosis, 268–270
Aortography, supravalvular aortic lumen stenosis, 20
Apical hypertrophic cardiomyopathy, 110–111
Apo A1, low levels in heart disease, 47
Apo E4, polymorphisms and reduction, 47
Arteriogram. *See* Coronary arteriogram
Aspirin, atrial fibrillation patient management, 68
Athlete's heart, diagnosis of, 8–9
Atorvastatin
    comparison with angioplasty, 2
    potency, 44
Atrial fibrillation
    anticoagulation therapy, 68
    chronic fibrillation with hypertension, 67–68
    classification, 38
    with digoxin toxicity, 97
    lone atrial fibrillation, 135
    mitral stenosis and systemic embolization, 226–227
    persistent condition management with pacemaker, 37–38
    pharmacotherapy, 38
    prevalence, 135
    recent-onset patients
        evaluation, 135
        findings, 134
        management, 135–136
    stroke risks, 68
    with thyroid storm, 35–36
    with Wolff-Parkinson-White syndrome, 77, 78
Atrial flutter, from hypomagnesemia, 91–92
Atrial remodeling, prevention, 38
Atrial septal defect
    associated syndromes, 143, 144
    management, 143, 144
    with mitral valve prolapse, 142–144
    with pericarditis, 10, 11
    types, 143
Atrial tachycardia
    diagnosis, 153, 154

Atrial tachycardia (*Cont.*)
  electrocardiography, 153, 154
  management, 154
AV block
  with digoxin toxicity, 20–21
  in Lyme disease, 286
  pacemaker indications, 40
  prosthetic infective endocarditis with first-degree block, 205–206
  with syncope, 29–30
  third-degree block and pacemaker management, 121–122
AV junction ablation, persistent atrial fibrillation management, 38
AV nodal reentrant tachycardia (AVNRT), 42, 99, 165
AV reentrant tachycardia (AVRT), Wolff-Parkinson-White syndrome type, 164–165

Barium swallow, chest pain work-up, 65
Bayes theorem, stress test interpretation, 257
Beta blockers
  acute myocardial infarction, 148
  atrial fibrillation with rapid ventricular rate, 36
  electrocardiogram effects, 23
  heat stroke association, 224–225
  thyroid crisis, 36
  ventricular fibrillation prevention, 23
Bezold-Jarisch reflex, 146
Body mass index (BMI), classifications, 49

Calcium channel blocker, Prinzmetal's angina management, 160
Cannon A waves, 113, 114
Carcinoid syndrome
  diagnosis, 208
  management, 208
  tricuspid regurgitation association, 207–208
Cardiac catheterization pressure measurement
  aortic insufficiency, chronic, 199, 200
  aortic stenosis, 245, 246
  pulmonary wedge pressure measurement error, 280
Cardiac tamponade
  causes of, 62
  echocardiography, 61, 62, 63, 284
  electrocardiography, 61, 62, 63
  management of, 62
  with pericardial effusion, 61–63, 283
Cardiomyopathy. *See also* Hypertrophic cardiomyopathy
  alcoholic cardiomyopathy, 14–15, 253–254
  dilated cardiomyopathies, 254, 255
  peripartum cardiomyopathy, 213–214
  with supraventricular tachycardia, 41–42
Cerebrovascular accident, electrocardiogram abnormalities, 89–90
Chest pain, differential diagnosis, 64–66
Chest trauma, 167
Chorda tendinea rupture, 232–233
Chronic obstructive pulmonary disease (COPD)
  with cor pulmonale, 100–101

Chronic obstructive pulmonary disease (COPD) (*Cont.*)
  differential diagnosis, 17
  multifocal atrial tachycardia, 101
Coarctation of the aorta
  chest film, 239, 240
  clinical features, 239, 240
  repair, 240
  sequelae, 240
Cocaine
  management of acute toxicity, 133
  myocardial infarction precipitation, 132–133
  norepinephrine reuptake inhibition, 133
  pheochromocytoma and cardiac complications, 133
Colonoscopy, management of mitral valve prosthesis patients, 228–229
Congestive heart failure
  in alcoholic cardiomyopathy, 14, 15, 253, 254
  anemia as cause, 52
  aortic valve homograft degeneration with, 51–52
  heart transplantation for, 184–185
  high output failure secondary to thyrotoxicosis, 249–250
  obese patient management, 238
Constrictive pericarditis, 222–223
Coronary arteriogram
  anatomy anomalies, 179–180
  syndrome X, 103–104
  thrombolysis follow-up, 171
Coronary artery anomalies
  benign anomalies, 180
  with ischemia, 180
  left coronary artery origin, 179–180
Coronary artery bypass graft (CABG)
  comparison with angioplasty, 2
  comparison with medical therapy, 2
  indications, 2, 3
Cor pulmonale
  with chronic obstructive pulmonary disease, 100–101
  diagnosis, 101
  diastolic dysfunction as cause, 210
  management, 101
  with pulmonary fibrosis, 16–17
Corrigan's pulse, 200, 244
C-reactive protein, cardiovascular risks, 47
Cyanosis
  ductus arteriosus with Eisenmenger's syndrome, 215, 216
  with Ebstein's anomaly, 115–116
  in tetralogy of Fallot, 234, 235
Cystathione beta-synthase deficiency, 188

D-dimer, pulmonary embolism testing, 220
de Musset's sign, 200, 244
Deep vein thrombosis, with heparin-induced thrombocytopenia, 201–202
Diabetes, management of coronary artery disease, 48–49
Diastolic dysfunction
  diagnosis, 209–210
  management, 210

Diffuse esophageal spasm, diagnosis of, 65
Digoxin
   kidney metabolism, 21, 97
   magnesium level effects, 91–92
   quinidine interactions, 97
   toxicity
      arrhythmias with, 97
      atrial tachycardia, 154
      AV block, 20–21
      incidence, 97
      nonparaoxysmal junctional tachycardia with AV dissociation, 96–97
      symptoms, 96, 97
Dissecting aneurysm, with supravalvular aortic lumen stenosis, 20
Distributive shock, 266
Ductus arteriosus
   closing following birth, 216
   with Eisenmenger's syndrome, 215–216
   treatment, 216
Duroziez's sign, 200

Early repolarization, electrocardiography, 87, 88
Ebstein's anomaly
   cyanosis with, 116
   electrocardiography, 115, 116
   management, 116
   pulmonary stenosis with, 116
Echocardiography. *See also* Transesophageal echocardiography
   acute mitral regurgitation, 82
   amyloid cardiomyopathy, 196, 197
   aortic insufficiency, chronic, 274, 275, 27
   atrial thrombi, 226, 227
   cardiac tamponade with pericardial effusion, 61, 62, 63, 284
   dissecting aneurysms, 19
   early mitral valve closure in aortic insufficiency, 243, 244
   Ebstein's anomaly, 116
   infective endocarditis, 206
   Marfan syndrome, 247, 248
   mitral stenosis complicated by pregnancy, 271, 272
   mitral valve prolapse, 193, 194, 195
   mural thrombus, 73
   peripartum cardiomyopathy, 213, 214
   prosthetic valvular stenosis, 268, 269, 270
   right bundle branch block follow-up, 126
   stress test, 94, 257, 258
   tricuspid stenosis and regurgitation from carcinoid syndrome, 207–208
   tricuspid valve endocarditis, 189, 190
   ventricular septal defect, 204, 235
   ventricular septal rupture, 218
Eisenmeger's syndrome
   with ductus arteriosus, 215–216
   management, 216
   tetralogy of Fallot differential diagnosis, 235, 236
Electrocardiography (EKG)
   alcoholic cardiomyopathy, 14, 15

Electrocardiography (EKG) (*Cont.*)
   amyloid cardiomyopathy, 196, 197
   antiarrhythmic agent effects, 23
   apical hypertrophic cardiomyopathy, 110, 111
   athlete's heart, 8–9
   atrial fibrillation, 10, 11
   atrial tachycardia, 153, 154
   AV block with digoxin toxicity, 20–21
   AV reentrant tachycardia, 42, 99, 164, 165
   calcium imbalances, 56, 57
   cardiac tamponade, 61, 62, 63
   cardiomyopathy secondary to supraventricular tachycardia, 41–42
   cerebrovascular accident abnormalities, 89–90
   chronic obstructive pulmonary disease with cor pulmonale, 100, 101
   cor pulmonale with pulmonary fibrosis, 16–17
   early repolarization, 87, 88
   Ebstein's anomaly, 115, 116
   false-positive stress test, 256–258
   hypercalcemia, 57, 108–109
   hyperkalemia, 56–57, 118, 119
   hypertrophic cardiomyopathy, 69–70
   hypokalemia, 4–5
   hypomagnesemia changes, 91, 92
   hypothermia, 151, 152
   idiopathic hypertrophic subaortic stenosis, 24–25
   infective endocarditis, 205, 206
   inferior posterior myocardial infarction with right ventricular infarction, 128, 129
   left bundle branch block
      anterior myocardial infarction with, 130–131
      infarction diagnosis with, 12, 13
   lidocaine indications, 147–148
   limb lead reversal, 168–169
   Lyme disease with complete heart block, 285, 286
   mitral valve prolapse, 33–34
   myocardial infarction following noncardiac surgery, 261, 262
   myocardial infarction with homocystinuria, 187
   myxedema with stable angina, 155, 156
   pericardial effusion, 284
   pericarditis, acute, 157, 158
   premature ventricular beats, 74
   Prinzmetal's angina, 159, 160
   propafenone and QRS complex widening, 22–23
   prosthetic infective endocarditis with first-degree block, 205, 206
   pulmonary embolism, 219–220, 221
   Q wave abnormalities without coronary disease, 163
   sick sinus syndrome, 140, 141
   stress test, 94, 126
   supraventricular tachycardia with left bundle branch block, 98, 99
   T wave changes, 34
   unstable angina, 53, 54, 58
   ventricular tachycardia, 112–114
   Wolff-Parkinson-White syndrome, 26–28, 76–77, 162–163

Endotoxic shock
  clinical features, 265, 266
  management, 266, 267
  myocardial depression with, 266, 267
  pathophysiology, 266
Ergonovine challenge, spasm induction, 65
Esophageal spasm, chest pain with, 65, 66
Estrogen replacement therapy, cardiovascular benefits, 49

Fat intake, hypercholesterolemia management, 44, 45

Gemfibrozil
  clinical trials, 2
  high-density lipoprotein elevation, 7, 49
Glycoprotein IIb/IIIa receptor inhibitors, unstable angina treatment, 54, 55, 59, 60
Grape juice, heart disease prevention, 44

Heart transplantation
  ages of donors and recipients, 185, 186
  contraindications, 185
  coronary artery disease following
    diagnosis, 241, 242
    incidence, 242
    risk factors, 242
    surveillance, 242
  indications, 184–185
  number of operations, 185
  outcomes, 185, 186
  rejection, 185, 186
Heat stroke
  beta blocker association, 224–225
  complications, 225
  management, 225
  onset, 225
Hemochromatosis
  cardiac dysfunction with, 252
  clinical features, 251, 252
  diagnosis, 252
  management, 252
Henoch-Schönlein purpura (HSP), cardiac abnormalities, 26, 27
Heparin-induced thrombocytopenia (HIT)
  with deep vein thrombosis, 201–202
  incidence, 202
  management, 202
  monitoring, 202
  types, 202
Hibernating myocardium
  clinical features, 230, 231
  diagnosis, 15, 231
  differential diagnosis, 231
  mechanisms, 231
High-density lipoprotein (HDL)
  coronary artery disease association with low levels, 7
  diet effects, 44
  functions, 7
  management of low levels, 6–7, 49
Hill's sign, in aortic insufficiency, 200

Homocysteine
  genetics of elevation, 188
  myocardial infarction with homocystinuria, 187–188
  reduction of levels, 47, 188
Hypercalcemia
  coma with, 108–109
  conditions with, 109
  electrocardiography, 57, 108–109
  management of severe disease, 109
Hypercholesterolemia
  coronary artery disease prevention management, 43–45
  diet, 44, 45
  screening recommendations, 44, 45
Hypereosinophilic syndrome
  causes of, 124
  diagnosis, 123–124
  endocardial damage, 124
  management, 124
Hyperfibrinogenemia, cardiac risks and treatment, 47
Hyperkalemia
  causes of, 119, 120
  electrocardiography, 56–57, 118, 119
  management, 119, 120
Hypertension
  with chronic atrial fibrillation, 67–68
  with coarctation of the aorta, 240
  with pheochromocytoma, 191–192
  pulmonary edema association, 209–210
Hypertriglycidemia, cardiovascular risks, 49
Hypertrophic cardiomyopathy (HCM)
  apical hypertrophic cardiomyopathy, 110–111
  classification, 111
  electrocardiography, 69–70, 110
  forms, 70
  heredity, 70
  management, 70
  prognosis, 111
  sudden death in, 70
Hypocalcemia, electrocardiography, 56–57
Hypokalemia
  cardiac effects, 5
  causes of, 5
  electrocardiography, 4–5
Hypomagnesemia, drug induction, 91–92
Hypotension, with heat stroke, 225
Hypothermia
  electrocardiography, 151, 152
  etiology, 152
  physiological response, 152
  treatment, 152
Hypothyroidism, cardiac manifestations, 156

Ibutilide, atrial fibrillation management, 135
Idiopathic hypertrophic subaortic stenosis (IHSS)
  diagnosis of, 25, 70
  electrocardiography findings, 24–25
Implantable cardioverter defibrillator (ICD), use in sudden cardiac death patients, 107
Infective endocarditis
  echocardiography, 206

Infective endocarditis (*Cont.*)
   from intravenous drug abuse, 189–190
   prophylactic antibiotics, 206, 229
   prosthetic infective endocarditis, 205–206
International normalized ratio (INR), 227
Intravenous drug abuse
   aortic insufficiency with, 243–244
   infective endocarditis with, 189–190
   septic pulmonary embolism with, 189–190

Japanese hypertrophic cardiomyopathy. *See* Apical hypertrophic cardiomyopathy

Kawasaki's disease
   with acute myocardial infarction, 175–176
   aneurysms with, 176
   fever management, 176
   findings, 176
Kussmaul's sign, 223

Left anterior descending artery (LAD)
   lesion management, 2
   Prinzmetal's angina involvement, 160
Left anterior superior fascicular block (LAFG), pacemaker management with anterior myocardial infarction, 40
Left bundle branch block (LBBB)
   anterior myocardial infarction with, 130–131
   myocardial infarction diagnosis with, 12, 13
   prognosis, 126
   with supraventricular tachycardia, 98, 99
Left ventricular hypertrophy, athlete's heart comparison, 9
Lidocaine
   use with pacing catheter, 40
   for premature ventricular beats with acute inferior infarction, 147–148
Low-density lipoprotein (LDL)
   statin management in prevention, 44
   subclasses, 47
Low-molecular-weight heparin (LWMH), unstable angina treatment, 54, 55, 59, 60
Lutembacher's syndrome, 142–144
Lyme disease
   with complete heart block, 285, 286
   management, 286
   stages, 286

Marfan syndrome
   aortic cystic medial necrosis, 248
   aortic dissection with, 85, 86
   chronic aortic insufficiency with left ventricular dysfunction, 274–276
   clinical features, 247, 248
   echocardiography, 247, 248, 274
   homocystinuria differential diagnosis, 188
Mitral regurgitation
   acute causes, 233
   afterload reduction therapy, 82, 233
   chorda tendinea rupture, 232–233

Mitral regurgitation (*Cont.*)
   ischemia induction, 82–83, 218
   pulmonary edema with, 81–83
   repair, 82, 233
Mitral stenosis
   classification, 272
   management, 272, 273
   in pregnancy, 271–273
   right heart failure from pulmonary hypertension, 277–278
   with systemic embolization, 226–227
Mitral valve prolapse (MVP)
   clicks and murmurs, 34, 194
   clinical findings, 193, 194, 195
   echocardiography, 193, 194, 195
   electrocardiography, 33–34, 194
   incidence, 194
   management, 194
   prognosis, 194, 195
   with atrial septal defect, 142–144
Mitral valve prosthesis
   patient management for colonoscopy and polypectomy
      anticoagulation, 229
      case features, 228
      endocarditis prophylaxis, 229
   prosthetic infective endocarditis, 205–206
Mobitz I AV block, with digoxin toxicity, 20–21
Mucocutaneous lymph node syndrome. *See* Kawasaki's disease
Multifocal atrial tachycardia (MAT), with chronic obstructive pulmonary disease, 101
Myocardial contusion, 167
Myocardial infarction
   acute inferior infarction with pulmonary edema, 81–83
   following noncardiac surgery
      electrocardiography, 261, 262
      incidence, 262
      onset, 262
      peripheral revascularization surgery, 262
      risk factors, 262
   with homocystinuria, 187–188
   inferior posterior myocardial infarction with right ventricular infarction, 128–129
   Kawasaki's disease in children, 175–176
   left bundle branch block
      anterior myocardial infarction with, 130–131
      infarction diagnosis with, 12, 13
   lidocaine for premature ventricular beats with acute inferior infarction, 147–148
   pacemaker management with bifascicular block, 40
   ventricular aneurysm, 72–73
   with ventricular septal rupture, 217–218
Myxedema
   cardiac manifestations, 156
   management, 156
   with stable angina, 155–156
Myxoma
   epidemiology, 150
   left atrial myxoma symptoms, 149, 150

Myxoma (Cont.)
  surgical management, 150
  transesophageal echocardiography, 149–150
  transient ischemic attack from, 149–150

Neurocardiogenic syncope, 32, 146
Niacin, lipid profile effects, 7, 49
Niaspan, high-density lipoprotein elevation, 7
Non-Q-wave infarction. *See* Unstable angina
Nonparaoxysmal junctional tachycardia with AV dissociation, digoxin toxicity, 96–97

Obesity
  cardiac effects, 238
  coronary artery disease risk, 49
  with left ventricular dysfunction, 237, 238
Osborn's wave, in hypothermia, 152

Pacemaker
  anterior myocardial infarction with bifascicular block management, 39–40
  AV block management, 121–122
  coding system, 122
  indications in anterior infarction, 40
  lidocaine use with pacing catheter, 40
  persistent atrial fibrillation management, 38
Papillary muscle
  ischemia and rupture, 82
  rupture and acute mitral regurgitation, 82–83, 218
Pericardial effusion
  with cardiac tamponade, 61–63
  diagnostics, 283, 284
  with hypothyroidism, 156
  with metastasis, 260
Pericardiocentesis, 260, 284
Pericarditis
  acute pericarditis
    electrocardiography stages, 157, 158
    findings, 157–158
    management, 158
  with atrial septal defects, 10, 11
  constrictive pericarditis
    findings, 222, 223
    laboratory tests, 223
Peripartum cardiomyopathy
  epidemiology, 214
  findings, 213, 214
  management, 214
  prognosis, 214
  types, 214
Peripheral revascularization surgery, myocardial infarction risks, 262
Pheochromocytoma
  cardiac complications of cocaine use, 133
  catecholamine effects, 192
  diagnosis, 192
  with hypertension and pulmonary edema, 191–192
  malignancy, 192
  origins, 192
Pneumonitis, amiodarone induction, 263–264

Polymorphic ventricular tachycardia
  electrocardiography, 79, 80
  torsade de pointes. *See* Torsade de pointes
Polypectomy, management of mitral valve prosthesis patients, 228–229
Positron emission tomography (PET), hibernating myocardium, 231
Postmicturition syncope
  findings, 145
  pathophysiology, 146
Pregnancy. *See also* Peripartum cardiomyopathy
  cardiac demands, 273
  mitral stenosis in, 271–273
Premature ventricular beats (PVBs)
  dietary management, 75
  electrocardiography, 74
  exercise induction, 75
  in healthy persons, 74–75
  lidocaine with acute inferior infarction, 147–148
Prinzmetal's angina
  calcium channel blocker management, 160
  electrocardiography, 159, 160
  pathophysiology, 160
  vessel disease epidemiology, 160
Procainamide, Wolff-Parkinson-White syndrome management, 77, 78
Propafenone, QRS complex widening, 22–23
Prosthetic valves. *See also specific heart valves*
  classification and durability, 269
  echocardiographic analysis, 269, 270
  mechanical failure mechanisms, 269
  stenosis, 268–270
Pulmonary capillary wedge tracing, holosystolic murmur, 82, 83
Pulmonary edema
  cerebrovascular accident association, 90
  hypertension association, 209–210
Pulmonary embolism
  clinical features, 219, 220
  D-dimer testing, 220
  electrocardiography, 219–220, 221
  management, 220
  ventilation-perfusion mismatches, 220, 221
Pulmonary fibrosis, with cor pulmonale, 16–17
Pulmonary hypertension
  diagnosis, 211, 212
  histopathology, 212
  management, 212
  prognosis, 212
  right heart failure from mitral stenosis, 277–278
  valve replacement surgery risks, 278
Pulmonary wedge pressure
  catheter wedging in measurement error, 280
  goal values in shock, 280
Pulsus paradoxus, 62, 63, 284

Quincke's pulse, 200
Quinidine
  digoxin interactions, 97
  torsade de pointes induction, 80

Quintuple auscultatory cadence, with Ebstein's anomaly, 116

Raloxifene, cardiovascular benefits, 49
Red wine, heart disease prevention, 44
Reteplase, clinical trials, 138
Rheumatic fever
    acute disease features, 181–182
    epidemiology, 182, 183
    Jones criteria, 182, 183
    management, 182
    pathophysiology, 182
    valvular disease with, 182, 183
Right bundle branch block (RBBB)
    with atrial septal defect, 143, 144
    etiology, 126
    follow-up tests, 126
    pacemaker management with anterior myocardial infarction, 40
    prognosis, 126

SA Wenckebach exit block, 141
Sensitivity, stress tests, 257
Septic pulmonary embolism, from intravenous drug abuse, 189–190
Shock
    endotoxic shock, 265–267
    mechanisms, 266
    pulmonary wedge pressure, 280
Sick sinus syndrome (SSS), 122
    electrocardiography, 140, 141
    management, 141
    SA Wenckebach exit block, 141
Sinus of Valsalva aneurysm
    aortic insufficiency with, 244
    findings of rupture, 173–174
    management, 174
Smoking, high-density lipoprotein depression, 7
Sodium nitroprusside, toxicity, 281–282
Specificity, stress tests, 257
Stable angina. *See also* Syndrome X
    clinical presentation, 1, 2
    evaluation, 2, 3
    with myxedema, 155–156
    revascularization versus medical therapy, 2, 3
    thallium stress test interpretation, 93–95
Statins
    potency of specific drugs, 44
    preventive utilization, 44, 45
Streptokinase, clinical trials, 138
Stress testing. *See also* Echocardiography; Electrocardiography; Thallium scanning
    false-positive stress test, 256–258
    interpretation of results, 257
Subarachnoid hemorrhage, electrocardiogram abnormalities, 89–90
Sudden cardiac death
    follow-up after resuscitation, 106–107
    implantable cardioverter defibrillator use, 107
    prognosis, 107

Supravalvular aortic lumen stenosis, 19–20
Supraventricular tachycardia
    atrial tachycardia, 153–154
    AV nodal reentrant tachycardia, 99
    with cardiomyopathy, 41–42
    from hypomagnesemia, 91–92
    with left bundle branch block, 98–99
    with Wolff-Parkinson-White syndrome, 77
Syncope
    AV block with, 29–30
    causes of, 30
    pharmacologic therapy, 32
    postmicturition syncope, 145–146
    symptoms of, 29, 30, 31
    tilt table testing for neurocardiogenic syncope, 32
Syndrome X
    angina with normal arteriogram, 103–104
    findings, 103–104
    management, 104
Systemic embolism, with mitral stenosis, 226–227
Systolic anterior motion (SAM), in idiopathic hypertrophic subaortic stenosis, 25

Tetralogy of Fallot
    clinical features, 234, 235
    Eisenmeger's syndrome differential diagnosis, 235, 236
    ventricular septal defect, 235, 236
Thallium scanning
    hibernating myocardium, 231
    obese patients, 238
    stress test
        accuracy, 257
        artery disease following heart transplantation, 241, 242
        indications for, 94, 95
        modes of, 94
        noninvasive test, 94
        rest testing, 94
        stable angina interpretation, 93–95
        vasodilators for testing, 94, 95
Thiocyanate toxicity
    clinical features, 281, 282
    management, 282
    sodium nitroprusside as source, 282
Thrombolysis. *See also specific agents*
    contraindications, 88
    coronary arteriography following therapy, 171
    indications, 13, 88
    outcomes, 171
    prevalence of use, 88
    reperfusion signs, 171
    selection of agent, 137–138
Thyroid storm
    with atrial fibrillation, 35–36
    beta-blocker therapy, 36
    causes of, 36
Thyrotoxicosis
    high output heart failure with, 249–250
    management, 250

Tilt table testing, neurocardiogenic syncope, 32
Tissue-type plasminogen activator (tPA), clinical trials, 138
Torsade de pointes
  electrocardiography, 79, 80
  induction by antimicrobial agents, 80
  management, 80
Transesophageal echocardiography (TEE)
  atrial thrombus detection, 68
  chorda tendinea rupture, 232, 233
  myxoma, 149–150
  pericardial metastasis, 260
  prosthetic valve evaluation, 269, 270
  supravalvular aortic lumen stenosis, 19
Tricuspid valve
  Doppler interrogation of regurgitation, 277, 278
  endocarditis with septic pulmonary emboli from intravenous drug abuse, 189–190
  repair, 190
  stenosis and regurgitation from carcinoid syndrome, 207–208
Tumor. *See also* Carcinoid syndrome; Myxoma; Pheochromocytoma
  pericardial metastasis, 260

Unstable angina
  cause of, 54, 59
  electrocardiography, 53, 54, 58
  prognostic factors, 54
  risk stratification, 54, 59
  signs and symptoms, 59
  treatment, 54, 59, 60

Variant angina. *See* Prinzmetal's angina
Vaughn Williams classification, antiarrhythmic agents, 23
Ventricular aneurysm
  anterior infarction association, 73
  diagnosis, 72–73
  management, 73
  with mural thrombi, 73
Ventricular septal defect (VSD)
  age at detection, 204
  echocardiography, 204, 235
  findings, 203–204
  surgical repair, 204, 235
  in tetralogy of Fallot, 235, 236
Ventricular septal rupture, with myocardial infarction, 217–218
Ventricular tachycardia
  management, 113, 114
  wide QRS tachycardia, 112–114
Ventriculophasic sinus arrhythmia, 21
Vitamin E, heart disease prevention, 44

Warfarin
  atrial fibrillation patients, 68
  mural thrombus management, 73
Wellens' criteria, 113
Wenckebach AV block, with digoxin toxicity, 20–21
Wolff-Parkinson-White syndrome
  AV reentrant tachycardia, 164–165
  electrocardiography, 26–28, 76–77, 162–163
  incidence, 77
  inferior infarction differential diagnosis, 162–163
  management, 77
  types, 27, 77, 163